Psychiatric Rehabilitation

Psychiatric Rehabilitation

2nd edition

Carlos W. Pratt

Kenneth J. Gill

Nora M. Barrett

Melissa M. Roberts

DEPARTMENT OF PSYCHIATRIC REHABILITATION
SCHOOL OF HEALTH RELATED PROFESSIONS
UNIVERSITY OF MEDICINE AND DENTISTRY OF NEW JERSEY
SCOTCH PLAINS, NEW JERSEY

ELSEVIER

AMSTERDAM • BOSTON • HEIDELBERG
LONDON • NEW YORK • OXFORD • PARIS
SAN DIEGO • SAN FRANCISCO • SINGAPORE
SYDNEY • TOKYO

Academic Press is an imprint of Elsevier

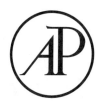

Elsevier Academic Press

30 Corporate Drive, Suite 400, Burlington, MA 01803, USA
525 B Street, Suite 1900, San Diego, California 92101-4495, USA
84 Theobald's Road, London WC1X 8RR, UK

This book is printed on acid-free paper. ∞

Library of Congress Cataloging-in-Publication Data
APPLICATION SUBMITTED

British Library Cataloguing in Publication Data
A catalogue record for this book is available from the British Library

ISBN 13: 978-0-12-564431-0
ISBN 10: 0-12-564431-0

For all information on all Elsevier Academic Press publications visit our Web site at www.books.elsevier.com
Printed in United States of America

06 07 08 09 10 9 8 7 6 5 4 3 2 1

*This book is dedicated to people with psychiatric disabilities and
to the psychiatric rehabilitation professionals who strive to
improve the quality of their lives and promote their recovery.*

Contents

Foreword   *xiii*
Acknowledgments   *xvii*

Part I   Understanding the Nature of Severe and Persistent Mental Illness

Chapter 1   The Experience of Mental Illness: An Introduction to Psychiatric Rehabilitation

Introduction   4
The Story of Paul   4
The Serious Mental Illnesses   9
Psychiatric Disability   10
The Stigma of Severe Mental Illness   13
Psychiatric Rehabilitation   14
Summary   26
Class Exercise   27
References   27

Chapter 2   Symptoms and Etiology of Severe and Persistent Mental Illness

Introduction   32
Symptoms   32
The Symptoms of Schizophrenia   33
Mood Disorders   42
Relevance to Psychiatric Rehabilitation   46
Dual Diagnosis   47
Etiology   50
The Story of Dara   53
Obsolete Etiological Theories   62
Summary   64
Class Exercise   64
References   65

Chapter 3 Course, Treatment, and Outcome of Severe and Persistent Mental Illnesses

Introduction   70
Course   72
Do Rehabilitation Services Matter?   78
Treatment   79
Biological (Somatic) Treatments   79
Psychosocial Treatments   93
Maria's Story   96
Understanding Course, Treatment, and Outcome: What the Staff and Consumers
    Don't Know *Can* Hurt Them!   97
Summary   101
Class Exercise   102
References   102

Part II   Psychiatric Rehabilitation Principles and Methodology

Chapter 4   Goals, Values, and Guiding Principles of Psychiatric Rehabilitation

Introduction   110
The Concept of Recovery   111
Goals, Values, and Guiding Principles   112
Guiding Principles of Psychiatric Rehabilitation   119
Psychiatric Rehabilitation Ethics   126
The Future of Psychiatric Rehabilitation Thought and Practice   133
Summary   134
Class Exercise   134
References   135

Chapter 5   Psychiatric Rehabilitation Methods

Introduction   140
Consumer Choice   141
Psychiatric Rehabilitation Readiness   142
Rehabilitation Diagnosis   144
Rehabilitation Plan   147
Rehabilitation Interventions   147
The Story of Paul (Continued from Chapter 1)   147
Skill Acquisition and Development   149
Resource Development   155
Evaluating Rehabilitation Progress   156
Summary   158

Class Exercise   159
References   160

Part III   Applications of Psychiatric Rehabilitation Principles and Methodology

Chapter 6   Psychiatric Rehabilitation Day Programming

Introduction   166
The Origins of Day Programming in the United States   167
The Story of Jill, Affinity House Member   171
Partial Hospitalization   173
Milieu Therapy   175
Components of a Psychiatric Rehabilitation Day Program   176
Evaluating Psychiatric Rehabilitation Day Programs   180
State-of-the-Art Psychiatric Rehabilitation Day Programming   183
Summary   186
Class Exercise   187
References   188

Chapter 7   Assertive Community Treatment and Case Management

Introduction   192
The Need for Continuity of Care   193
Awareness of the Need for Care Coordination at the National Level   196
Case Management   196
Models of Case Management   199
The Story of Micky   201
Evaluating Case Management   203
The Development of Assertive Community Treatment   204
Assertive Community Treatment: An Evidence-Based Practice   208
The Future of ACT and Case Management Approaches   214
Summary   215
Class Exercise   215
References   216

Chapter 8   Dual Diagnosis: Substance Abuse and Mental Illness

Introduction   220
History of Dual Diagnosis Treatment   221
Fundamental Treatment Strategies in Providing Integrated Dual Disorders: Stages of Treatment   225
Stages of Change: A Case Study Applying Motivational Interviewing   227
Principles of Treatment for People with Dual Diagnoses   228
Integrated Services: An Evidence-Based Practice   230

Roger's Story   234
Summary   238
Class Exercise   238
References   240

Chapter 9   *Vocational Rehabilitation*

Introduction   244
Barriers to Employment   245
Developing Vocational Services   250
Vocational Service Modalities   255
Supported Employment   258
Carl's Story   260
Models of Supported Employment   264
Other Vocational Preparation Services   267
Supported Employment: An Evidence-Based Practice   268
Summary   269
Class Exercise   270
References   271

Chapter 10   *Supported Education*

Introduction   276
Benefits of Supported Education   276
Barriers to Education   277
History of the Supported Employment Model   280
Definition and Models of Supported Education   283
Jose's Story   287
Applying Psychiatric Rehabilitation Principles to Supported Education   289
Research in Supported Education   291
Dissemination of Supported Education   295
Future Directions in Supported Education   295
Summary   298
Class Exercise   298
References   299

Chapter 11   *Residential Services and Independent Living*

Introduction   304
Barriers to Housing   304
History of Residential Services   307
Rehabilitation Treatment Facilities as Residential Providers   312
Stigma and Residential Treatment Programs   312

Emergence of the Linear Continuum Paradigm   313
The Story of Joanna: An Experience of the Linear Continuum
    Approach   315
Supported Housing: A New Approach to Residential Services   318
The Independent Living Movement   323
Housing First   326
Summary   330
Class Exercise   330
References   331

Chapter 12   *Self-Help and Peer-Delivered Services*

Introduction   336
Defining Self-Help and Peer Support   336
History of the Self-Help Movement   338
Self-Advocacy and the Ex-Patient/Consumer/Survivor Movement   339
Collaboration between Consumers and Provides   342
Self-Help for Persons with Dual Diagnoses   345
Access to Self-Help   346
The Story of David   347
Beyond Self-Help: Categories of Peer-Provided Services   349
Research on the Effectiveness of Self-Help and Peer-Provided Services   352
Challenges for Peer Providers   358
Supports and Professional Development   362
Other Influential Roles for Consumers   364
Summary   366
Class Exercises   367
References   367

Chapter 13   *The Role of the Family in Psychiatric Rehabilitation*

Introduction   374
Working with Families and Psychiatric Rehabilitation Principles   375
Kevin's Story: A Confidentiality Issue   381
The Burdens of Family Living for the Person with Mental Illness   386
Family Interventions   387
Family Psychoeducation: An Evidence-Based Practice   392
Other Family Psychoeducation Approaches   394
The Concept of Family Recovery   395
The Story of NAMI   396
Familial Strengths and Resilience   399
Summary   399
Class Exercise   400
References   401

Chapter 14   Psychiatric Rehabilitation in Hospital Settings

Introduction   406
Functions of State Psychiatric Hospitals   410
Stan's Story   412
Julie's Story   414
Challenges in the Hospital Environment   416
Psychiatric Rehabilitation Models within Hospitals   420
Case Study of a Hospital Implementing Individualized Psychiatric
    Rehabilitation   422
Is Hospitalization Always Necessary?   423
Summary   425
Class Exercise   426
References   426

Glossary   *429*
Index   *437*

Foreword

Psychiatric rehabilitation is no longer a new field. As you will discover in this text, many people date the field as beginning in the mid-1970s, although some of the principles and values of the field date back more than 150 years. As we conceive of it today, psychiatric rehabilitation is based on a vision of recovery, meaning that a rich and meaningful life is possible for people who have been diagnosed with a mental illness—including individuals who have difficulties significant enough to merit the term "disability." This idea of recovery goes back many years, although research documenting the fact of recovery is relatively recent. Philosophical roots of the recovery vision include the idea that people with a mental illness can improve with exercise, fresh air, and meaningful activity, and the idea that social support and connections to other people promote good mental health. Psychiatric rehabilitation also has political roots, and has been powerfully influenced by people who have been diagnosed with a mental illness and who have taken a stand against traditional treatments and systems that have infringed on their civil and human rights.

My own interest in the field of psychiatric rehabilitation began with an appreciation of some of these humanistic ideals and philosophies, but was quickly consolidated through contact with some very outspoken advocates. I was fortunate to learn early on that the people who use mental health services have clear opinions of what works and what doesn't, and need to be involved in determining how those services are provided. I learned that politics affects service delivery in more ways than through funding (or lack of funding). Sadly, I also learned that some professionals who provide mental health services hold attitudes at least as negative as those of the general public who know little or nothing about psychiatric disorders.

Over its short lifetime, psychiatric rehabilitation has become increasingly mainstream and is recognized as a valuable and effective approach to helping people with psychiatric disabilities gain the homes, the work, and the relationships that we all desire. In spite of its increasing acceptance as a useful constellation of services, psychiatric rehabilitation remains too seldom a career choice among professionals with advanced academic training. Psychiatric rehabilitation needs more than advanced professionals, however. The need for non-degreed professionals—people with training but not graduate degrees—remains high. In addition, the field desperately needs workers from diverse backgrounds, because the profile of the majority of psychiatric rehabilitation workers does not match the increasingly diverse profile of people who need and use psychiatric rehabilitation services.

This textbook presents information on psychiatric rehabilitation in an accessible way, making it invaluable for introducing people to the field. Having this information so well organized and so clearly presented provides a resource that will help meet the training needs of people working or planning to work in psychiatric rehabilitation.

In addition to being "user friendly," this textbook presents a broad view of the many perspectives, interventions, and developments that have expanded psychiatric rehabilitation. One of the strengths of the book is its lack of exclusive focus on any one perspective, technique, or program model. The professional organization for people who work in psychiatric rehabilitation, the U.S. Psychiatric Rehabilitation Association, has clearly stated the importance of offering a variety of program models.

In addition, this textbook integrates background information on history, leaders, and philosophy, while providing a picture of mental health services and systems as they exist today. Understanding the process by which the current mental health systems have come into being can help us recognize the complexity of changing the services offered, and can also prove that change is possible. Having watched the changes in the field during the past 30-plus years, and having studied the history predating me and most of my colleagues, I find that an appreciation of history helps me continue to work to change the system, while recognizing that real change on a large scale can take a long time.

Having worked with the authors of this text, I appreciate both their personal and professional qualities. Who they are and what they do have both contributed to the production of this textbook. As professionals, the authors are active drivers of the movement to improve the quality of psychiatric rehabilitation service delivery. They go beyond their roles as committed educators, and have contributed substantially to the increased professionalism in the field. All together, they have invested countless hours to improving training, to raising standards, and to increasing communication among people in the field.

I have had the good fortune to work on some projects with each of the textbook authors. They are, individually and as a group, warm, open minded, and welcoming of collaboration. Their integrity is obvious in the degree to which they really live the values and principles of psychiatric rehabilitation in their own work. I have been impressed with the ease with which they incorporate new ideas into their understanding of and teaching in psychiatric rehabilitation.

The new edition provides an example of incorporating new ideas and research. For example, the recent identification of evidence-based practices in psychiatric rehabilitation is now described in the text. Program effectiveness research is updated, and expanded information is included for some program models, such as integrated treatment for people with both a psychiatric disorder and substance abuse and supported education. New information has been incorporated with a reminder of how the basic principles of psychiatric rehabilitation related to current program models, making this edition both up to date and timeless.

Although some readers may be surprised to see a chapter in a book on psychiatric rehabilitation devoted to hospital-based services, this edition does address the reality that many public psychiatric inpatient facilities still exist. The authors recognize the conflict between principles and practices raised by focusing on such services, but point out that if such inpatient facilities *do* remain (regardless of whether they "must" or should remain), then integrating psychiatric rehabilitation into these facilities will surely be of benefit.

The need for a second edition of this text within 7 years of the publication of the first edition shows the rapid growth of the field of psychiatric rehabilitation. It is exciting to imagine what changes might be included in future editions, if this dramatic pace continues. We have come a long way, and we have a long way to go. People with psychiatric disabilities deserve respect and support, and have demonstrated that a mental illness does not need to be a barrier to a rich and successful life. Hopefully, services and systems will improve, and will more actively involve the people who use them. I hope that this textbook continues to inspire readers to enter the field of psychiatric rehabilitation and to contribute to the change, growth, and service improvements that are needed in the years to come.

Patricia B. Nemec
Boston University
March 2006

Acknowledgments

Psychiatric rehabilitation has gone through some important changes since the publication of this textbook's first edition in 1999. We hopefully have captured many of these new developments. One thing that has not changed is the generosity of our colleagues in the psychiatric rehabilitation field, who have provided us with their critical judgment and sage advice. Without this support our task would have been much more difficult and the final result much less complete. The following individuals contributed time and effort to this project: Annette Backs, Gary Bond, Patrick Corrigan, Robert Drake, Rusty Foster, Patti Holland, Stephen Jakubowycz, Carol Mowbray, Kim Mueser, Pat Nemec, Phyllis Solomon, Russell Smith, Anne Sullivan-Soydan, Peggy Swarbrick, and Tony Zipple.

Part I

Understanding the Nature of Severe and Persistent Mental Illness

Chapter 1

The Experience of Mental Illness:
An Introduction to Psychiatric Rehabilitation

Introduction 4

The Story of Paul 4

Discussion of Paul's Story 8

The Serious Mental Illnesses 9

The Symptoms of Mental Illness 10

The Causes of the Severe Mental
Illnesses 10

Psychiatric Disability 10

**The Stigma of Severe Mental
Illness 13**

Psychiatric Rehabilitation 14

What Does the Term "Psychiatric
Rehabilitation" Mean? 14

The Emergence of Psychiatric
Rehabilitation 15

Deinstitutionalization 15

Psychiatric Rehabilitation Terminology and
Language 17

Developing Psychiatric Rehabilitation
Knowledge 19

Psychiatric Rehabilitation: A Science or an
Art? 20

Evidence-Based Practices 22

Scientific Literature and Meetings 24

Standards for Creating Psychiatric
Rehabilitation Professionals 25

Summary 26

Class Exercise 27

References 27

Chapter 1 begins with the story of Paul, a young man diagnosed with a severe mental illness, schizophrenia. After reading about Paul you will cover basic definitions of severe mental illness, disability, and stigma. Most importantly, this chapter will introduce you to the field of psychiatric rehabilitation, an evolving set of methods, strategies, and concepts for the community treatment of persons with severe mental illness. The final section of the chapter discusses how psychiatric rehabilitation knowledge is developed, the identification of evidence-based practices, and the sources of that knowledge for professionals and students.

This chapter will answer the following questions:

1. What are some of the symptoms and problems that might afflict a young person stricken with a severe mental illness?

2. What are severe mental illnesses and how are they defined?

3. *What is psychiatric rehabilitation?*
4. *How and when did the practice of psychiatric rehabilitation begin?*
5. *What is the state of psychiatric rehabilitation today?*

Introduction

Psychiatric rehabilitation, sometimes referred to as psychosocial rehabilitation, is a comprehensive strategy for meeting the needs of persons with severe and persistent mental illness. A true understanding of psychiatric rehabilitation (PsyR) begins with awareness and sensitivity to the personal experience of severe and debilitating mental illnesses.

Unlike many diseases with predictable symptoms and outcomes, the experience and consequences of mental illness vary considerably from person to person. This is true even for individuals diagnosed with exactly the same condition. Take for example two persons both diagnosed with schizophrenia, undifferentiated type. One may be experiencing auditory hallucinations (hearing voices), while the other person is plagued by paranoid ideas but experiences no auditory hallucinations. The history or course of mental illness may also differ from person to person. One person may have frequent relapses, while another will have additional acute episodes only occasionally. In addition, each person may adjust and respond to his or her illness differently. One person may be severely disabled throughout the course of his or her life, while another may cope well and overcome the disability.

The Story of Paul

Like any person's story, Paul's is unique. At the same time, in many respects, Paul's story resembles millions of similar situations that unfold every year throughout our country and around the world. Each of us has ideas and attitudes about mental illness that we get from personal experience, from the media, or from speaking with others. Some of these ideas are accurate. Others are half-truths and myths. Some are just plain wrong. As you read about Paul's experience consider the attitudes and ideas you have about mental illness. Also, consider the following questions:

1. Why did Paul become ill when he did? Were there any events or situations that might have led to Paul's illness?
2. What kinds of things did Paul experience as he became ill? Did the disease itself cause all of these things?
3. Could Paul's illness have been predicted or even avoided?
4. How did Paul's family handle the situation? Should they have done something differently?
5. Are there any clues as to how Paul will respond to treatment?

Paul began to realize something was wrong when he couldn't follow the lectures in his college classes. Almost anything could become a distraction. A crack in the blackboard or the inflection of a particular word would seem as important to him as what the professor was saying. Even in his favorite class, macroeconomics, with a professor he really liked, he couldn't keep his attention on the material. Nineteen years old, a college freshman, living away from home for the first time in his life, Paul found that school was becoming a nightmare. An A−/B+ student in high school, now halfway through his first college semester, Paul was losing his ability to concentrate. He strained to listen and take good notes but his thoughts were confused. He could not seem to maintain his focus. Instead, he would hear a particular word, his thoughts would go off on a tangent, and he would lose the focus of the lecture. After class, he would struggle to summarize the main points, but nothing seemed to stand out. Everything was of equal importance. At first, Paul felt mainly frustration, but as his inability to focus continued, his anxiety increased and he began to feel frightened.

In high school Paul hung around with a group of college-bound, but not particularly motivated students. Blessed with a moderately high IQ, Paul could usually get above-average grades by paying attention in class and cramming for his finals. His one love was business. He could spend hours reading books about successful businessmen like Michael Dell and Bill Gates or books describing how successful companies like Microsoft and Ben and Jerry's were created, developed, and managed. He dreamed of one day developing and becoming the CEO of his own company. For Paul, the business environment seemed to offer opportunities for creativity and self-expression. While not interested in the personal contact necessary for a sales career, Paul was attracted to the problem solving and planning required of a successful executive. Paul's neighbor, Nancy, was his love interest during high school. Like Paul, Nancy was on the quiet side and they got along well together. Paul and Nancy would ride bikes, go to the movies, play computer games, and study together. They were best friends and talked about getting serious. Paul viewed it as a tragedy when she moved out of state with her family the summer after their sophomore year. At first, they wrote to each other weekly, but the connection grew weak and after about 6 months they hardly corresponded at all.

Paul played right field on the junior varsity baseball team during his sophomore year in high school. The coach saw him as a mediocre player and Paul only played when the team was ahead. He didn't go out for baseball again as a junior. Instead, he joined the computer club and began spending most of his time surfing the Internet and following stocks. Likable but shy, Paul spent a lot of his free time with his computer during his junior and senior years.

Paul's friend Kevin was also a member of the computer club and spent many hours hacking, surfing the Internet, and adjusting his imaginary stock portfolio to compete with Paul's. As they became friendlier, Paul felt safe confiding in Kevin. They often talked about their hopes and dreams for the future and their pet likes and dislikes. Although they weren't considered popular, Paul and Kevin were liked by most of their high school peers. Kevin was really serious about computers. He planned to be a math and computer science major in college, and his motivation to get the grades he needed to pursue his goal rubbed off on Paul.

Childhood had been a happy time for Paul. The oldest child in his family, he always got plenty of attention and love from his parents and a lot of encouragement. He thought of his family as an on-going source of friendship, love, fun, and support. His father worked as a personnel manager for a large manufacturing company. He liked his job, loved his family, and usually had a kind word for everyone. Paul's mom worked as a medical technician at the local laboratory. She was proud of this job because it required technical skill. She also liked it because she could schedule her own hours to make time when her family needed her. It was no secret that her family came first. Paul's sister Alice was a junior in high school and his younger brother Ted was in the eighth grade.

Going away to college had seemed like a great adventure to Paul. During orientation he met his future roommate Ira, who came from out of state. A psychology major, Ira shared Paul's interest in computers and surfing the Internet. An instant friendship emerged. At first, as classes started Ira had the same positive effect on Paul's study habits as his friend Kevin. Ira, like his mother whom he looked up to, wanted to pursue a Ph.D. in psychology. Being very organized, he made sure that he and Paul set aside a block of time each evening to be used only for studying. Ira and Paul joked about becoming nerds, but Paul was secretly glad for the discipline.

Several weeks after he noticed he was having trouble focusing on lectures, Paul found himself feeling both suspicious and angry with Ira. Whenever Ira said something to him, Paul would become suspicious of what he meant or what he might be up to. He felt that Ira was only being friendly with him in order to take control of their relationship. He began to refuse to speak with Ira so that he would not feel like he was being manipulated. But, keeping distant only made him feel rejected and angry and he blamed that on Ira as well. He found that no matter how much he wanted to mend their relationship, he was not really able to be friendly with Ira. When he tried to communicate, he felt manipulated and controlled. When he withdrew, he felt angry and rejected.

At the same time he noticed that he was having trouble relating to his professors. He felt they were manipulating him as well. Studying every night had given Paul a real edge in his classes and early on his professors thought of him as one of the brighter students. Now, after an excellent start, his apparent total reversal came as a real shock to his professors. Several of them asked to speak with Paul after class, asking if everything was all right. Paul denied any problems while wondering why they were singling him out, since he still had a good average. Paul decided that he was being held to a stricter standard than the other students and that the school was closely observing him. After several of these inquiries, Paul found it harder and harder to get to class. His inability to concentrate made it seem pointless anyway. Instead, he spent his time alone in his dorm room playing computer games. Finally, with failing grades in every class, Paul left for home before finals.

His parents were worried and confused by Paul's behavior. Telephone conversations with Paul had alerted them that something was wrong but left them puzzled. Paul talked about isolation, people manipulating and controlling him, and being "observed" by the school. Their first thought was that Paul was using drugs. They knew Paul had experimented with marijuana in high school but that had not seemed to be a problem at the time. When they asked Paul about drugs he adamantly denied it and showed none of the telltale signs. When he got home it was obvious to his parents that something else was wrong. Both parents were very upset and after a long discussion, they decided to ask Paul to see Dr. Williams, the family doctor. Paul had always liked Doc Williams and he was clearly fond of Paul. Ashamed of his poor performance at school and confused by his own thoughts and feelings, he agreed to see him the following week.

Home in a safe place and feeling less suspicious, Paul was able to tell Dr. Williams everything that had been happening to him. As he conveyed his story, he felt that much of what he told the doctor made no sense. Why had he mistrusted his new friend? Why wasn't he able to concentrate in class? Why had he started cutting classes? All the behaviors, thoughts and feelings he reported seemed strange as if they had happened to someone else. Dr. Williams listened to Paul's story and reassured him that it was not uncommon for students going away to college for the first time to have an anxiety reaction. He suggested that Paul see a colleague of his with special training to work with these types of problems, a psychiatrist named Dr. Kline.

During the week he had to wait before his appointment with Dr. Kline, Paul started to become withdrawn and suspicious of his family. During evening meals he heard a voice telling him that he wasn't his mother's child. His parents tried to hide their own anxiety by accepting Paul's odd behavior. When he saw Dr. Kline he was so suspicious that he had trouble relating his story. Dr. Kline suggested that in addition to some medication, Paul might consider signing himself into a hospital for a period of observation and treatment. He assured Paul that this was the best course of action and that he would be able to leave if he ever changed his mind. Feeling very distrustful, Paul refused the hospital as well as the medication Dr. Kline prescribed. Paul stayed home throughout that winter and into the spring. He became progressively more withdrawn and uncommunicative. Most of the time, he stayed in his room listening to music. During June, Paul told his mom that Dr. Kline was giving him orders by broadcasting thoughts to him telepathically. As these symptoms increased, Paul became agitated and threatening. Finally, at Dr. Williams's suggestion, his parents took him to the local private psychiatric hospital where he stayed for 2 weeks.

After 2 weeks in the hospital, Paul felt like he wasn't ready to be discharged. He was still hearing voices, feeling withdrawn, and on a high dose of injectable medication, but the nurses assured him that living at home and going to the community mental health center would be much better for him. Paul visited the mental health center before he was discharged. His intake staff worker gave him a tour of a special program for people with problems like his. People there seemed friendly and the program looked interesting but he still wasn't sure. His parents were both hopeful and concerned about Paul's return. At the suggestion of the hospital social worker, they told Paul that if he were going to live at home he would have to agree to attend the program at the community mental health center.

His first week at the program was difficult. He still wasn't sure what was wrong with him. His doctors at the hospital had been vague about his condition. When he thought about being mentally ill he became really scared, tried to think about something else or decided he was just suffering from stress. While he and a staff person at the program were filling out his initial treatment plan, the staff person told him that he should expect to be at the program for a long period of time, his diagnosis was schizophrenia.

Paul wasn't exactly sure what that meant. But, at the same time it was what he had dreaded all along. He felt fear growing in the pit of his stomach. His old life was over; he felt that the worker was telling him that he was insane.

Discussion of Paul's Story

Paul's story raises a number of important issues about mental illness that you will learn more about as you read this book. Many of these issues are controversial. Throughout this text you will see that, depending on training and orientation, theorists, researchers, and mental health professionals often have very different answers to these questions.

One important issue involves questions of *etiology*, or the cause(s) of such illnesses. What caused Paul's illness? Could someone have predicted that Paul would become ill by observing his development, and could the illness have been prevented? Partly because there is still a great deal we do not know about the etiology of the severe mental illnesses, this is an area of great controversy and heated debate. Some professionals believe that aspects of Paul's personal history, environment, and family life may help us to understand the cause of his illness. Others feel that these issues have little or no bearing on the disease because its cause is essentially biological rather than environmental. Most importantly, the different etiological beliefs held by professionals, family members, and people like Paul lead to choices of specific treatment strategies.

Another important issue that is raised is the question of *prognosis* or the probable course or outcome of the disease. Will he recover with medication and treatment? Or, will he become progressively more confused, alienated, and withdrawn over time? Can the prognosis of such a disease even be established? Although there is increasing agreement among professionals on the prognosis of these diseases given correct medication and services, there is still great variability between people with the same illness.

The final and most important issue remains: What is the best way to help Paul and other people like him? As you will see, there are many aspects to the care of mental illness. Specific beliefs about the etiology of these diseases lead to specific treatment strategies. *Treatment* is usually considered to be any action designed to cure a disease or reduce its symptoms. *Rehabilitation*, on the other hand, is usually defined as any action intended to reduce the negative effects of the disease on the person's everyday life.

To help explain this difference, let's consider a woman who has had a stroke and has lost her ability to walk. A doctor might prescribe anticoagulants, blood pressure medication, change in diet, and regular exercise to help reduce the probability of future strokes. These prescriptions would be considered treatment. The doctor might also prescribe physical therapy to help return the patient to the highest level of physical mobility after the deficits caused by the stroke. This therapy aimed at returning the patient to normal or near-normal functioning would be considered rehabilitation. Finally, a rehabilitation professional making a home visit might recommend that a ramp be built to the front door, that doorknobs be changed to levers, and that the bathroom be fitted with hand bars. These modifications to the patient's environment would also be considered part of the rehabilitation process.

The differences between treatment and rehabilitation seem clear for the woman who had a stroke. But for the person with mental illness, like Paul, the difference between treatment and rehabilitation is not always clear. Indeed, some professionals believe that it is a mistake to make a distinction between the *treatment* of mental illness and a process of *rehabilitation*. In fact, researchers have found evidence that the rehabilitation process itself has a direct and positive effect on the disease (Bond et al., 2001; Lysaker et al., 2001). Most PsyR professionals believe that treatment and rehabilitation are complementary processes.

The importance of the differences and similarities between treatment and rehabilitation will become evident as you move through this text. This issue is vital when considering questions such as "Who provides treatment? Who provides rehabilitation? What is the role of the psychiatric rehabilitation practitioner? What kinds of services should be provided?"

This textbook will provide you with answers to many of these questions. Real people, like Paul, and his loved ones are dependent on the answers. You will also learn about new, challenging, and complicated issues that address the best ways to help persons with severe mental illness.

The Severe Mental Illnesses

Serious and persistent mental illnesses, like the one that struck Paul, affect many people in our society and around the world. In the United States approximately 2.1% to 2.6% of the population have a mental illness that is severe enough to reduce their ability to perform living and working tasks effectively (International Association of Psychosocial Rehabilitation Services [IAPSRS], 2001). This translates to 5,250,000 to 6,500,000 people in the United States. The President's New Freedom Commission on Mental Health puts the estimate somewhat higher, saying 5% to 7% of adults in the United States have a serious mental illness, which would be 15 to 20 million people (President's New Freedom Commission for Mental Health, 2003).

For society as a whole, schizophrenia, which strikes an estimated 1% of the population, is by far the most devastating and the most feared mental illness. In addition, several other mental illnesses also cause untold suffering and disability. The *Diagnostic and Statistical Manual of Mental Disorders*, fourth edition, text revision (DSM-IV-TR), of the American Psychiatric Association (2000) recognizes recurring depressive disorders, bi-polar and unipolar disorders (commonly known as manic depressive disorders), schizoaffective disorder, and organic brain syndromes among others as serious mental illnesses that can become long term, cause psychosis, and lead to psychiatric disability.

Today, there is increasing awareness that people who experience severe mental illness often suffer from other serious maladies as well. These "dually diagnosed" individuals may be coping with substance abuse problems, developmental disabilities, severe learning disabilities, and chronic physical illnesses at the same time they are struggling with their mental illness. As you might imagine, the problems raised when someone is suffering from more than one disorder at the same time can be very difficult. Which disorder should be treated first? Does the treatment of one disorder negatively affect the treatment of another disorder? Which disorder is causing the symptoms that are present? Special programs for people who are dually diagnosed are increasing around the country. These programs are staffed by professionals who are cross-trained to address multiple problems. The issue of dual diagnosis is covered in depth in Chapter 8.

The Symptoms of Mental Illness

Mental illnesses may present a wide variety of symptoms. The symptoms of the severe mental illnesses can be classified into two categories: positive symptoms and negative symptoms. Positive symptoms refer to what is added to the individual because of the disease. *Psychoses*, the faulty interpretation of reality due to incorrect sensory perceptions (*hallucinations*) or thoughts (*delusions*), are good examples of positive symptoms. Negative symptoms refer to things that the individual has lost because of the disease. Social withdrawal and an inability to experience pleasure, *anhedonia*, are typical examples of the kinds of negative symptoms someone with severe mental illness might experience. The great majority of persons experiencing these conditions are diagnosed with schizophrenia or a bi-polar disorder (manic depression). Chapters 2 and 3 will cover the cause, symptoms, and treatment of mental illness in more depth.

The Causes of the Severe Mental Illnesses

The pathological processes that cause these conditions are still poorly understood (Anthony & Liberman, 1986; Walker et al., 2004). Nevertheless, there is growing consensus that these conditions have a strong biological component (Dincin, 1990; Torrey, 2001). With the development of increasingly sophisticated soft tissue and metabolic imaging techniques such as CAT, PET, and MRI scans, researchers have been able to demonstrate actual changes in brain tissue and brain functioning corresponding with psychotic episodes (Taylor, 1987; Torrey, 2001; see also Andreasen, *The Broken Brain*, 1984). At the same time, researchers have looked at the contribution of genetics by comparing the life spans of individuals whose parents have schizophrenia with those whose parents do not have schizophrenia (Marcus et al., 1987) and studying identical and fraternal twins when one of the twins has the disorder (e.g., Torrey, 1994). These studies provide strong evidence that genetics play an important role when someone is stricken with a severe mental illness. Despite these advances, the causes of severe mental illness are not known. Chapters 2 and 3 will cover the symptoms, diagnosis, probable causes, probable courses, and outcomes of these illnesses in more detail.

Psychiatric Disability

Without effective rehabilitation, a severe mental illness can disable a person for life. Most often striking during the late teens and early twenties, life disruptions like the one Paul experienced are very common with these illnesses. When school, work, and family are disrupted, the individual cannot acquire the skills needed to cope with the demands of

---

BOX 1.1
**Biographical Sketches—
Early Theorists**

Emil Kraeplin (1856–1926)

An eminent German psychiatrist, Kraeplin is credited with establishing the first classification system for the severe mental illnesses. He was also the first clinician to recognize the difference between dementia praecox (schizophrenia) and manic-depressive illness. Receiving his M.D. degree from the University of Wurzburg in 1878, Kraeplin continued his neurological studies and studied with the "father" of the new field of psychology, Wilhelm Wundt. This work led to his publishing of *Compendium der Psychiatrie (Concise Summary of Psychiatry)* in 1883. Kraeplin divided mental illness into exogenous conditions, which were caused by external factors and were therefore treatable, and endogenous conditions, which he believed were caused by biological or hereditary factors and which he considered incurable. Using this classification strategy, Kraeplin saw manic-depressive illness as exogenous and therefore treatable and dementia praecox as endogenous and essentially incurable. Kraeplin believed dementia praecox stemmed from organic pathological changes in the brain. He is also credited with classifying three important subtypes of dementia praecox: catatonia, halted motor activity;

hebephrenia, regression to a vegetative state; and paranoia, delusions of persecution or grandeur.

Eugene Bleuler (1857–1939)

One of the most influential psychiatrists of his time, Bleuler is credited with introducing the term *schizophrenia* by combining two Greek words meaning "split" and "mind." Rather than the split personality of popular fiction, Bleuler believed that the "split" was usually between the person's cognitive (thinking) and affective (emotional) processes. A Swiss psychiatrist, Bleuler studied medicine at the University of Bern, was appointed professor of psychiatry at the University of Zurich and became director of the Burgholzli Asylum in Zurich. It was at Burgholzli, where he worked from 1898 to 1927, that he conducted his studies of schizophrenia. In 1911 he published his groundbreaking paper "Dementia Praecox oder Gruppe der Schizophrenien" ("Dementia Praecox: Or the Group of Schizophrenias"). Contrary to the professional wisdom of his day, Bleuler believed that the schizophrenias were actually several different diseases, that they were not necessarily incurable, and that the course of the disease was not always negative. During Bleuler's later career he was assisted by Freud's disciple Carl Gustav Jung. Under the influence of Freud's theories, Bleuler became convinced that schizophrenia could have psychological rather than biological causes and that it could be treated using psychoanalytic techniques.

---

modern life. Without these skills, which many take for granted, the individual cannot function successfully.

These conditions tend to be long lasting as well as severe and are referred to as "severe and persistent mental illness." Thus, they often disrupt and stunt normal intellectual, social, and vocational development or lead to conditions where acquired skills are lost due to disuse. This lack of ability, whether because skills were never acquired or were acquired and subsequently lost, is the hallmark of psychiatric *disability*. Although psychiatric symptoms can often be controlled by medication and therapies, disability secondary to the disease often persists. The analogy of a physical trauma may help to clarify this issue. A person who loses the use of his legs because of an automobile accident becomes disabled, because he has lost skills like walking and running. The damage from the accident persists or is permanent, while the physical danger has passed.

CONTROVERSIAL ISSUE
Schizophrenia or "Neurotransmitter/ Stress Syndrome"

Since Bleuler coined the term *schizophrenia* and distinguished it from dementia praecox, the term has been widely used in psychiatry. The DSM-IV-TR and its earlier editions have consistently used the term *schizophrenia*, modifying it with disease categories such as paranoid, catatonic, or undifferentiated. Today, literally millions of persons in the United States and around the world carry a diagnostic label of schizophrenia.

The term *schizophrenia* is widely used by the media and entertainment industries, where it is portrayed as the very essence of a severe mental illness. The paranoid schizophrenic label used by the media conjures up images of wild-eyed assassins who kill and maim for no apparent reason.

The term *schizophrenia* is also used to denote apparent contradictions in people, organizations, or policies. The Iran-Contra scandal was often labeled the product of a "schizophrenic" policy of selling arms to our enemies in order to raise money to support our allies. This misuse of the term also reinforces the common misconception that schizophrenia is a form of multiple personality disorder, which it is not.

The clear abuse of the term and increased understanding of these illnesses has prompted debate about the continued use of "schizophrenia" as a diagnostic label. Jerry Dincin, who served for many years as the executive director of Thresholds, a large psychiatric rehabilitation agency in Chicago, argued that the diagnostic label schizophrenia should be changed to "neurotransmitter/stress syndrome" (Dincin, 1990). This new diagnostic label captures both the biological basis (neurotransmitter) and the environmental vulnerability (stress) aspects of the severe mental illnesses. But more importantly, *"neurotransmitter/stress syndrome,"* or a similar term, does not necessarily carry the stigma and negative connotation of a label like schizophrenia. Dincin uses an analogy from the developmental disabilities field to make his point. The terms *"morons," "idiots,"* and *"imbeciles"* of 30 years ago (when they were used as diagnostic labels by professionals) have been replaced by terms with much less negative impact (Dincin, 1990). The probable relationship of neurotransmitters to severe mental illness will be discussed in more depth in Chapter 2.

The actual costs of changing such a label might be large. Besides the obvious changes in charts, records, and diagnostic manuals, a great deal of re-training would need to take place within the mental health delivery system and the systems that pay for treatment.

One might also consider the media's response to such a change. Popular culture would still need a label for "madness" since individuals with these labels supply the motivating force for many real and fictional stories of crime and violence. Could "neurotransmitter/stress syndrome" become the stigmatized label of the future?

Some PsyR theorists and researchers such as William Anthony and Robert Liberman cite evidence that the degree of psychiatric disability is related to the individual's premorbid skill level. The term *premorbid* refers to the period before the individual became ill. In this case, to what the individual's skill level was before the illness. In addition, Anthony and Liberman infer that higher skill levels can reduce the intensity of psychiatric illness. We will cover the contributions of these skill theorists in a later chapter.

Disability is an important medical and social concept. The Americans with Disabilities Act of 1990, which is discussed in Chapter 7, defines disability as a substantial limitation in a major life activity (Lawn & Meyerson, from Liberman, 1992). Another important medical body, the World Health Organization, defines *disability* as an inability to participate or perform at a socially desirable level in such activities as self-care, social relationships, work, and situationally appropriate behavior.

Most importantly for Americans, the Social Security Administration has outlined four key areas of psychiatric disability: (1) activities of daily living (ADLs) (e.g., grooming, hygiene, maintaining a household, managing finances); (2) social functioning (with family, friends, community, and in the workplace); (3) concentration, pace, and task persistence (ability to function for 6 to 8 hours without supervision); and (4) the ability to tolerate competitive work (Lawn & Meyerson, from Liberman, 1992). Duration of disability is also an important factor. To meet the Social Security Administration's definition the disability has to be continuously present for at least 12 months.

The Stigma of Severe Mental Illness

When someone has a severe mental illness, the diagnosis itself can cause serious problems. As Hall, Andrews, and Goldstein (1985) point out "Schizophrenia is . . . a sentence as well as a diagnosis." The person labeled *schizophrenic* carries a powerful stigma to which other people may react with fear and rejection. Because the symptoms of these diseases can affect how a person thinks, feels, behaves, and communicates, the effects of the diseases are often apparent to other people. Unlike common symptoms such as coughing, sneezing, or running a fever, psychiatric symptoms are often not attributed to a disease. Sometimes, since they are so little understood, psychiatric symptoms are attributed to supernatural, spiritual, or demonic causes.

Mental illness is so frightening that healthy persons often refer to people with mental illness using the name of their mental illness. Someone with schizophrenia may be labeled a "schizophrenic" by some of the people with whom they have regular contact. Someone with paranoid schizophrenia may be called a "paranoid." By contrast, the individual suffering from diabetes is less frequently referred to as a *"diabetic"* by friends and acquaintances and usually only when it is pertinent such as when meals are being planned. E. Fuller Torrey, M.D., a psychiatrist who treats, researches, and writes on schizophrenia believes that persons experiencing schizophrenia are treated like the lepers of the 20th century (Torrey, 2001). The term *stigma* originally referred to the ancient practice of physically marking (scarring) villains so that others would know that they were criminals and be on their guard. Many persons today react in the same way when they meet a person they think is mentally ill.

Peoples' reaction to stigma refers to what Coleman (1986) called "the dilemma of difference." Most people accept that individuals are different in many ways. When some differences are deemed unacceptable, people with undesirable characteristics or differences may be stigmatized. What a given society chooses to stigmatize is somewhat arbitrary. In the past, some societies considered persons who today might be diagnosed with schizophrenia, as higher beings who were specially gifted and able to commune with God. Saint Francis of Assisi was known to speak with the animals, which was considered proof of his saintly nature. Today, our first reaction might be to consider such behavior as evidence of a psychotic process.

Much of the stigma surrounding mental illness has its roots in ignorance and fear. This is not surprising since until very recently there was little scientific evidence to support any theory explaining serious mental illness. Some scholars even questioned the very existence of mental illness. In his writing, Thomas Szasz suggested that mental illness is simply a learned behavior that, for some people, is a realistic reaction to modern society. Today, as we are beginning to get a clearer understanding of mental illness, we can begin to combat the stigma left by centuries of ignorance and fear.

The ignorance that has surrounded mental illness since the beginning of history is being lifted by modern psychiatry with the advent of imaging techniques such as CAT, PET, and MRI scans, genetic research, the development of new drugs, and other breakthroughs. While we fear cancer and have compassion for those who are stricken, medical science has increased our understanding of the disease and reduced the stigma cancer patients once experienced. Recent progress in the treatment of AIDS is helping to reduce the stigma associated with that condition. In the same way, future citizens educated about mental illness may fear the disease but not the person.

In addition to knowledge about the disease, contact with individuals who successfully cope with it can eradicate the stigma it carries. Actual contact with persons who have these serious mental illnesses has been shown to decrease stigma (Corrigan et al., 2003).

The community treatment of mental illness also has the potential to reduce stigma. Treating persons experiencing severe and persistent mental illness in the community means that at one time or another everyone may come in contact with them.

This exposure to persons with mental illness is a powerful tool for reducing the stigma that surrounds the disease. As most psychiatric rehabilitation staff will tell you, persons with mental illness are no different from you and me, except for their disease. Keeping these persons in institutions adds to the stigma surrounding the disease. Accepting them into the community helps to eliminate stigma because living and working in the community on a daily basis highlights their basic humanity not their disability.

Psychiatric Rehabilitation

What Does the Term "Psychiatric Rehabilitation" Mean?

In the helping professions, the term *rehabilitate* means to restore to an optimal state of constructive activity. Of course, what is "optimal" is relative to the individual. An individual's "optimal" level of constructive activity depends on several factors. How well a person functions depends on how severe the illness is at the time, the severity of the disability, the abilities he or she still possesses, the outside supports that are available, and what some theorists call the "stage of recovery." *Stage of recovery* refers to the individual's level of progress in his or her ability to cope with the disease and disability and his or her self-image as a functioning person. The concept of recovery will be dealt with in some depth in Chapter 4. Psychiatric rehabilitation refers to efforts to restore persons with psychiatric disabilities to optimal states of constructive activity. The degree of disability a person experiences is often variable. Some persons with severe and persistent mental illness may be disabled in many aspects of their lives. Other persons may be disabled in only one area, while otherwise being generally free of disability.

Numerous definitions of PsyR exist, reflecting a range of philosophical and technical differences among practitioners (Anthony, 1979; Anthony & Liberman, 1986; Carson, B. E., & Chambers, C. in Rutman 1994; Hughes, 1994; Rutman, 1994). Ruth Hughes (1994), former executive director of IAPSRS, provided an excellent definition that most PsyR practitioners can agree with:

> The goal of psychiatric rehabilitation is to enable individuals to compensate for, or eliminate the functional deficits, interpersonal barriers and environmental barriers created by the disability, and to restore ability for independent living, socialization and effective life management. (p. 11)

In 1992 the *Psychosocial Rehabilitation Journal* asked its readers to submit definitions of PsyR. The following definition of PsyR, which received an honorable mention in the contest, captures both the humanity and the hope inherent in the rehabilitation process:

"Psychosocial rehabilitation means that a person who before was afraid to go into a store to order an ice cream soda can now be an ice cream store manager" Martha Green (in Rutman, 1994).

The Emergence of Psychiatric Rehabilitation

Practitioners of PsyR are united in believing that persons with severe and persistent mental illness can achieve greater independence and a better quality of life with the help of psychiatric rehabilitation services. This assumption, that persons with psychiatric disabilities can participate in a successful rehabilitation process, is in marked contrast to the beliefs of many mental health professionals only a few generations ago and some today. Until the late 1970's and early 1980's, the conventional wisdom about severe mental illness was that it took an insidious downward course with little or no hope of recovery. Prior to 1987, the DSM-III (*Diagnostic and Statistical Manual of Mental Disorders*, third edition) published by the American Psychiatric Association (1980) stated that the most common course of schizophrenia consisted of acute episodes followed by "increasing residual impairments" (p. 185). In contrast to this pessimistic view, recent research has demonstrated that, even for those with severe psychiatric disability often labeled as "backward" patients, the long-term *prognosis* is positive (DeSisto, Harding, McCormack, Ashikaga, and Brooks, 1995; Harding, Brooks, Ashikaga, Strauss, and Breier, 1987; Torrey, 2001).

Another positive development is the work researchers, practitioners, and consumers of PsyR services are doing to develop the concept of *recovery* from psychiatric disability. Even though some of the disabilities and residual symptoms may be life-long, the field of PsyR is rapidly learning and defining what it means to "recover" from major mental illness (Anthony, 1993, 2000; Deegan, 1988). The concept of recovery will be discussed in greater detail in Chapter 4.

Deinstitutionalization

The emergence of PsyR as a unique enterprise can be directly traced to the *deinstitutionalization* movement that began in the 1960s and early 1970s. Between 1960 and today, approximately 90% of the persons in long-term state psychiatric institutions were discharged into the community. Based on current population estimates, to date some 900,000 persons experiencing severe and persistent mental illness have either been discharged from psychiatric hospitals or not institutionalized (Torrey, 2001). When the policy of deinstitutionalization began, literally thousands of patients who had been institutionalized for much of their adult lives were discharged into the community for treatment. Given their traditional mental health training, many, if not most, of the community mental health staff workers were unprepared for this challenge (Stern & Minkoff, 1979; Farkas, O'Brien, and Nemec, 1988). In many areas of the United States, persons who were deinstitutionalized were deemed to be "inappropriate" for the existing community services in place at that time. This despite the fact that the major impetus for the nationwide federal funding of community mental health centers begun in 1963 was specifically designed to care for this population. Workers trained to provide individual psychotherapy for persons with supposed psychodynamic problems tended to classify these people as not being good "treatment cases." Marianne Farkas, of the Center for Psychiatric Rehabilitation, Boston University, found that this newly deinstitutionalized population had low "patient" status because they were not highly verbal and did not demonstrate high rates of treatment success (Farkas et al., 1988). As a result, many persons with chronic mental illness were relegated to programs staffed by less educated persons with non-traditional academic degrees and by paraprofessionals (persons without academic credentials).

Torrey (2001) asserts that only about 5% of the 789 federally funded community mental health centers (CMHCs) accepted the challenge of providing appropriate services to the deinstitutionalized population. The majority of the centers focused their efforts on providing counseling, psychotherapy, consultation, and education in the broader area of mental illness. Mostly because CMHC staff members were ill equipped to deal with them, persons with severe mental illness became increasingly isolated and remained underserved in the community.

The academic preparation of mental health professionals was very slow to adjust to the needs of the deinstitutionalization movement. This poor academic response was caused by a lack of recognition of the plight of this population as well as a lack of awareness of the treatment strategies necessary to aide them. A review of introductory undergraduate psychology textbooks carried out as late as 1992 revealed that lobotomy (brain surgery to relieve symptoms) was written about more than psychiatric rehabilitation (Halter, Bond, & De Graaf-Kaser, 1992). None of the 28 introductory textbooks mentioned common PsyR approaches such as the Clubhouse Model (e.g., Fountain House, Horizon House, etc.), the National Institute of Mental Health's Community Support System, or social skills training. In addition, hospital treatment was given much more coverage than community treatment at a time when hospital stays were being reduced and large psychiatric hospitals being closed.

In addition to the textbooks, in many cases the clinical focus of undergraduate curricula has remained focused on the more traditional psychodynamic, cognitive, and behavioral treatment models. Graduate education curricula have often sidestepped the issue of treating persons with major mental illness by stating that this population is not appropriate for the treatment strategies they are training their students to use (e.g., psychotherapy).

BOX 1.2
Choosing Words with Dignity

The words we choose to use to portray people with mental illness reflect our attitudes and beliefs about the value, dignity and worth of people with disabilities. Our words influence the public perception and acceptance of people with disabilities. People with disabilities are people first and foremost, who also happen to have a disability, or a different set of abilities.

Progressive mental health systems use, at all times, descriptive words that emphasize the person's worth and abilities, not the disabling condition. They understand that people may have a disorder or disability but the people are not the disability. They also recognize that people are diminished when they are described by diagnosis (e.g., "schizophrenic," "paranoid," "borderline"), by slang (e.g., "psychos," "schizos"), and by phrases that negatively categorize them (e.g., "the mentally ill," "the chronically mentally ill," "young chronics," "retarded," "dually diagnosed"). Medical terms such as "patient" are not used in these systems to refer to people who are not in medical settings, because they are inconsistent with rehabilitation and community support philosophy.

IAPSRS (2003) proposed use of the term "people in recovery," in an attempt to reflect the fact that many, if not all persons with severe and persistent mental illnesses are engaged in an active process of recovery. This terms reflects the "person first" thinking, but actually begs the question of whether all people with mental illness are recovering or not. Assuming everyone is in recovery, in a way, trivializes the process of recovery. It's almost like saying all living people are "breathing."

It should be the written and public policy of all systems and agencies working with people with disabilities not to use labels like "the seriously mentally ill" or use terms like "he is a bi-polar disorder." It should be the policy of all programs to consult with consumers and ex-patients in their states to identify a phrase or phrases that are respectful of individual dignity and reflect the preferences of the majority of individuals. Some phrases with general growing acceptance are "people with psychiatric disabilities," "persons with severe and persistent mental illness," "ex-patients," or "consumers." All current and future documents should reflect this policy.

Developing Psychiatric Rehabilitation Knowledge

Early practitioners of psychiatric rehabilitation learned their trade by experience through a trial-and-error process. The typical community-based mental health center was originally designed for persons with less severe conditions. When the national policy of deinstitutionalization began, community workers and services were confronted with a large group of individuals being released from psychiatric institutions who did not respond well to existing treatment modalities, medications, and services. It soon became apparent that neither the existing community services nor the types of services previously offered in the psychiatric hospitals were helping this new group adapt to the community environment. In response, many of the community mental health staff assigned to work with this population began devising new strategies and services to meet their needs. These pioneer staff struggled to develop treatment philosophies consistent with the goals of community treatment. They often had to design programs for this new population where none had existed. Without recourse to references or handbooks, using emerging concepts such as least restrictive treatment environment, client involvement, and normalization as guidelines, innovative programs and services were created. These new services were evaluated by their success or failure. Of course, many of these solutions failed or were later discarded as better solutions were developed.

Some successful models already existed in places like Fountain House in New York City and Horizon House in Philadelphia. These successful programs, which we will deal with in greater depth in Chapter 6, served as models for the services that were being developed in communities around the country.

Since very little, if any, formal education about psychiatric rehabilitation existed at the time, programs tended to hire bright, young, motivated individuals and teach them psychiatric rehabilitation on the job as it was practiced at that setting. Much of what was known was handed down from supervisor to supervisee, and the staff from individual programs tended to share the same ideas and philosophy. Knowledge was also picked up at the yearly conferences of emerging PsyR professional associations, or from journal articles on PsyR that appeared infrequently in publications dedicated to other disciplines.

The process of developing new programs and services based on emerging philosophical concepts made psychiatric rehabilitation an exciting and very creative profession in the 1970s and 1980s. Without models or reference points, program staff members were free to create programs in many forms, and they did. Psychiatric rehabilitation services today cover a wide range of styles, types, and philosophies. This wealth of program types and designs has provided excellent opportunities for testing and refining PsyR theories and practices. Like other emerging fields, PsyR periodically experiences a "shaking out" of some of these ideas as new knowledge is acquired and agreement is reached on which ideas are the most effective (producing positive results) and efficient (producing results economically). More effective strategies are retained while others are discarded. The recent identification of some psychiatric rehabilitation strategies as evidence-based practices (EBPs), which will be covered extensively in this text, is ushering in just such a "shaking out."

Psychiatric Rehabilitation: A Science or an Art?

Brainstorming sessions, sometimes with staff and consumers combined, to develop creative strategies for achieving PsyR goals and objectives are a far cry from the systematic precision required for scientific research. Creating new programs and strategies can be an art and some of the creations are ingenious; for example, using consumers as job coaches to help other consumers learn and keep regular jobs in the community. Or, helping consumers learn about their illnesses by participating in discussion groups where they read and discuss research literature from PsyR journals, such as the *Psychiatric Rehabilitation Journal* and the *American Journal of Psychiatric Rehabilitation*.

The developments of strategies like these are often serendipitous. New strategies and techniques are also developed by improving on the ideas of others. A previous executive director of a very large rehabilitation agency known for developing innovative programming once stated that he really is not that intelligent, he mainly "steals" or adopts other people's ideas and then improves on them. Of course, we can judge the intelligence of this strategy by observing the effectiveness of the programs he developed.

Many of these creative solutions work, as the staff and consumers who utilize them will attest. But what is it about these strategies that works and what should another PsyR program do to ensure that the same strategies will work for them? Many of the solutions that appear to be effective to staff and consumers alike, in fact, are not. A common mistake, for example, is crediting a new strategy with rehabilitation gains when the improvement is actually caused by what is known as a "Hawthorne effect." You may have heard about the experiments at the Hawthorne plant of the Western Electric Company in Cicero, Illinois, during the 1930s. In one experiment, researchers found that no matter how they manipulated the lighting intensity in the work rooms (higher, lower, or no change), production went up. After much consideration, they concluded that instead of responding to the intensity of the lighting, the workers were responding to being studied by the researchers. In the case of PsyR, a Hawthorne effect implies that the consumers' improvements or gains may actually be caused by the attention they are getting because they are using the new strategy, rather than by the strategy itself. This might also be the case with staff members who strive harder when they are enthusiastic about a new program and convey their optimism to the consumers they are working with.

Is PsyR a science, an art, or some combination of both? The three goals of any scientific inquiry are (1) description (What is the process or phenomenon?), (2) explanation (How does it work?), and (3) prediction (What will happen in the future?). These principles can be applied to severe mental illness. In that case we would like to (1) describe the effects of severe mental illness, (2) explain why mental illness has these effects, and (3) predict the course and outcome of these illnesses. The same set of principles can be applied to PsyR interventions. We need to (1) describe a PsyR intervention, (2) explain how the intervention works, and (3) predict what the outcome of the intervention will be. Many dedicated PsyR practitioners believe that approaching the task from this technical-scientific perspective will produce the best results for their clients. In fact, it is just this formulation that is behind the advent of evidence-based practices (Gill & Pratt, 2005).

Research produces knowledge. Scientific PsyR knowledge is developed through rigorous systematic research based on the scientific method of observation, description, control, and replication. For PsyR this means that, in general, if we apply the same treatment to the same population under the same conditions, we expect to get approximately the same results. To foster this type of scientific knowledge, several research centers focusing specifically on PsyR and the community treatment of persons with severe mental illness have received public funding. Notable among these research centers are the Center for Psychiatric Rehabilitation at Boston University; the New Hampshire-Dartmouth Psychiatric Research Center; the Center for Psychiatric Rehabilitation at the Illinois Institute of Technology; the Mendota Mental Health Research Center, Madison, Wisconsin; and Thresholds, Chicago, Illinois. Additionally, the National Institute for Disability and Rehabilitation Research (NIDRR) funds Rehabilitation Research and Training Centers (RRTC) at Boston University, the University of Pennsylvania, and the University of Illinois at Chicago to develop and disseminate new knowledge. Many of these RRTCs deal with aspects of the rehabilitation of severe mental illness. These research centers strive to increase our knowledge of how to provide effective services for persons with severe mental illnesses. Recent work identifying specific EBPs holds great promise for improving services.

Evidence-Based Practices

From its earliest beginnings, psychiatric rehabilitation has sought, usually by trial and error, to develop effective services for persons with severe mental illness. This process has led to the existence of a large number of essentially idiosyncratic services, some of which are effective and some not. The adoption of an evidence-based practice approach is addressing this problem. The EBP process employs controlled clinical trials to identify effective services and define the critical elements that produce positive outcomes.

The Implementing Evidence-Based Practice Project

As the PsyR research and knowledge base grew, it became clear that some practices and strategies were superior to others at producing desired outcomes for persons. This situation was clearly demonstrated by the recommendations of the Schizophrenia Patient Outcome Research Team (PORT) project (Lehman & Steinwachs, 1998). The PORT study, which made recommendations for the treatment of schizophrenia, also found that in many cases individuals with schizophrenia were not provided with proper treatment and services. Additionally, there was increasing recognition by researchers and administrators that service providers and programs were slow to adopt new research findings to usual practice, indicating a large lag between research findings and implementing those findings in the field.

To address this issue, in 1998 the Robert Wood Johnson Foundation sponsored a meeting of researchers, clinicians, administrators, consumers, and family members to begin the process of identifying evidence-based practices for PsyR. This group, dubbed the Implementing Evidence-Based Practices Project, was charged with identifying interventions that were backed up by reliable research results. Through an extensive review of the research literature this group was able to identify six potential evidence-based practices.

Identifying an Evidence-Based Practice

A number of important steps must be carried out to establish an EBP. Most EBPs started from a service innovation. Such innovations (e.g., assertive community treatment [Chapter 7], supported employment [Chapter 9]) typically come about through the trial-and-error efforts of dedicated professionals trying to improve services. After an innovation shows promise, the next step is to carefully and objectively define the service including carefully explaining just how the service is performed, who performs it, for how long, and so forth. The definition of the service becomes the service model that will subsequently be field tested.

The service model of a potential EBP must be studied using multiple *controlled clinical trials.* This type of research, which typically involves random assignment of participants

BOX 1.3
Robert E. Drake

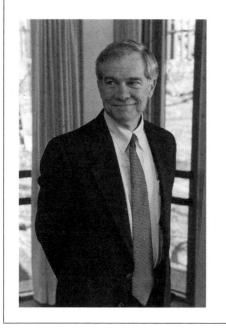

Robert E. Drake, M.D., Ph.D., is the Andrew Thomson Professor of Psychiatry and Community and Family Medicine at Dartmouth Medical School. He is also the director of the New Hampshire-Dartmouth Psychiatric Research Center. Dr. Drake has been a long-term contributor to the psychiatric rehabilitation knowledge base through his work developing and evaluating innovative community programs for persons with severe mental disorders. He is one of the recognized leaders in the development of evidence-based practices for PsyR. He is well known for his work in integrated dual disorders treatment (substance use disorder and severe mental illness), supported employment services, and assertive community treatment, among other work. Dr. Drake's many books and more than 300 papers cover diverse aspects of adjustment and quality of life among persons with severe mental disorders and those in their support systems. Educated at Princeton, Duke, and Harvard universities, he has worked for many years as a clinician in community mental health centers. Dr. Drake is a sought-after speaker in the United States and internationally regarding his work on improving services for people with severe mental illness.

to experimental and control groups, has the advantage of allowing researchers to make causal inferences between the variables under study. For example, a researcher may determine that a specific educational strategy helps consumers learn about their illness, or that a specific medication reduces a specific category of symptoms. In addition, controlled clinical trials greatly reduce the possible effects of bias on the results. A good example of bias reduction in research is the use of "blind" evaluators. In an experiment comparing, let us say, consumer quality of life in different housing situations, the "blind" evaluator would not know which experimental condition (e.g., experimental group or control group), in this case which housing type, was represented by the consumers she was evaluating. In this way, the evaluator is protected from unconsciously biasing the evaluations and hence the research results. Evaluators might also be blind to the hypothesis being studied or the exact form of the research design.

The evidence to support an EBP must be in the form of *reliable, objective evidence.* Of course, we have just stressed that controlled clinical trials are designed to produce reliable, objective evidence if it is present. Still, the reliability of data and the objectivity of data can and should be independently assessed. In addition, such research needs to be repeated in different settings, by different researchers, and produce similar corroborating results. This replicability is one of the hallmarks of science.

If the model for the EBP, refined by the research results, proves to effectively produce specific desirable outcomes for persons with severe mental illness its elements are converted into a *fidelity scale*. Think of this fidelity scale as a blueprint for how the service should be provided as well as a rating scale that determines how close a service comes to replicating the model. The fidelity scale of an EBP is used to determine how well other programs are providing the same service. In short, how much fidelity to the EBP model do they demonstrate? Research findings suggest that services with higher fidelity to the EBP model produce better outcomes (e.g., Bond, 2004).

Current Evidence-Based Practices

To date six EBPs, each of which will be described in some detail in this textbook, have been identified:

1. Medication management
2. Assertive community treatment (ACT)
3. Supported employment (SE)
4. Illness management and recovery education
5. Family education
6. Integrated treatment for dual disorders (Dixon et al., 2001; Drake et al., 2001; Mueser, Torrey, Lynde, Singer, & Drake, 2003; Torrey et al., 2001).

Each of these EBPs has been shown to have a positive impact on one or more aspects of these disorders. Specifically, multiple controlled clinical trials of the six EBPs just listed have been shown, among other things, to produce:

- Symptom improvement (especially for positive symptoms)
- Less hospital utilization
- Fewer and less severe relapses
- Higher rates of competitive employment
- Improved quality of life
- Increased community involvement
- Better control of substance abuse problems (Dixon et al., 2001; Drake et al., 2001; Mueser et al., 2003; Torrey et al., 2001).

Scientific Literature and Meetings

Starting from a small group of psychiatrists, psychologists, social workers, and other professionals working and publishing in related areas, PsyR research has come into its own during the last three decades. The first regular issue of *Schizophrenia Bulletin*, a quarterly journal of the National Institute of Mental Health, was published in 1974. This journal was dedicated to facilitating "the dissemination and exchange of information about schizophrenia." In 1977 the IAPSRS and the Boston University Center for Psychiatric Rehabilitation launched the *Psychosocial Rehabilitation Journal*, today called the *Psychiatric Rehabilitation Journal*. This quarterly journal has been the primary source for PsyR research, evaluation, and ideas. *Psychiatric Rehabilitation Skills*, today called the *American Journal of Psychiatric Rehabilitation*, published by the Illinois Institute of

Technology and the University of Medicine and Dentistry of New Jersey, is dedicated to publishing PsyR research from around the world. Several other journals regularly carry PsyR research and evaluation reports, such as *Psychiatric Services*, an American Psychiatric Association journal, and *Community Mental Health Journal*, the journal of the National Council of Community Mental Health Centers. Articles about PsyR also appear in journals from the fields of psychology, psychiatry, social work, vocational rehabilitation, and other disciplines.

International, national, and local PsyR conferences are excellent places for discussing PsyR research, evaluation, and ideas. Initially, these conferences provided the opportunity for PsyR professionals to get together with others doing the same work to share ideas. Today's conferences include consumers and family members and take in a broad spectrum of issues and interests. The United States Psychiatric Rehabilitation Association (USPRA, formerly IAPSRS), which holds a yearly conference at a major city in the United States, has chapter organizations in more than 40 states. These state organizations also sponsor conferences, meetings, and institutes on special topics. The World Association for Psychosocial Rehabilitation (WAPR) sponsors a congress of PsyR professionals approximately every 2 to 3 years at a major world city. WAPR congresses are genuine multi-lingual, multi-cultural events with presentations by PsyR professionals representing countries from the Americas, Europe, Asia, Africa, and Australia.

These worldwide conferences help to emphasize the global nature and impact of severe mental illness. With some slight variations, the incidences of diseases such as schizophrenia are constant both around the world and over time. The plight of persons experiencing severe and persistent mental illness in Third World countries is especially troubling. At the 1989 WAPR congress, Dr. Vijay Nagaswami of the Schizophrenia Research Foundation in Madras, India, stated that "In developing countries . . . the mentally ill continue to languish and can be considered lucky if they receive even medication" (1989, p. 20). The international PsyR movement is actively promoting the sharing of knowledge and ideas to meet this challenge.

Standards for Creating Psychiatric Rehabilitation Professionals

USPRA, formerly known as IAPSRS, the largest organization of psychiatric rehabilitation professionals in the United States, has taken the initiative in establishing PsyR as a profession. This effort includes the establishment of a national test-based professional certification, the Certified Psychiatric Rehabilitation Practitioner, and accredited program standards through the Council on the Accreditation of Rehabilitation Facilities (CARF) and the Council on Accreditation (COA). In addition, IAPSRS had established practice guidelines for the assessment, evaluation, and interventions of psychiatric rehabilitation (IAPSRS, 2001). As of this writing (2006), these guidelines are undergoing revision. Finally, IAPSRS had outlined a Code of Ethics for PsyR professionals (IAPSRS, 1996).

Like other professions such as doctors, lawyers, and public school teachers, official recognition of one's professional status requires being licensed by the state where the professional provides services. To be licensable by states, a profession needs to have very clear guidelines spelling out who practitioners are, what special knowledge they have, what services they provide, and their professional standards and ethics. In short, defining who is qualified to provide what type of services to the public.

The Certified Psychiatric Rehabilitation Practitioner (CPRP)

Efforts to define the professional role of the psychiatric rehabilitation practitioner has advanced significantly during the last several years. In 2000–2001, IAPSRS sponsored a role delineation study (IAPSRS, 2001). More than 300 PsyR experts contributed to a multi-step project in which they identified both the knowledge and the skills required to be a minimally competent practitioner. More than 90 tasks, each with several pieces of knowledge and skills, were identified. Later these tasks were ranked in terms of how frequently they are used, how important they are for helping people with mental illness, and how critical they are for avoiding harm to persons with mental illness. The seven broad domains that were identified are ranked here in terms of their overall importance, criticality, and frequency as rated by PsyR experts (IAPSRS, 2001):

1. Interpersonal competencies
2. Interventions
3. Assessment, planning, and outcomes
4. Community resources
5. Professional role
6. Systems competencies
7. Diversity

This role delineation report was used to develop the test questions contained in the Certified Psychiatric Rehabilitation Practitioner (CPRP) examination. This standardized exam, which serves as a demonstration of competence, is combined with an assessment of level of education, amount of experience, and professional references to designate an individual a Certified Psychiatric Rehabilitation Practitioner. A listing of all the individuals who are certified PsyR professionals is published by USPRA on the World Wide Web at http://www.uspra.org/certification. The certification program, now overseen by the Commission on the Certification of Psychiatric Rehabilitation, is a major development in the definition of PsyR professionals. The written test is now used on an international basis to evaluate PsyR knowledge. The first exam was offered in 2002 in the United States and Canada. Singapore is using the certification program and New Zealand is considering it.

By 2005, 12 U.S. states had passed legislation recognizing the CPRP as identifying individuals qualified to deliver these services in their state. Several states are considering a license based on this credential. The Canadian Province of Nova Scotia and the country of Singapore have also recognized the CPRP credential.

Summary

Being struck with a major mental illness can be a devastating experience affecting a person's entire life. Particularly because they tend to strike during the late teen/early adult years, these diseases often cause severe disabilities. Despite the extreme personal and societal costs of these conditions, we are still unclear as to their cause. With the advent of modern diagnostic tools it has become clear that these conditions are biologically based. An additional major source of disability is the stigma attached to these diseases. Increased knowledge and education are helping to reduce stigma, but we still have a long way to go in this respect.

Psychiatric rehabilitation encompasses the community treatment and rehabilitation of persons with severe mental illness. Psychiatric rehabilitation in its present form began in response to the deinstitutionalization movement in the late 1960s. Initially through trial and error and later through systematic clinical research, services are increasingly becoming more refined. Psychiatric rehabilitation is emerging as a unique discipline with its own body of research, journals and publications, and professional organizations and conferences. The major U.S. organization, USPRA, is actively working toward the professionalization of PsyR personnel and practices.

Class Exercise
Knowledge and Attitudes about Severe Mental Illness

Imagine that you are a case worker in a psychiatric rehabilitation program. A new client, diagnosed with schizophrenia, and recently assigned to your case load asks you the following questions. How would you respond?

1. Why did I become ill? What causes this disease?
2. I feel O.K. right now. Will I get sick again?
3. How long will I have this condition? Will I ever get better?
4. Will I be able to have a "normal" life?

References

American Psychiatric Association. (1980). *Diagnostic and statistical manual of mental disorders* (3rd ed.) Washington, DC: Author.

American Psychiatric Association. (2000). *Diagnostic and statistical manual of mental disorders* (4th ed., text revision). Washington, DC: Author.

Andreasen, N. C. (1984). *The broken brain.* New York: Harper Collins.

Anthony, W. A. (1979). *The principles of psychiatric rehabilitation.* Baltimore, MD: University Park Press.

Anthony, W. A. (1993). Recovery from mental illness: The guiding vision of the mental health service system in the 1990's. *Psychosocial Rehabilitation Journal, 16*(4), 11–23.

Anthony, W. A. (2000). A recovery-oriented service system: Setting some system level standards. *Psychiatric Rehabilitation Journal, 24*(3), 11–23.

Anthony, W. A. (1993). Recovery from mental illness: The guiding vision of the mental health service system in the 1990's. *Psychosocial Rehabilitation Journal, 16*(4), 11–23.

Anthony, W. A., & Liberman, R. P. (1986). The practice of psychiatric rehabilitation: Historical, conceptual and research base. *Schizophrenia Bulletin, 12*(4), 542–559.

Bond, G. R. (2004). Supported employment: Evidence for an evidence-based practice. *Psychiatric Rehabilitation Journal, 27*(4), 345–359.

Bond, G. R., Resnick, S. R., Drake, R. E., Xie, H., McHugo, G. J., & Bebout, R. R. (2001). Does competitive employment improve nonvocational outcomes for people with severe mental illness? *Journal of Consulting and Clinical Psychology, 69*, 489–501.

Coleman, L. M. (1986). Stigma: An enigma demystified. In S. C. Ainlay, G. Becker, & L. M. Coleman (Eds.), *The dilemma of difference* (pp. 211–232). New York: Plenum Press.

Corrigan, P., Thompson, V., Lambert, D., Sangster, Y., Noel, J. G., & Campbell, J. (2003). Perceptions of discrimination among persons with serious mental illness. *Psychiatric Services, 54*, 1105–1110.

Deegan, P. E. (1988). Recovery: The lived experience of rehabilitation. *Psychosocial Rehabilitation Journal, 11*(4), 11–19.

Dell Orto, A. (2001). Editor, special issue on psychiatric rehabilitation education. *Rehabilitation Education, 15*(2).

DeSisto, M. J., Harding, C. M., McCormack, R. V., Ashikaga, T., & Brooks, G. W. (1995). The Maine and Vermont three-decade studies of serious mental illness. *British Journal of Psychiatry, 167*, 331–342.

Dincin, J. (1990). Speaking out. *Psychosocial Rehabilitation Journal, 14*(2), 83–85.

Dixon, L., McFarlane, W. R., Lefley, H., Lucksted, A., Cohen, M., Falloon, I., et al. (2001). Evidence-based practices for services to families of people with psychiatric disabilities. *Psychiatric Services, 52*(7), 903–910.

Drake, R. E., Goldman, H. H., Leff, H. S., Lehman, A. F., Dixon, L., Mueser, K. T., et al. (2001). Implementing evidence-based practices in routine mental health service settings. *Psychiatric Services, 52*, 179–182.

Farkas, M. D., O'Brien, W. F., & Nemec, P. B. (1988). A graduate level curriculum in psychiatric rehabilitation: Filling a need. *Psychosocial Rehabilitation Journal, 12*(2), 53–66.

Gill, K. J. (2001). Editor, special issue on psychiatric rehabilitation education. *Psychiatric Rehabilitation Skills* (3).

Gill, K. J., and Pratt, C. W. (2005). Clinical decision making and the evidence-based practitioner. In R. E. Drake, M. R. Merrens, & D. W. Lunde (Eds.), *Evidence-based mental health practice.* New York: Ww. Norton & Company.

Hall, W., Andrews, G., & Goldstein, G. (1985). The cost of schizophrenia. *Australian and New Zealand Journal of Psychiatry, 19*, 3–5.

Halter, C. A., Bond, G. R., & De Graaf-Kaser, R. (1992). How treatment of persons with serious mental illness is portrayed in undergraduate psychology textbooks. *Community Mental Health Journal, 28*(1) 29–42.

Harding, C. M., Brooks, G. W., Ashikaga, T., Strauss, J. S., & Breier, A. (1987). The Vermont longitudinal study of persons with severe mental illness I: Methodology, study sample and overall status 32 years later. *American Journal of Psychiatry, 144*, 718–726.

Hughes, R. (1994). Psychiatric rehabilitation: An essential health service for people with serious and persistent mental illness. In IAPSRS, *An Introduction to Psychiatric Rehabilitation*. Columbia, MD: Author.

International Association of Psychosocial Rehabilitation Services. (1996). *Core principles of psychiatric rehabilitation*. Columbia, MD: Author.

International Association of Psychosocial Rehabilitation Services. (2001). *Role Delineation Study of Psychiatric Rehabilitation Practitioner*. Morrisville, NC: Columbia Assessment Services.

International Association of Psychosocial Rehabilitation Services. (2003). *Language Guidelines*. Morrisville, NC: Columbia Assessment Services.

Lehman, A. F., & Steinwachs, D. M. (1998). Translating research into practice: The schizophrenia Patient Outcome Research Team (PORT) treatment recommendations. *Schizophrenia Bulletin, 24*, 1–10.

Lehrman, N. S. (1961). Do our hospitals help make acute schizophrenia chronic? *Diseases of the Nervous System, 22*(9), 489–493.

Liberman, R. P. (Ed.). (1992). *Handbook of psychiatric rehabilitation*. Boston: Allyn and Bacon.

Linn, M. W., Caffey, E. M., Klett, C. J., Hogarty, C. E., & Lamb, H. R. (1979). Day treatment and psychotropic drugs in the aftercare of schizophrenic patients. *Archives of General Psychiatry, 36*, 1055–1066.

Lysaker, P. H., Evans, J. D., Kim, H. W., Marks, K. A., Meyer, P. S., Tunis, S. L., et al. (2001). Symptoms and work performance in schizophrenia. *Schizophrenia Research, 49*, 139.

Marcus, J., Hans, S. L., Nagler, S., Auerbach, J. G., Mirsky, A. F., & Aubrey, A. (1987). Review of the NIMH Israeli kibbutz-city study and the Jerusalem infant development study. *Schizophrenia Bulletin, 13*(3), 425–437.

Mueser, K. T., Glynn, S. M., Corrigan, P. W., & Baber, W. (1996). A survey of preferred terms for users of mental health services. *Psychiatric Services, 47*(7), 760–761.

Mueser, K. T., Torrey, W. C., Lynde, D., Singer, P., & Drake, R. E. (2003). Implementing evidence-based practices for people with severe mental illness. *Behavior Modification, 27*(3), 387–411.

Nagaswami, V. (1989). Community based rehabilitation of persons suffering from chronic psychoses in developing countries. In *Proceedings of the II Congress of the World Association for Psychosocial Rehabilitation* (p. 20). Barcelona, Spain.

Pratt, C. W. (2005). Editor, special issue on Psychiatric Rehabilitation education and credentials. *American Journal of Psychiatric Rehabilitation, 8*(2).

President's New Freedom Commission on Mental Health. (2003). *Final report.* Available online at http://www.mentalhealthcommission.gov/reports/FinalReport/

Ridgway, P., & Zipple, A. M. (1990). The paradigm shift in residential services: From the linear continuum to supported housing approaches. *Psychosocial Rehabilitation Journal, 13*(4), 11–31.

Rutman, I. D. (1994). What is psychiatric rehabilitation. In IAPSRS, *An Introduction to Psychiatric Rehabilitation.* Columbia, MD: Author.

Schmieding, N. J. (1968). Institutionalization: A conceptual approach. *Perspectives in Psychiatric Care, 6*(5), 205–211.

Stern, R., & Minkoff, K. (1979). Paradoxes in programming for chronic patients in a community clinic. *Hospital & Community Psychiatry, 30*(9), 613–617.

Taylor, E. (1987). The biological basis of schizophrenia. *Social Work*, March–April, 115–121.

Torrey, E. F. (1994). *Schizophrenia and manic depressive disorder: The biological roots of mental illness as revealed by the landmark study of identical twins.* New York; Basic Books

Torrey, E. F. (2001). *Surviving schizophrenia.* New York: Harper Collins.

Torrey, W. C., Drake, R. E., Dixon, L., Burns, B. J., Flynn, L., Rush, A., et al. (2001). Implementing evidence-based practices for persons with severe mental illnesses. *Psychiatric Services, 52*(1), 45–50.

Walker, E. F., Sabuwalla, Z., & Huot, R. (2004). Pubertal neuromaturation, stress sensitivity, and psychopathology. *Development and Psychopathology 16*(4), 807–824.

Chapter 2

Symptoms and Etiology of Severe and Persistent Mental Illness

Introduction 32

Symptoms 32

Persistence of Symptoms over Time 33

The Symptoms of Schizophrenia 33

Positive and Negative Symptoms 34

Delusions 34

Hallucinations 36

Thought Disorders 37

The Experience of Symptoms 37

Lack of Awareness of One's Own
Symptoms as a Symptom 39

Phases of Schizophrenia 40

How the Phases of Schizophrenia Affect
Consumers' Lives 41

Mood Disorders 42

How Are Schizophrenia and Mood
Disorders Different? 45

**Relevance to Psychiatric Rehabilitation
46**

Dual Diagnosis 47

Mental Illness and Developmental
Disability 48

Mental Illness and Substance Abuse 49

Etiology 50

Physiological Evidence of the Disease Process
in the Brain 50

The Story of Dara 53

Neurotransmitters 54

Neurotransmitters and Mental Illness 55

The Role of Genetic Factors 55

Risk among Biological Relatives 56

Fetal Development and Early Infancy 58

The Role of Stress 59

The Stress/Vulnerability/Coping/Competence
Model 61

Etiology Summary 62

Obsolete Etiological Theories 62

The Myth of the Myth of Mental Illness
63

Summary 64

Class Exercise 64

References 65

People with a variety of serious and persistent mental illnesses can benefit from psychiatric rehabilitation services. The most common diagnoses of the people in psychiatric rehabilitation programs are from the schizophrenia and mood disorder categories. The symptoms of these major mental illnesses are often catastrophic in their impact, threatening the integrity of the person's thoughts, feelings, and sense of self. Today, we understand that these illnesses are brain disorders that have severe physiological, psychological, and social consequences. The causes of mental illness seem to be related to an interaction of heredity and environment. Being vulnerable to these disorders appears to be, in large part, genetic; that is, inherited. This genetic vulnerability apparently interacts with environmental and developmental factors to provoke the onset of these disorders. This chapter and the next include brief vignettes about individuals with mental illnesses. All are factually based, but they often represent only a brief interval in, or a single aspect of, the life of a person with a severe and persistent mental illness.

This chapter will answer the following questions:

1. *What are the most common symptoms of the severe and persistent mental illnesses?*
2. *What are the current scientific theories about the etiology (cause) of these conditions?*
3. *How does stress affect people who have severe mental illnesses?*

Introduction

The goal of psychiatric rehabilitation is to help individuals recover from the catastrophe of serious mental illness. The disabling nature of these disorders is a result of both their severity and their persistence. Psychiatric rehabilitation programs serve people with a variety of disorders, primarily individuals recovering from psychoses, as discussed in Chapter 1. In a study of 13 PsyR programs, 65% of the individuals served had schizophrenic disorders, 25% had mood disorders (bipolar disorder, major depression, etc.), and 10% had a variety of other conditions (Arns, 1998). Therefore, this chapter will focus primarily on schizophrenia, with some attention paid to the major mood disorders.

Symptoms

Symptoms are literally signs or indicators of an illness or disease. They are also a cause of suffering for the individual with the disease. According to the traditional medical model, observing symptoms, or patterns of simultaneously occurring symptoms, leads to the diagnosis of the underlying disorder. An example is a young child who has the sniffles, is cranky, tugs at his or her ear, and has a fever. The doctor examines the middle and inner ear and sees that it is red. All of these are symptoms or indicators of the illness commonly known as an ear infection. The earache, while a symptom of an infection, is also causing suffering for the child. The treatment is usually to provide antibiotics to stop the infection, which also relieves the child's pain.

The symptoms of mental illness, as discussed in Chapter 1, involve the senses, emotions, and cognition (thinking). These symptoms shape how the person perceives, thinks about, and reacts to the world around him or her. Besides indicating a serious illness, like the child's earache, these symptoms can become a preoccupying and consuming experience in the person's life. In the case of the earache, with treatment the situation is temporary and specific. In the case of the most serious mental illnesses, the severity and the persistence of symptoms may be all encompassing and disruptive to the person's functioning at home, school, work, and in the community in general.

Persistence of Symptoms over Time

One of the most devastating features of mental illness is that psychiatric symptoms often reoccur and persist, in one form or another, sometimes for the entire life of the individual. Indeed, these illnesses used to be referred to as *chronic* mental illnesses.

Individuals who experienced these disorders were often insensitively referred to as "chronics." Fortunately, this terminology has fallen out of favor for the following reasons: First is the emergence of person-first language (e.g., "a person with schizophrenia" rather than "a schizophrenic"); second is that "chronic," which simply means "lengthy," has gradually become equated with "low functioning" and "hopeless." The overall negative associations with this label turned out to be not only inaccurate, but also very harmful (Harding, Zubin, & Strauss, 1992). In Chapter 3 we will discuss evidence about the inaccuracy of the "chronic" label.

Nevertheless, the fact that psychiatric symptoms may persist, despite treatment, is one of the most important challenges of PsyR. In short, how can we help persons recover and live meaningful, productive lives despite the continuing presence of psychiatric symptoms?

The Symptoms of Schizophrenia

Schizophrenia is the most common disorder of persons who utilize psychiatric rehabilitation services (Arns, 1998). Diagnosing schizophrenia is difficult and takes time, in part because the symptoms of schizophrenia are so varied and numerous. As yet, there is no single definitive sign that indicates schizophrenia is present. Other serious disorders must be ruled out first. For example, many drug reactions look strikingly like schizophrenia during the acute phases of the illness, hence the term, psychedelic drug, which refers to a class of drugs that causes psychotic-like symptoms. Unlike the symptoms of schizophrenia, these drug-induced conditions are short lived and have a very different impact on the individual.

The symptoms of severe and persistent mental illness are ongoing rather than transient experiences. In the case of schizophrenia, an individual's most serious symptoms may last several days to many years, waxing and waning in intensity. As of yet, there are no laboratory tests and no direct outward physical signs of mental illness. While there are some subtle physiological signs, they are not diagnostic in themselves. For example, as we will discuss later in this chapter, some people with schizophrenia and other mental illnesses have a smaller head size, perhaps due to difficulties in their prenatal development.

Positive and Negative Symptoms

According to the official manual of the American Psychiatric Association (APA, 2000), *Diagnostic and Statistical Manual of Mental Disorders,* fourth edition, text revision (DSM-IV-TR), the characteristic symptoms of schizophrenia can be categorized into two broad groups: positive symptoms and negative symptoms. The positive symptoms appear to reflect an excess or distortion of normal functions, whereas the negative symptoms appear to reflect a diminution or loss of normal functions (APA, 2000, p. 299). It is important to note that negative symptoms are considered much more difficult to treat and are oftentimes much more disabling than positive symptoms. Positive and negative symptoms are described and illustrated in the following paragraphs; they are also summarized in Box 2.1.

We will consider negative symptoms first. Clearly, all of the symptoms of schizophrenia are "negative" in the sense that they are harmful. However, this class of symptoms is referred to as "negative" because it is characterized by the absence of something that is normally present. For example, avolition and anhedonia are common negative symptoms. In these terms "a" is similar to "anti" and literally means "not." Thus, avolition is the lack of willpower or motivation. Anhedonia means not in pursuit of pleasure and the term refers to an inability to experience pleasure. Both are common negative symptoms experienced by people recovering from psychotic disorders. Many mental health professionals mistake these symptoms, which are common among people with severe and persistent mental illness, as simply a choice not to be motivated. Consider the experience of Pete, a newly hired psychiatric rehabilitation staff person:

> *I went to the rooms throughout the program and then to the work units, but it was all the same. Most of the time, it seemed members of the program were sitting around, doing nothing, staring into space. Some staff were really good at engaging the members, but the members had a hard time sustaining activity. People seemed to move slowly; they were slow to smile. He thought to himself, why are these people so negative and down, so unwilling to do anything?*

In contrast, positive symptoms, such as hallucinations, delusions, and most thought disorders, are, in a sense, more blatant signs of a mental illness. They are known as positive symptoms because they are added to the individual's experience as a result of the disease. For example, when someone with schizophrenia, or another mental illness, hears voices it is defined as a positive symptom, because these auditory hallucinations are something added by the disease.

Sometimes people who have serious mental illnesses appear distracted, mumbling or talking to themselves, bewildered, or "in their own world." These are behaviors that are secondary to positive symptoms, such as auditory hallucinations or other internal stimuli, which are described in detail later in this chapter.

Delusions

Among the most common positive symptoms of psychosis (defined in Chapter 1) are delusions—bizarre beliefs or ideas that the person cannot be "talked out of." A common

---

BOX 2.1

Positive and Negative Symptoms of Schizophrenia

The positive symptoms of schizophrenia include distortions or exaggerations of:

1. Thinking and ideas (delusions)
2. Perception and sensations (hallucinations and illusions)
3. Language and communication (disorganized or bizarre speech)

4. Behavioral self-control (grossly disorganized or catatonic behavior).

Negative symptoms include losses or deficits in:

1. The range and intensity of emotional expression (flat affect)
2. The fluency and productivity of thought and speech (alogia)
3. The initiation of goal-directed behavior (avolition).

---

type of delusion is the feeling that one's actions are under the control of others. Consider this example:

> *Sal was a bright man who formerly worked as a teacher. Since developing schizophrenia, he thought that two individuals were controlling his actions, "Marlboro Man" and "Frank." These were not their real names, he said, but code names, aliases. They were real people, cousins of Sal's, but Sal thought they were controlling his life, intervening to make him fail, talking to his students (when he still had students), and talking to his employers, who would then fire him. Sal thought "Marlboro Man" and "Frank" caused his other symptoms, polluted his water, and contaminated his bathroom. Once, Sal started teaching at a day program, helping his fellow consumers learn Spanish. When the students had the normal difficulties, making mistakes, confusing pronunciation, etc., Sal gave up. In explanation, he said, "It's no use, it's Marlboro Man and Frank interfering again." In the early phases of Sal's illness he talked about the two men, but in the active phase he was totally preoccupied with them. Even when he was relatively well, they were always in his thoughts.*

Another category of delusions, grandiose delusions, involves believing one has great worth, power, knowledge, a special identity, or a special relationship with God or a famous person. Typical grandiose delusions include believing one is God or Jesus Christ. Other typical delusions involve believing oneself to be especially famous, beautiful, or influential.

> *Louise, a plain-looking person, average in many ways, arrived at her day program one day saying, and believing, that she was a famous designer of clothes and that a new perfume had been named after her.*

Other types of delusions might include believing there are evil or negative forces targeting one's self or a loved one. Examples include believing the Mafia is harassing you or the CIA or FBI has you under surveillance. These delusions can also take the form of ideas of reference, in which an individual believes special messages are being sent to them by the radio, television, computer, or even in an everyday remark.

Carol, a middle-aged woman with schizophrenia, had not been hospitalized for many years. She was concerned because she thought television programs were sending her special messages and she knew this was a bad sign. She wished to reassure her caseworker (and herself) that she was not getting ill. She called her caseworker on the phone and said she had something to tell her. Carol's comment was, "Oh, no, I won't let the TV bother me."

The impact of delusions on an individual's behavior can be extreme, with the individual taking specific actions in response to a belief. Uncontrolled emotional responses such as inappropriate laughter and crying occasionally occur. Delusions may occur by themselves or simultaneously with the next major symptom we will discuss: hallucinations.

Hallucinations

Hallucinations are incorrect sensory information that the individual experiences as real. The individual must deal with heightened internal stimulation (often in the form of a hallucination) or exaggerated experiences of external stimuli (illusions). The most common hallucinations, which are usually the worst during the active phase of illness, are auditory in nature. Poor concentration and attention span seem to be a natural outgrowth, in part, of these sensory experiences. As discussed later, there may be other reasons for distractibility, including various types of thought disorders.

Auditory hallucinations may include any variety of experiences, such as a voice that keeps a running commentary on one's actions or thoughts, or multiple voices conversing with each other. These hallucinations can take the form of:

- Voices speaking one's thoughts aloud, as one man said, "I have very loud thoughts."
- Two or more voices arguing, as one woman said:

  I heard the voices of the staff here at the program yelling at each other. It started as two voices, later more voices were added, including yours. Later, it was like eighteen voices or something like that. It was so overwhelming I stayed in bed and never got out.

- Voices commenting on one's actions; for example, consider Ralph's predicament:

  Ralph did not like walking around his neighborhood. It was pleasant and safe enough, except he could not stand the chatter of his neighbors commenting on his behavior. He could hear their voices as he passed their homes.

- A voice or voices telling or ordering the individual to do a specific thing. These hallucinations, called *command hallucinations,* can have dangerous consequences. A woman, who had jumped from a bridge into the river, later reported that voices had been telling her to jump for several days before she complied.

Thought Disorders

In addition to delusions and hallucinations, individuals may experience thought disorders, which are symptoms associated with cognition or thinking (i.e., the processing of information). In schizophrenia, the cognitive symptoms are quite prominent and include thought disorders, thought broadcasting, thought insertion, and racing thoughts. Consider the story of Betty, who experienced thought broadcasting:

> *For years, I could never understand why people acted certain ways, especially why they never responded to me when I sent them messages. Then I went to a psychoeducation group in which I learned that not everybody thought as I did. For a long time, I believed people could hear my thoughts. I could hear theirs. At first, I didn't believe that people could not hear my thoughts, because as far as I'm concerned I still hear others' thoughts.*

Other individuals complain of very intrusive thoughts being put into their heads (thought insertion) or not under their control.

> *Elise believed that her parents and doctors conspired against her by arranging to have a surgical procedure performed on her while she was asleep. She thought the procedure involved the insertion of "metal patterns" in her brain that controlled many of her thoughts and actions. This delusion system provided an explanation for Elise who experienced some of her thoughts as being intrusive and inconsistent with her thinking prior to the onset of her illness.*

Other people experience racing thoughts, such as Tommy who stated:

> *My thinking is all messed up; it moves really fast and makes me nervous because I can't keep up with it.*

The Experience of Symptoms

Sometimes it is difficult to tell specifically which symptoms someone is suffering from. At the same time, it is apparent that the person is currently experiencing one type of psychotic symptom or another.

> *In a meeting with her doctor, Andrea told her that she was no longer taking her medicine. When her doctor asked why, Andrea responded, "Because God told me not to take it." The doctor tried several different ways to persuade Andrea to take her medicine, including saying to her "God helps those who help themselves," but Andrea just kept repeating, "God told me not to take it." Almost exasperated, the doctor said, "Andrea, God told me to tell you to take the medicine." The doctor was very startled when Andrea said, "OK."*

Was this evidence of a grandiose or religious delusion, that God was sending direct messages, or was it an auditory hallucination? After all, if you were hearing a disembodied voice, where would you think it was coming from?

The effect of symptoms on the person can vary markedly, with younger individuals at higher risk for acting in response to both hallucinations and delusions.

> *Rachel, a meek and mild, middle-aged woman, who has suffered from schizophrenia for most of her life, recalled how she lost the custody of her children more than 10 years ago because she responded to a delusion. She thought her crying infant son had been sent by the devil, so she threw him out of the window. Fortunately, he survived, but she lost custody of all three of her children. Since that time she not has committed any violent acts. Over the years she has developed a good, but generally long-distance, relationship with her children. She has held several jobs and has some close friends. In retrospect, she could not believe what she had done, particularly since she rarely acts in response to her symptoms now. Today, occasionally she feels hostile, angry, or a bit suspicious, but she knows that this is often a sign that she needs some assistance.*

Rachel's experience provides an extreme example of a bizarre and violent act committed is response to a hallucination or delusion. While such an event is quite dramatic, it is also rare, in that most individuals who experience these symptoms do not act in such a manner.

Some individuals have adapted to their symptoms quite well and while they certainly would prefer not to have them, they experience a relatively peaceful coexistence with them.

> *When it was Catherine's turn to speak about the experience of auditory hallucinations at a psychoeducation group, this generally cantankerous 70-year-old said with a grin, "Yeah, sure, I hear voices, but what the hell? I argue with them, put them in their place, and that's the end of it. I don't let them bother me."*

While experiencing severe symptoms, the self-regulation of one's behavior becomes more difficult, as was evident in Rachel's experience. Often, however, along with the psychotic symptoms the individual will have some self-awareness, as Catherine's comments indicate. Consider this vignette:

> *Andrew had not been doing well lately. He hid from the outreach workers when they came to his home. One day, he became convinced that his voices would abate if he jumped in the river; that is, they would be "washed away." Andrew went down to the polluted river in his city and jumped in. In the water, he felt his nostrils fill with water and realized he was drowning. He swam to safety. Sopping wet, he walked to the local mental health center where he was a client and asked for help.*

Although his behavior seemed very bizarre and dangerous, Andrew was not totally out of touch with reality and had some awareness of his actions. Perhaps, like Catherine, he might be able to develop a proactive stance toward his symptoms and self-regulate his behavioral responses accordingly in the future.

Were Andrew's actions in response to a delusional belief? Did voices tell him to jump in the river? Or was it a thought disorder, an example of concrete thinking, the "washing away" idea, taken too literally? Andrew's own description of his experience was not clear enough to ascertain what symptoms prompted his behavior. In a sense, the answers to these questions are not what was really important at the time. Behavior is often the result of an array of symptoms rather than a response to one symptom. What was very important is that both Andrew and his helpers recognized that he was in the acute or active phase of the illness and that his behavior had become unpredictable.

It is very important to understand that many individuals who experience severe psychotic symptoms, such as hallucinations or delusions, still manage to care for themselves and others. Many maintain their own homes, hold jobs, or attend school despite their symptomatology.

Lack of Awareness of One's Own Symptoms as a Symptom

Although not explicitly included as one of the symptoms of schizophrenia or other severe and persistent mental illnesses, a lack of awareness of the symptoms themselves by the persons with the disorder seems to be a common characteristic of the illness. This is especially evident during the acute phase of the disorder. Individuals seem unaware of the fact that their symptoms are, in fact, symptoms of an illness. It seems that the disordered brain, attempting to make sense of its own state, interprets its disordered functioning as normal. Xavier Amador and his colleagues have investigated this phenomenon at length.

Borrowing a term from neurology, Amador has studied anosognosia (the lack of knowledge of knowledge, or not knowing you do not know). Sometimes mistaken for denial or lack of insight, an individual confabulates or makes up explanations that apparently make sense to him or herself, but seem absurd to others (Amador & Paul-Odouard, 2000). An extreme example is a person who has been blinded due to a brain injury, who seems apparently unaware of the fact that he or she is blind and explains his or her difficulties by saying the lighting is bad, furniture has been moved, and so forth.

An example of an individual with schizophrenia's lack of awareness comes from earlier in our chapter. You will recall Andrea, who believed God was speaking to her. She was not aware of the fact that these were auditory hallucinations. In fact, Andrea believed she was not sick at all and did not require intervention. Andrea's physician cleverly did not try to contradict her beliefs, or label them as denial, but employed an intervention that was consistent with her frame of reference and her reality at the moment.

Even Dr. Amador, a professional psychologist, who has a family member affected by mental illness and is a consumer himself, was unaware of his own depression for a time. It was not until, for practice, he completed a research questionnaire for a colleague. The colleague, after scoring the form, spoke to Dr. Amador and pointed out that he may be depressed.

The title of Amador's book sums up the idea: *I Am Not Sick, I Do Not Need Help* (Amador & Johanson, 2000). The book suggests that many people with mental illness, instead of being in irrational denial of their illnesses, rationalize discrepant information that they perceive and logically conclude there is no evidence of illness and thus no need to pursue help. This could be a large contributing factor to the high rate of medication noncompliance that will be discussed in Chapter 3. Why take medication if you believe you are not sick? Traditionally, this has been referred to as lack of insight, but Amador prefers the term *anosognosia*.

Recovered consumers commonly report recognizing this lack of awareness or not knowing what you do not know. That is, when not acutely ill, consumers report that during the acute stages of their illness, they were, in fact, unaware they were sick. Equally startling is that sometimes, having recovered from a relapse, the consumer who previously acknowledged the presence of illness, once again loses awareness of the fact that he or she has a mental illness.

> *Jerry, when well, could describe the antecedents of his illness, the various symptoms, and the restlessness and desire to wander aimlessly. He knew the antecedents were indicators of a relapse coming soon. Yet the next couple of times Jerry relapsed, while others could see it coming, he could not. Eventually, he did learn that when he started to wander, an early warning sign for him, he should seek help. However, Jerry still did not directly connect his "wandering" to his psychiatric illness or its symptoms. He did associate it with "upcoming trouble," but did not see it as part of a psychiatric illness when he was in the midst of experiencing this problem.*

Amador strongly suggests that direct confrontation is rarely a useful approach. Rather, it is better to communicate that you understand the person's frame of reference, in order to build rapport. Then, when the opportunity arises, gently raise doubt about inconsistencies the individual might be experiencing. This is the beginning of the often gradual process of motivating the individual to see things differently, want changes in his or her own life, and pursue active treatment.

Phases of Schizophrenia

The duration (see Box 2.2, Criterion C) of an episode of schizophrenia must persist for at least 6 months for an accurate diagnosis to be made (APA, 2000). The symptoms a person experiences during an episode may vary considerably depending on which "phase" of the illness is present.

The *prodromal phase* (before the full syndrome) is a period of deterioration in functioning and increase of symptoms, both positive and negative. In "The Story of Paul," from Chapter 1, Paul's inability to focus on college lectures, his suspicious feelings about his roommate and professors, and his increasingly withdrawn behavior were all indicative of the prodromal phase of schizophrenia.

The *acute* or *active phase* is the period with the most severe and extreme symptoms. Positive symptoms are most prominent during this phase. In "The Story of Paul," hearing voices, increased suspicion and withdrawal, and the belief that his doctor was giving him orders by broadcasting thoughts to him telepathically, occurred during the active phase of Paul's illness.

During the *residual phase,* symptoms become milder. Both positive and negative symptoms decrease, but negative symptoms are more likely to persist. Paul's story left off when he was most likely nearing the end of the active phase of the schizophrenic episode. In a few months, as Paul entered the residual phase of the illness, his symptoms would

---

BOX 2.2

Diagnostic Criteria for Schizophrenia Excerpted from DSM IV-TR (APA, 2000, p. 312)

A. Characteristic symptoms: Two (or more) of the following, each present for a significant portion of time during a 1-month period (or less if successfully treated):

(1) Delusions (i.e., bizarre beliefs or ideas)
(2) Hallucinations (usually auditory, i.e., "hearing voices")
(3) Disorganized speech (e.g., frequent derailment or incoherence)
(4) Grossly disorganized or catatonic behavior
(5) Negative symptoms (i.e., flat affect, alogia, or avolition).

Note: Only one Criterion A symptom is required if delusions are bizarre or hallucinations consist of a voice keeping up a running commentary on the person's behavior or thoughts, or two or more voices conversing with each other.

B. Social/occupational dysfunction: For a significant portion of the time, since the onset of the disturbance, one or more major areas of functioning such as work, interpersonal relations, or self-care are markedly below the level achieved prior to the onset (or when onset is in childhood or adolescence, failure to achieve expected level of interpersonal, academic, or occupational achievement).

C. Duration: Continuous signs of the disturbance persist for at least 6 months. This 6-month period must include at least one month of symptoms (or less if successfully treated) that meet Criterion A (i.e., active phase symptoms) and may include periods of prodromal or residual symptoms. During these prodromal or residual periods, the signs of the disturbance may be manifested by only negative symptoms or two or more symptoms listed in Criterion A present in an attenuated form (e.g., odd beliefs or unusual perceptual experiences).

[Additional criteria caution the diagnosing clinician to rule out other physical and psychiatric disorders as well as considering the presence of preexisting developmental disorders of childhood].

---

probably have decreased, and while he still might have been withdrawn and felt mistrustful, his auditory hallucinations would likely have decreased in frequency and intensity.

How the Phases of Schizophrenia Affect Consumers' Lives

To experience the phases of a schizophrenic episode only once would be very disruptive to one's life. Unfortunately, many individuals experience this dreaded sequence of phases repeatedly, resulting in numerous and unpredictable disruptions to their lives. Persistent negative symptoms during long residual phases with occasional bursts of positive symptoms may dominate the person's existence, making it difficult to concentrate or focus, even on simple day-to-day tasks. Functional deficits associated with the disorder interfere with goal-directed behavior involving one's career and lifestyle. Thus, a disproportionately large number of people with schizophrenia are chronically unemployed, have not finished their education, do not reside in their own homes, are unmarried, and are estranged from their relatives. Later in this book we will address how the interventions of psychiatric rehabilitation can help these individuals to cope more effectively, regain control over their lives, and pursue goals such as employment and independent living.

Mood Disorders

More common than schizophrenia, mood disorders are estimated to affect from 5% to 20% of the general population. Compared to schizophrenia, mood disorders affect a smaller proportion (about 25%) of persons served in psychiatric rehabilitation programs (Arns, 1998). This is probably because mood disorders cover a wide spectrum of symptoms and functional deficits. Some individuals experience relatively mild or moderate symptoms that do not have a significant negative effect on their day-to-day functioning and therefore do not require PsyR services. Others have occasional bouts of mood swings intermixed with long periods of good mental health. It is also common for people with other serious disorders to experience mood disorders as well.

The most serious mood disorders are episodic, recurrent, and cause significant functional deficits. Three types of episodes are associated with mood disorders (APA, 2000). Keep in mind that every individual with a mood disorder does not necessarily experience each type of episode.

Depressive episodes are characterized by extreme sadness or emptiness lasting most of the day, everyday, for a period of 2 weeks or longer. *Manic episodes* are marked by an elevated mood, in which the person feels excessively "up" or "high," and occasionally excessively irritable, for a period of a week or more. In a *mixed episode*, a person meets the criteria for both types of episodes, cycling through depressive and manic phases of the illness. When an individual experiences one or more recurrent episodes of depression, he or she may be diagnosed with major depression, recurrent (APA, 2000). Individuals who experience more than one instance of two out of the three types of episodes may have what is known as *bipolar disorder*, formerly called *manic-depression*. Both major depression and bipolar disorder may or may not have some of the psychotic features described earlier, such as hallucinations and delusions.

Most people know what it is like to be "down in the dumps" for a day or two. Some have had longer bouts of feeling sad, perhaps accompanied by insomnia or a change in appetite. By contrast, consider the following:

> *Marian has a mid-management position in a large company. She generally enjoys her work, but she has not made it in to the office for almost 3 weeks. She cannot rouse herself in the mornings. When she finally does get up, close to noon, she has trouble getting anything done, even a load of laundry. It seems to take an eternity to get herself out of bed, walk to the kitchen, and make herself a cup of coffee. She feels sadder then she can remember, except perhaps when her father died 4 years ago. But this seems worse, because at least after her father's death friends could distract her and she could forget her sorrow for brief periods. Her current sadness has a different quality, like she is at the bottom of a pit, with no hope of getting out, or ever feeling happy again. She finds herself crying for hours at a time, but she cannot figure out why she is weeping. Marian knows she needs help, but cannot motivate herself to even make a phone call.*

Marian is experiencing a major depressive episode. While some of her symptoms may have been experienced by many people not diagnosed with a severe mental illness, Marian's symptoms are more severe and of longer duration. In fact, she is experiencing a severe and persistent mental illness that is extremely disabling. The criteria for making this diagnosis are outlined in Box 2.3.

The symptoms of a manic episode are almost literally the opposite of those of a depressive episode. They are outlined in Box 2.4. Consider the experiences of Mark, a fairly average, married, middle-age man who recalls his earlier manic episodes with a mixture of amusement, embarrassment, and regret.

> *It is pretty wild being in that state; there is even some fun, if you don't get into too much trouble. You have a great feeling of self-confidence. You don't so much as feel that you are the president, but feel you have pull with him. I'd always get my hands on a really big, fancy car, which I would rent or even buy. I would head for another state, spending wildly until my credit got cut off. Somehow, I would have a pretty girl on my arm, at least some of the time. The stuff I did! I can't believe my wife didn't divorce me. She almost did, more than once, even though she was coming to realize that, bizarrely enough, all this was due to an illness.*

BOX 2.3
Criteria for Major Depressive Episode
(APA, 2000, p.356)

A. Five or more of the following symptoms have been present during the same 2-week period and represent a change from previous functioning; at least one of the symptoms is either (1) depressed mood or (2) loss of interest or pleasure.
Note: Do not include symptoms that are clearly due to a general medical condition, or mood-incongruent delusions or hallucinations.

(1) Depressed mood most of the day, nearly every day, as indicated by either subjective report (e.g., feels sad or empty) or observation made by others (e.g., appears tearful). *Note:* In children or adolescents, can be irritable mood.

(2) Markedly diminished interest or pleasure in all, or almost all, activities most of the day, nearly every day (as indicated by either subjective account or observation made by others).

(3) Significant weight loss when not dieting or weight gain (e.g., a change of more than 5% of body weight in a month) or decrease in appetite nearly every day. *Note:* In children, considerable failure to make expected weight gains.

(4) Insomnia or hypersomnia [excessive sleep] nearly every day.

(5) Psychomotor agitation [excessive movement] or retardation [slowed movement] nearly every day (observable by others, not merely subjective feelings of restlessness or being slowed down).

(6) Fatigue or loss of energy nearly every day.

(7) Feelings of worthlessness or excessive or inappropriate guilt (which may be delusional) nearly every day (not merely self-reproach or guilt about being sick).

(8) Diminished ability to think or concentrate, or indecisiveness nearly every day (either by subjective account or observed by others).

(9) Recurrent thoughts of death (not just fear of dying), recurrent suicidal ideation without a specific plan, or a suicide attempt, or a specific plan for committing suicide.

B. The symptoms do not meet the criteria for a mixed episode.

C. The symptoms cause clinically significant distress or impairment of social, occupational, or other important areas of functioning.

[Criteria D and E caution clinicians to rule out substance use, other medical conditions and simple bereavement].

BOX 2.4
Criteria for Manic Episode (APA, 2000, p. 362)

A. A distinct period of abnormally and persistently elevated mood lasting at least 1 week (or any duration if hospitalization is necessary).

B. During the period of mood disturbance, three (or more) of the following symptoms have persisted (four if the mood is only irritable) and have been present to a significant degree:

(1) Inflated self-esteem or grandiosity.
(2) Decreased need for sleep (e.g., feels rested after only 3 hours of sleep).
(3) More talkative than usual or pressure to keep talking.
(4) Flight of ideas or subjective experience that thoughts are racing.
(5) Distractibility (i.e., attention too easily drawn to unimportant or irrelevant external stimuli).

(6) Increase in goal-directed activity (either socially, at work or school, or sexually) or psychomotor agitation (extreme restlessness).
(7) Excessive involvement in pleasurable activities that have a high potential for painful consequences (e.g., engaging in unrestrained buying sprees, sexual indiscretions, or foolish business investments).

C. The symptoms do not meet criteria for a mixed episode.

D. The mood disturbance is sufficiently severe to cause marked impairment in occupational functioning, usual social activities, or relationships with others, to necessitate hospitalization to prevent harm to self or others, or the presence of psychotic features.

E. The symptoms are not due to the direct physiological effects of substance use (e.g., a drug of abuse, a medication or other treatment) or a general medical condition (e.g., hyperthyroidism).

Another individual, Robert, with a history of manic phases put it this way:

I would set out, say, to hitchhike to Hawaii. Yeah, hitch rides, leave the East Coast, and ignore the fact that the Pacific Ocean was in the way, even if I got across the country. Of course, I had to hitch hike, I had already cracked up my car, left my job, stopped paying my mortgage, lost my condo. But I would have big plans for myself.

Both men also described very dark periods. Robert said:

I'd get so I would lose my confidence, not get out of bed, not shower for weeks or change my clothes. The mornings were the worst. Nighttime was not so good either. I'd be in bed, not asleep, not wanting to get up.

Mark noticed a cycle or pattern that was seasonal.

It got so I dreaded the fall, the short days before winter set in. Even on medication, I still feel the changes in myself according to the time of year.

Of course, what is so remarkable are the extremes in symptoms within the same individuals—the two opposite poles, thus the term *bipolar disorder*.

Many individuals only experience depressive episodes, such as Marian, described earlier, or Ann who reported:

In a way, everything stopped. I didn't take care of anything, anybody, my husband, my kids, no one, not even myself. I mostly did nothing. I thought a lot about death, even suicide, but I did not even have the energy to do anything about it.

While individuals in manic phases are at risk for harming themselves or others, through their impulsive and sometimes dangerous behavior, people in depressive phases, are at greater risk for suicide.

> *Una had made many attempts on her life, so many it was not taken very seriously. These attempts were called gestures. But she knew for certain she wanted to die. During her last depressive episode, as she was getting better, she started to make plans. She was tired of it all and of all the medications that never really gave her relief. This time she succeeded in slitting both her arms and bleeding to death before she could be found.*

How Are Schizophrenia and Mood Disorders Different?

While schizophrenia is characterized by its psychotic symptoms, and a mood disorder is characterized by its emotional or affective symptoms, the distinction between the two diagnostic categories is not always so clear. For example, both Robert and Mark who were diagnosed with bipolar disorders experienced grandiose delusions. They said their thoughts raced quickly, and Mark said that at times he heard voices. Consider what happened to Dave:

> *Dave had racing thoughts, imagined he was a Mafiosi and, at other times, a saint. He spoke quickly and incoherently. At times he would suddenly become sullen and withdrawn. He was treated with antipsychotic medication for many years, without much improvement and many side effects. He died in the state hospital. Later on, when his daughter was diagnosed with bipolar disorder, manic type, it occurred to the other members of the family that their father may have been incorrectly diagnosed as having schizophrenia and, therefore, improperly treated all those years.*

Many individuals exhibit the symptoms of both schizophrenic and mood disorders. Their diagnosis does not fit neatly into either category. Consider the story of Tara:

> *Tara's mental health workers believed she had schizophrenia because when she became ill she heard voices, had mixed-up thoughts, paced constantly, and believed aliens controlled her. When not sick, she was often cheerful and vivacious. Recently, she sounded sort of hopeless and said "I can't do anything." Her caseworker was so used to hearing so many clients say that, she barely noticed. Then, Tara began to stop her usual social and volunteer activities. Her personal hygiene became very poor. She stared off into space, and basically stopped talking.*

Does Tara really have schizophrenia? Does she have another type of psychosis? Is she someone who has schizophrenia, but now is also experiencing a depressive episode? Are these the signs of a catatonic episode, perhaps the most bizarre form of schizophrenia, in which movement stops altogether?

Tara's flat affect (the lack of expression of emotions), her withdrawal, and her poor concentration are indicative of a variety of illnesses (see DSM IV-TR; APA, 2000). Too often mental health professionals, including psychiatrists, jump to conclusions about a person's diagnosis. The risks associated with an incorrect diagnosis are great, because the choice of psychotropic medication is, in large part, based on the diagnosis. The wrong medications are not only unhelpful, they can be directly harmful because of side effects and the potential aggravation of other symptoms. For example, antidepressant medication can increase symptoms of psychosis and antipsychotic medication can bring on depressive symptoms. Issues about medications will be discussed further in Chapter 3.

The symptoms of mood disorders and schizophrenia resemble each other and in some cases may even be identical. Indeed, many individuals meet the criteria for both schizophrenic and mood disorders at different times throughout their lives or, occasionally, even at the same time. Individuals who have schizophrenic symptoms and also meet the criteria for one of these mood disorders are classified as having schizoaffective disorder, which has two subtypes, bipolar and depressed (APA, 2000).

Relevance to Psychiatric Rehabilitation

This brief overview of psychiatric symptomatology among persons with severe and persistent mental illness is intended to help the reader grasp the highly disruptive nature of these disorders. The symptoms of these disorders are far more serious than the ups and downs of everyday life. They are also not transient like the effects of experimenting with drugs or alcohol. The impact of these symptoms can be all encompassing, causing extreme distress and disrupting the living, working, and learning of individuals who experience these illnesses. It is important for PsyR professionals to have a clear understanding of what consumers are up against and dealing with everyday. Hopefully, some understanding of the nature of symptoms allows us to feel empathy for someone struggling with a severe mood or thought disorder.

Professionals who have knowledge of symptoms can also help consumers learn about, monitor, and cope with the phases of their illness. In addition, this knowledge is sometimes useful in assisting individuals to communicate with their psychiatrist. However, it is important to understand that most psychiatric rehabilitation interventions do not directly address the symptoms of these illnesses; rather, they address the impairments caused by the disruptiveness, severity, and persistence of the symptoms. PsyR professionals emphasize and build on the healthier features of the person: his or her strengths and interests.

Unfortunately, many professionals have a tendency to overemphasize symptoms, sometimes even missing alternative and simpler explanations. For example, social withdrawal is a common behavioral symptom of persons with severe and persistent mental illness. The extreme, of course, is the individual who does not speak at all or does not seek the company of others, like Eva described next. Is Eva withdrawn because of her illness?

> *Eva spoke rarely, if at all, uttering occasional words in a thick Italian accent. Her psychiatrists and caseworkers must have written a thousand times in her chart "socially withdrawn." One day, a thought occurred to her caseworker. The caseworker went to another member of the program who spoke Italian and asked him to talk to Eva. When he did, Eva's face brightened immediately. She then produced long, coherent sentences in Italian. The consumer-translator said, "She speaks Italian, definitely a southern dialect, but I understand her, although she murders a beautiful language."*

Clearly, her social withdrawal was not the symptom that the staff members had assumed it to be.

Similarly, there is a tendency for some mental health professionals to not only overemphasize symptoms, but dwell on crises and bizarre behavior, perhaps because they make for juicy "war stories." The strengths and personal interests of mental health consumers are sometimes overlooked due to this bias on the part of professionals.

> *Leonard was a young, lanky fellow who wore a leather jacket and talked to himself in a combination of tough, street language and apparent gibberish, which was referred to as a thought disorder and even described as a "word salad," a jumble of apparently incoherent words, sentences, phrases, and ideas. It was difficult to communicate with Leonard and engage him in any activities. Sometimes he would try to speak to people. One day all he would say was "LBJ, Sam Rayburn, US Senate" and the like. Because of his incoherent speech, all of this was attributed, by a staff person, to delusions of grandeur, mixed with a good dose of thought disorder. She assumed that Leonard believed he spoke to or knew great statesman of our country. However, one day, this staff person asked Leonard to talk more slowly and repeat himself more clearly. The staff person soon found out that Leonard was quite a history and politics buff. His facts were accurate and he did not believe he was talking with great historical figures. Leonard's difficulty expressing himself, directly related to the symptoms of his illness, obscured a great interest of his.*

The psychiatric rehabilitation professional working with Leonard had found an interest around which to engage Leonard, and perhaps a strength on which to build. In subsequent chapters we will explore how psychiatric rehabilitation helps consumers utilize their strengths, overcome functional deficits, and ultimately achieve their goals.

The description of dire symptoms in this chapter might lead one to conclude that the outlook is hopeless, but this is far from the case. Indeed, many of the individuals described above who experienced serious problems have continued to struggle with their disorders and achieve successful lives. Chapter 3 will address the long-term outcomes of these conditions.

Dual Diagnosis

The term *dual diagnosis* refers to the presence of two coexisting conditions. The two dual diagnoses most often encountered in PsyR services are mental illness and substance abuse (i.e., drug or alcohol) and mental illness and developmental disability. In both cases, the presence of a dual diagnosis has historically been a complicating factor in receiving adequate and appropriate services. Mental health providers often knew little about drug abuse or developmental disability and may have either declined to provide services to someone with a dual diagnosis or provided mental health services without addressing the coexisting disability. Similarly, substance abuse service providers and developmental disability service providers often either addressed only the issues with which they were familiar or declined to provide services altogether. Recently the presence of coexisting conditions, and the ways in which those conditions affect each other, have received greater attention.

Advances in the treatment and rehabilitation of individuals with mental illness and a substance abuse disorder will be examined in depth in Chapter 8.

Mental Illness and Developmental Disability

The term *developmental disability* encompasses a number of conditions including cognitive disabilities (i.e., mental retardation), autism, cerebral palsy, epilepsy, brain injury, and spina bifida. A developmental disability is a severe, disabling condition that arises in infancy or childhood, persists indefinitely, and causes serious problems in language, learning, mobility, and the capacity for independent living (New Jersey Developmental Disabilities Council, 1997/1998, p. 1).

Since the mid-1800s, when the first segregated schools were developed for children with mental retardation, most people with severe developmental disabilities have been institutionalized for most of their lives. The first segregated schools were designed to be small, personal, individualized, and temporary, offering services designed to develop the skills necessary for success in the community. Segregated schools quickly became large institutions designed to "protect" society from children with retardation who might grow up to be depraved and dangerous adults (Mauch, 1991, p. 3). In a further attempt to "protect" society, the eugenics movement, begun at the turn of the century, encouraged the sterilization of people with developmental disabilities.

During the 1950s, parents of people with developmental disabilities began to demand a greater focus on educational and developmental approaches to services. The idea of institutions as the only service option was rejected and some parents began to keep their children with developmental disabilities at home. Parental organizations such as the Association for Retarded Children (ARC) emerged. ARC, which later changed its name to the Association for Retarded Citizens and more recently became simply The Arc (Roberts, 1996), became strong advocates for family members. During the 1960s and 1970s, litigation and advocacy led to the establishment of rights for people with developmental disabilities, such as public education and services in the least restricted environment (Mauch, 1991). The work of many people such as Wolfensberger, who articulated the principle of normalization (discussed in Chapter 4), and Marc Gold, who demonstrated that people with the most severe cognitive disabilities could learn complex skills, fueled the growing dissatisfaction with institutional care. These new ideas about the rights and abilities of people with disabilities ultimately led to the development of supported employment (discussed in Chapter 9) and other community-based supports for people with developmental disabilities. During the last few decades, we have seen the downsizing and closing of state institutions as more and more people with developmental disabilities are being supported in their efforts to live, learn, work, and socialize in the community (Mauch, 1991; Schwartz, 1992; Torrey, 1993).

Incidence of Mental Illness and Developmental Disability

Studies of people with developmental disabilities living in the community suggest that among these individuals 20% to 35% experience a coexisting mental illness (Parsons,

May, & Menolascino, 1984; Torrey, 1993). However, Parsons and colleagues caution that these studies include many children under the age of 12 and, therefore, should not be considered a true reflection of incidence among adults. More recently, Szymanski et al. (1998) reported an incidence rate for schizophrenia, other psychotic disorders, and mood disorders among people with developmental disabilities that is similar to that found in the general public. They further reported that the incidence of personality disorders, among people with developmental disabilities, appears to be higher than usual, but suggested that this may be "related to maladaptive personality traits resulting from negative social experiences" (p. 14). Furthermore, the full range of mental illnesses has been identified among people with developmental disabilities (Torrey, 1993).

Diagnosing mental illness in a person with a developmental disability can be a difficult task. The diagnostic process includes self-report of thoughts, feelings, and symptoms. For individuals with significant communication impairments, this may be difficult, if not impossible. Often, in these situations, a diagnosis is based on reported behavior such as an increase in aggression, self-injury, tearfulness, and withdrawal. These same behaviors, can also be indications of physical illness, psychological stress, or dissatisfaction (Stark, McGee, Menolascino, Baker, & Menousek, 1984; Torrey, 1993).

The potential for misdiagnosis is clearly great. A misdiagnosis brings with it the possibly unnecessary or incorrect use of medication, which is of great concern to people with disabilities, their families, and advocates.

Individuals with developmental disabilities and mental illness have great difficulty receiving adequate services. Often the services that are available are provided by different systems that are funded by different sources. Programs designed for mental illness often consider individuals with a dual diagnosis to have mental retardation as the primary diagnosis, and programs designed for developmental disorders often consider persons with a dual diagnosis to have a mental illness as the primary diagnosis. PsyR practitioners have to make an effort to work across programs, with people from different disciplines and programs.

Mental Illness and Substance Abuse

The dual diagnosis of mental illness and substance abuse refers to the presence of a severe psychiatric disorder and abuse of or dependence on alcohol or drugs. This dual diagnosis is referred to in a number of ways, for example, dually diagnosed, dually disordered, MICA (mentally ill chemical abuser), MISA (mentally ill substance abuser), or CAMI (chemical abuse and mental illness) (U.S. Department of Health and Human Services, 1995).

Incidence of Mental Illness and Substance Abuse

Individuals with both a mental illness and a substance-related disorder appear to make up an astounding percentage of the overall population of people with severe mental illnesses. Studies indicate that between 17% and 63% of individuals diagnosed with a serious mental illness also abuse substances (Drake, McLaughlin, Pepper, & Minkoff, 1991;

Sciacca & Thompson, 1996). Drake and colleagues suggest that the factors contributing to this high incidence are deinstitutionalization and changing societal norms. In short, because people who have a mental illness now spend more time in the community than in hospitals, they have increased access to drugs and alcohol. At the same time, society in general has increased its acceptance of the use of drugs and alcohol.

For many people with this dual diagnosis, the substance abuse predates the onset of mental illness and the reasons for using seem to be the same reasons given by people without disabilities who abuse substances. Some researchers hypothesize that the drug use precipitates or induces the mental illness. For other individuals the reasons for using drugs and alcohol may include self-medication to alleviate psychiatric symptoms, to medicate side effects, to be liked by their peers without disabilities, or to increase their level of comfort in social interactions (Drake et al., 1991).

Further complicating this phenomenon, the group of people identified as having a dual diagnosis is not homogenous. Individuals who have both a mental illness and a substance abuse problem differ from each other in psychiatric diagnosis and severity, type and level of substance abuse, and extent of the impact either disability has on life functioning (Weiss, Mirin, & Frances, 1992). Luke, Mowbray, Klump, Herman and Boots-Miller (1996) identified seven clusters of individuals by examining the type and level of substance abuse and the impact on medical needs, employment, legal involvement, family/social problems, psychiatric problems, and others.

This topic is covered in more detail in Chapter 8, which is devoted exclusively to psychiatric rehabilitation interventions addressing the dual disorders of serious mental illnesses and addictions.

Etiology

What is the origin of the strange symptoms described in this chapter? Why are some people affected by severe mental illnesses such as schizophrenia? What is the source of the vulnerability for these disorders?

While the jury is still out on these questions, we are much closer to a final verdict today than anytime in the past. The evidence continues to grow that the root cause of these devastating illnesses is biological in nature rather than psychological or *psychodynamic* (i.e., theoretically rooted in past events and the unconscious). Interestingly, much of this progress can be directly attributed to the development of high-speed computers that have made high-definition medical imaging possible.

Physiological Evidence of the Disease Process in the Brain

Many persons with schizophrenia and their families attribute the illness to psychological stress alone, a conclusion that is *inconsistent* with psychiatric research (Holzinger, Kilian, Lindenbach, Petscheleit, & Angermeyer, 2003). However, why would we assume that individuals who experience or observe a condition would necessarily know its origins? Does being bald give you insight into the hormonal changes that have taken place to bring about hair loss? Certainly not.

Summarizing all available evidence on the etiology of schizophrenia, Walker, Kestler, Bollini, and Hochman (2004) reached the conclusion that both genetic and prenatal factors can influence vulnerability to this illness. The same can be said for mental illnesses in general. Subsequent processes, including brain development, that occur during adolescence and exposure to stressful events can trigger the onset of what is known as a major mental illness.

The evidence is overwhelming that schizophrenia and similar conditions are due to changes in the structure and functioning of the brain (Buchanan & Carpenter, 1997; Frith, 1997; Walker et al., 2004). Today, very sophisticated neuroimaging techniques, such as magnetic resonance imaging (MRI), computerized axial tomography (CAT) scans, and positron emissions tomography (PET) scans, provide a window for viewing living, working brains. Developed with the help of high-speed computers, MRI and CAT scans provide pictures of the brain's structure, whereas PET scans provide snapshots of its functioning.

Using these various brain scans, the living brains of people with serious mental illnesses have been compared to other individuals, of the same age and sex, without mental illnesses. Based on the differences found between people with serious mental illnesses and those without them, it has become increasingly clear that the brains of people who have a serious mental illness have both a different neuroanatomy and different neural functioning than people who do not have a major psychiatric disorder (Buchanan & Carpenter, 1997).

An MRI scan provides images of the tissue, structure, and spaces (ventricles and sulci) in the brain. In the MRI scans shown in Figure 2.1, the lighter gray areas are the brain tissue cells, or neurons, and the darker gray areas are the ventricles. The ventricles are large fluid-filled enclosures and the sulci are the spaces or folds in the brain's cortex. These are part of the normal anatomy or structure of the brain. Normally, ventricles and sulci become enlarged as part of the aging process. In the MRI scans pictured in Figure 2.1, note that the person with schizophrenia, on the right, has less brain tissue and enlarged ventricles compared to the peer of the same age, on the left.

People diagnosed with schizophrenia, compared to others their own age, often have larger spaces in their brain in the form of enlarged ventricles and sulci, indicating they have less brain tissue (Gur & Pearlson, 1993). MRI and CAT scans have consistently found that these spaces are enlarged in the brains of people with schizophrenia (Heckers, 1997). Based on this evidence, it appears that some people with schizophrenia have suffered a type of physical dementia (e.g., enlarged ventricles), perhaps as early as adolescence or young adulthood.

The brains of people with schizophrenia, and perhaps other mental illnesses, have other significant structural differences when compared to people of the same age and sex, and even differ from those of their family. People with schizophrenia have a significantly smaller brain region, known as the hippocampus, in comparison to their peers (Schulze et al., 2003). Studies have shown that reductions in the size of the hippocampus occur during the first psychotic episode. In addition, there are differences in the frontal and temporal lobe regions of the brains of people with schizophrenia. Parts of the temporal and frontal lobes have less volume and are smaller than they should be (Conklin & Iacona, 2002; Kurachi, 2003a, 2003b). Raine and colleagues (2002) found that there are also

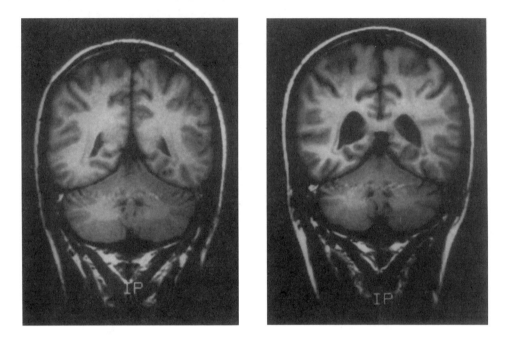

Well twin   Affected twin

FIGURE 2.1   MRI scans of 28-year-old identical twins discordant for schizophrenia, showing enlarged cerebral ventricles in the affected twin. (Courtesy of Dr. E. Fuller Torrey and Dr. Daniel Weinberger, Clinical Brain Disorders Branch, National Institute of Mental Health.) OK.

frontal lobe differences in persons with schizophrenia spectrum disorders, that is, individuals with symptoms similar to schizophrenia who do not experience severe episodes of psychosis. Many of the problems people with schizophrenia experience, such as problems with auditory (hearing) processing in the form of hallucinations, understanding concepts and abstract ideas, and other cognitive or thinking problems, are associated with these regions of the brain. Differences can also be seen in a nearby region known as the amygdala.

The causes for the differences in brain structure are not known but a number of theories are emerging. One involves neurotrophins, which are the hormone-like growth factors that help neurons to grow, arrange themselves properly, and develop synaptic connections with other neurons. People with schizophrenia have an abnormally low level of neurotrophins. One major neurotrophin, brain-derived neurotrophic factor (BDNF), has been found to be significantly lower in people with schizophrenia (Pitiladar, Gonul, Taneli, & Akdeniz, 2004). These abnormal levels lead to abnormal neuronal development and abnormal development of both the dendrites (branches of brain cells) and synapses (small spaces where different brain cells meet).

Another theory is based on the evidence that the stress response of persons who have serious mental illnesses, which is the release of a set of brain hormones called glucocorticoids, is poorly regulated. The response to stress is therefore unduly prolonged. Glucocorticoids are known to interact with the hypothalamus–pituitary axis (HPA). The hypothalamus is a brain structure associated with many human appetites and drives. It is directly connected to a very important gland, the pituitary. High levels of glucocorticoids and prolonged response to stress have been found among people who have a serious mental illness. This prolonged stress reaction may lead both to the experience of escalating symptoms, relapses, and the deterioration of certain brain structures (Cotter & Pariante, 2002). In animal studies, the prolonged release of glucocorticoids is associated with the development of a smaller hippocampus, a problem specifically found in schizophrenia.

The Story of Dara

Besides demonstrating an important point about the physiological basis of severe mental illness, Dara's experience provides a good illustration of the importance of educating families and consumers. As you read the following story, consider what the family should have known and what effect their not knowing had on their attitude about Dara's chances for recovery.

Dara's family was upset enough about her latest "episode" as they called it. A 54-year-old, married woman with two children, Dara had been ill for more than 25 years. Dara is a graduate of a two-year college and worked as an accounting clerk in an insurance agency. Suddenly, for no apparent reason, she stopped going to work. Then one day she jumped out into traffic. Fortunately, she was rescued by a police officer. When she was asked why she had jumped out into traffic, she said that voices had been telling her to do this for several hours and she had finally given in. Once in the traffic she got frightened and yelled for help. At the hospital, she said the president of the United States intervened to save her and had personally sent the police officer. Upon admission, the doctor ordered a CAT scan to rule out a dementia, such as early-onset Alzheimer's disease, that might have contributed to her seemingly bizarre behavior. She did have enlarged spaces (ventricles) in her brain. Her son said, "Oh my God, what could be worse, more bad news about mom!" Later, they learned, it was the same bad news they had already been living with for many years. Like many people with schizophrenia, she had significant changes in the structure of her brain, perhaps for most of her adult life.

PET scans provide colored pictures of the brain's activity, by measuring where the brain is metabolizing glucose. Thus, it detects how neural brain cells are using sugar, glucose in this case. More use of glucose is indicative of more nerve cell activity. Figure 2.2 provides some examples of PET scans. The brighter areas indicate more brain activity, the darker areas indicate less activity. During tasks requiring a great deal of concentration, the areas of the brain known as the frontal lobes become very active. Figure 2.2 compares the frontal lobe of a person with schizophrenia, on the right, with a person without

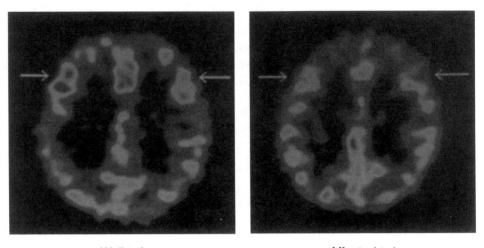

Well twin   Affected twin

FIGURE 2.2   PET scan study of 31-year-old identical twins discordant for schizophrenia. The well twin on the left shows evidence of more cerebral blood flow in the area of the frontal lobe (arrows). The twin with schizophrenia has less cerebral blood flow to the frontal lobe and is thus "hypofrontal." (Courtesy of Dr. E. Fuller Torrey and Dr. Daniel Weinberger, Clinical Brain Disorders Branch, National Institute of Mental Health.)

schizophrenia, of the same age, on the left. Both are working on the same task, yet the person with schizophrenia, as indicated by the darker frontal lobe area, has far less activity in that area than the other individual.

A variety of studies have shown that the frontal lobes are underactive in persons with schizophrenia (e.g., Buschbaum & Haier, 1987). Considering the behavioral functions that are mediated by the frontal lobes, underactivity in this area is likely to result in lack of energy, poor attention and concentration, poor emotional control, flat affect, and restlessness. These problems correspond closely to the negative symptoms of schizophrenia described earlier in this chapter.

Cerebral blood flow studies measure brain activity by tracing where the brain is using blood and oxygen. These studies have found results similar to those from the PET scan studies (Buschbaum & Haier, 1987). Once again, the frontal lobes were found to be underactive. The cerebral blood flow studies have also shown that other areas, such as the temporal and parietal lobes, are receiving more blood and oxygen, compared to people without schizophrenia, indicating overactivity in these areas. This overactivity may account for the experience of hallucinations, delusions, and the excessive internal stimulation reported by people with psychoses.

Neurotransmitters

The PET scan and cerebral blood flow studies imply that it is not just the structure of the brain that is different, but the neural functioning, or brain activity, which is disordered.

The brain is an electrochemical organ and neurotransmitters are literally the chemical messengers of the brain. Neurotransmitters ensure the proper functioning of the brain's electrical circuitry, which underlies all of our behavior. Even the simplest actions and thoughts are the result of the functioning of many neurons (cells of the nervous system) in many different areas and systems of the brain, working in collaboration to produce complex patterns of activity. One brain cell communicates with many other brain cells through the activity of one or more neurotransmitters. Indeed, neurotransmitters regulate all of this complex electrochemical interaction. As many as 30 to 40 different neurotransmitters may be involved. Each neurotransmitter is implicated in many different behaviors or functions. It is also true that the simplest of behaviors can involve numerous neurotransmitters. Some of the major neurotransmitters are as follows:

- *Dopamine:* Involved in all sorts of behavior, especially the regulation of movement, hearing, and perhaps planning.
- *Norepinephrine:* Also known as adrenalin, it is involved with the circulatory system, the heart, but also sleep, appetite, and sexual behavior.
- *Serotonin:* Involved in sleep, impulse control, regulation of body temperature, and other functions.
- *GABA:* Believed to be involved in anxiety.
- *Acetylcholine:* Involved in movement, also muscles, learning and memory, and normal intellectual functioning.

Neurotransmitters and Mental Illness

The systems of two of the neurotransmitters, dopamine and serotonin, seem to be involved in schizophrenia. In persons with this disease, dopamine appears to be overactive and serotonin underactive, although the full explanation for these actions is far more complicated. Nevertheless, the disorders in these systems lead directly to the symptoms of schizophrenia.

Two neurotransmitters, serotonin and norepinephrine, appear to be involved in mood disorders. This combination would account for the changes in sleep, appetite, and drive seen in individuals with these illnesses.

Brain development and brain chemistry are influenced by psychosocial and physical factors. Responses to stress may lead to changes in neurotransmitter functioning. A person who was already vulnerable for genetic or developmental reasons may have abnormal changes in his or her neurotransmitter system in response to an environmental insult or stressor. It is likely that a genetic vulnerability combined with a chain of biological events and environmental stressors may result in the onset of a mental illness. We will explore the role of genetic and environmental factors in the next subsection.

The Role of Genetic Factors

What causes the changes in neuroanatomy and neurotransmitter functioning just described? The evidence suggests that to a large degree these changes are inherited. For quite some time, based on simple observations of familial incidence of mental illnesses, many researchers, including Sigmund Freud, hypothesized that schizophrenia and the other severe mental illnesses were inherited. There is no doubt that the risk of developing schizophrenia is greatly increased if one's biological or "blood" relatives have the illness. Numerous studies have found that even if you have never had any contact with your biological relative who is affected by schizophrenia, and have never shared the same environment, you have an elevated chance of developing this disease (Kendler & Deihl, 1993).

Risk among Biological Relatives

The probable genetic component of these illnesses is illustrated by examining changes in the probability of developing these conditions. In the general population, for persons who do not have relatives with these conditions, the risk for schizophrenia ranges from about one-half of 1% to 1%. If one parent or sibling has the disorder, the risk is 10 times larger, jumping to 5% to 10% (Torrey, 2001). If both parents have the disorder, the probability of developing the illness can be nearly 50%. Research has demonstrated that these risk increases are independent of environmental factors.

The exact etiology of schizophrenia has remained one of the major mysteries surrounding this disease. In the past, much of this debate pitted environmental and hereditary factors against each other. Based on a unique environmental characteristic, the Israeli high-risk study (Marcus et al., 1987) attempted to help solve this problem. Many Israeli settlements, particularly in formerly unpopulated areas such as the Negev Desert, were built on the kibbutz model. One characteristic of a kibbutz is that all the children are raised together by child care workers rather than being raised in the family. This means that for the children raised in a kibbutz, the environment is basically similar. From a research perspective it was assumed that many environmental factors that might contribute to schizophrenia would also be held constant in the kibbutz. To investigate this phenomenon (among others), researchers identified 100 Israeli children: 50 children from the Kibbutz and 50 children from the city where they were brought up in traditional nuclear families. Half of the children from the Kibbutz (25) and half of the children from the city (25) had one or both parents with a diagnosis of schizophrenia. The other children had parents who were apparently free from mental illness. These children were studied over a 30-year period. Researchers periodically assessed these individuals' neurobiological signs, social adjustment, home life (parenting), and, ultimately, their mental health. One striking finding of this study was that all the children who went on to develop either schizophrenia or severe mental illness had a parent diagnosed with a mental illness. Whether the parent with mental illness raised the child or not, the probability of the child developing the disorder did not change. That is, those individuals whose biological parents had a mental illness were equally likely to develop the illness, whether or not they were raised by their parent who was mentally ill. Similar genetic studies in Europe, particularly in Scandinavia, have confirmed this finding. The Israeli high-risk study provides one example from the body of compelling evidence that genetics play a strong role in the etiology of schizophrenia.

Figure 2.3 illustrates in a "tree" or pyramid the nature of the risk factors that are associated with nine out of 100 individuals ultimately diagnosed with schizophrenia or a

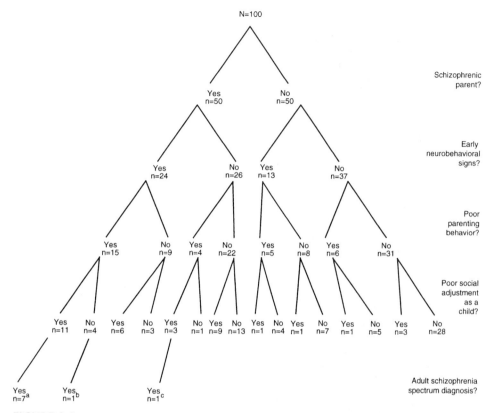

FIGURE 2.3 Decision-tree model for development of schizophrenia. Application to Israeli high-risk study data. Breakdown cases marked "a" = 1 residual-type schizophrenia, 3 paranoid schizophrenia, 2 schizoid personality disorders, and 1 mixed spectrum disorder. Breakdown case marked "b" = 1 residual-type schizophrenia. Breakdown case marked "c" = 1 schizoid personality disorder with dysthymic disorder. (From Marcus et al., 1987.)

related disorder, sometimes called the schizophrenic spectrum. *Yes* indicates the presence of the risk factor, *No*, the absence of the risk factor. The top of the diagram starts with 50 persons who have a parent with schizophrenia and 50 who do not, the bottom row shows the 9 persons who ultimately developed the disorder. Of the 9 who developed the disorder, note that all are in the "branch" that had a genetic relative with the disorder, but they also experienced other risk factors as well. In fact, they all had at least two of the following three risk factors: early neurobehavioral signs, poor parenting, and poor social adjustment. This illustrates that genetic factors while necessary were probably not sufficient to develop the disorder.

Attempts to identify a *genetic locus,* literally the genetic location that accounts for a significant proportion of cases of schizophrenia, have not met with success (Kato et al., 2002). Instead, researchers, using molecular genetic techniques, have identified an array of genes that may contribute to a portion of the population of individuals diagnosed with the disorder (Walker et al., 2004). Studies of twins have been particularly revealing with respect to the role genetics play in schizophrenia. Twins can be classified as either monozygotic, coming from one fertilized egg that later splits into two separate zygotes; or dizygotic, coming from two separate eggs fertilized at about the same time. Identical twins are monozygotic and have identical gene sets. Fraternal twins are dizygotic and have gene sets as similar (or different) as brothers and sisters born at different times.

When one of a pair of fraternal twins has schizophrenia, the concordance, or probability, that the other twin will develop the disease is similar to the rate for any siblings: 5% to 10%. For identical twins, with identical genetic heritage, the concordance rate jumps to 40% to 50% (Torrey, 2001). These figures show that while genetics play a key factor in the etiology of schizophrenia, genetics alone are not a sufficient cause of the disease. If people simply inherited the disorder genetically, the concordance rate between monozygotic identical twins would be 100%, since they have identical gene sets. Therefore, some developmental or environmental factors must account for why some identical twins do not become ill when their sibling has schizophrenia.

Fetal Development and Early Infancy

Events that occur *in utero* seem to be another factor that contribute to the development of schizophrenia. The importance of fetal development in the prenatal environment is highlighted by other findings from twin studies. When twins develop in the same *chorion,* that is, the same "sac" in their mother's womb, the concordance rate for schizophrenia is higher than when they develop in separate chorions. Birth during the winter months, maternal infections during the second trimester of pregnancy (a time of extensive brain development), lower birth weights, and complications in the delivery of the child are all associated with a higher incidence or likelihood of developing schizophrenia among those at genetic risk (Cannon, Jones, & Murray, 2002; Torrey, 2001).

Biological factors affect the risk of developing schizophrenia or other severe mental illnesses among people at genetic risk. Their genetic heritage may make the brain more vulnerable to viruses during fetal development or infancy. Obstetric delivery problems such as temporary deprivation of oxygen may be another of these potentially harmful events. All of these are referred to as insults to the fetus or infant. These insults, in turn, lead to abnormal development of brain structure or tissue, altering how the person's brain structure and brain chemistry evolves.

Three groups of complications are consistently associated with the development of schizophrenia: (1) complications of pregnancy: bleeding, diabetes, rhesus incompatibility; (2) abnormal fetal growth and development: low birth weight, congenital malformations, reduced head circumference; and (3) complications of delivery: asphyxia, emergency cesarean section. However, the degree to which any of these factors explains the incidence of schizophrenia is relatively small (Cannon et al., 2002). Among the general population these complications, which are rather common, double the chance of developing schizophrenia, from about 1% to 2%. Thus, most people who experience these complications *do not* develop schizophrenia; however, for those at genetic risk, they may be particularly significant.

CONTROVERSIAL ISSUE
The Chronological and Geographical Incidence of Schizophrenia

Research suggests that the prevalence rate of schizophrenia is affected by what month people are born in and where they live. These differences may or may not provide a clue as to the cause(s) of schizophrenia, but they apparently are not caused by chance. Researchers who believe that infectious agents in the environment, such as viruses, are implicated in schizophrenia have pointed to these differences as possible evidence for their theories.

People born in the winter or early spring have a higher likelihood of developing schizophrenia than persons born during other seasons (Torrey, 2001; Walker et al., 2004). This is true regardless of the hemisphere where the individual is born (when it is summer in the Northern Hemisphere, it is winter in the Southern Hemisphere). These seasonal varia-tions, which are probably not due to chance, may relate to diet, climate, or other seasonal changes.

Ireland has long been known to have an inordi-nately high rate of schizophrenia. Some reports found that Ireland had a higher rate of persons hospitalized for schizophrenia than any other country in the world (Torrey, 2001). Torrey, who has studied schizophrenia in Ireland, reported that there were large differences in the prevalence of the disease even between different regions in the country. By contrast, countries such as Ghana and Botswana in Africa and New Guinea and Taiwan in the Pacific have very low rates of the disease. How can we account for these differences in rates? Some obvious answers may involve how persons with schizophrenia are identified and counted in differ-ent settings. Another explanation may deal with the genetic heritage of different groups. Finally, differ-ences in geography related to climatic differences may provide us with a clue.

The Role of Stress

Despite what the public is encouraged to believe by the media, severe mental illness is not caused solely by the stress we encounter in our day-to-day lives. E. Fuller Torrey (2001), a psychiatrist and author who has done extensive research in this area, considers stress "a minor cause" at best. He points out that illnesses such as schizophrenia are not more prevalent in highly stressful times, such as during wars or large natural catastrophes such as floods, plagues, and famines. Nor do we see more schizophrenia in environments that are very stressful, such as prisons and concentration camps. Instead, stress may very well be "the straw that breaks the camel's back," as Torrey puts it. Apparently, when someone has the genetic vulnerability and has suffered the requisite biological insults, stress may push them over the edge and bring forth the disease (Torrey, 2001).

Psychosocial and environmental stress may play a part in brain development and brain chemistry. Responses to environmental and psychosocial stress always lead to changes in the brain's chemical messengers, neurotransmitters. However, in individuals who are already vulnerable for genetic or developmental reasons, abnormal changes in neurotrans-mitter functioning may take place. This is the basic premise of the *diathesis stress model* (see Figure 2.4), which proposes that a biologically vulnerable person, when exposed to a stress or trigger, then develops the disease (Anthony & Liberman, 1986).

Adoption studies have supported the diathesis stress model of etiology. Studying adopted people diagnosed with schizophrenia, that is those who did not grow up with a parent who had schizophrenia, Walker and colleagues (2004) found that the rate of

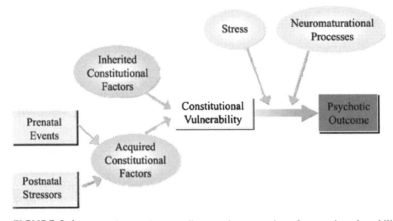

FIGURE 2.4   Stress factors that contribute to the expression of a genetic vulnerability, from Walker, E., Kestler, L., Bollini, A., and Hochman, K.M. (2004) Schizophrenia: Etiology and Course. *Annual Review of Psychology, 55,* 401–430. (Reprinted Courtesy of Annual Review of Psychology.)

psychoses and other severe disorders was significantly higher than in other adopted people. In disruptive family environments, however, an elevated rate of schizophrenia was found that was not seen among adoptees reared in healthy family environments. This suggests that stress may have played a role in the increased incidence of the disease.

Episodes of the illness can be triggered by various stressors, many of which may appear to be normal in their intensity, but which can lead to the catastrophic symptoms and events of mental illness. Stressors that have the potential to bring on an acute episode include personal losses, developmental transitions, and stressful life events such as marriage, graduation, and moving. Physical illness, injury, substance abuse, and other physiological factors such as sleep deprivation have also been associated with the onset of psychiatric symptoms. "Even in the absence of a time-limited stressor, vulnerable individuals can succumb to ambient levels of challenge, tension, or conflict in their environment . . . " (Anthony & Liberman, 1986 pp. 542–543).

The role of stress in the onset of major depression appears to be a significant but not a sufficient cause. The onset of an episode is typically preceded by a serious personal loss of a loved one, a job, a home, or other personal catastrophe. However, although stress has been established as a fairly strong contributing factor, it does not account for why some individuals respond to loss by experiencing a brief period of sadness and hopelessness and others develop a severe condition.

The most obvious example comes from examining responses to the death of a loved one. Most individuals have a period of what is known as *uncomplicated bereavement.* That is, their mood is depressed, they feel hopeless, they may even want to die for a time, are unable to sleep, or lack an appetite. Many people experience this for a period of weeks or even months, without it markedly affecting their social or occupational functioning. In sharp contrast, individuals suffering from major depression may experience a full-blown episode of depression that severely disrupts their normal functioning, as described in Box 2.3.

Stressful life events also play a role in the onset of episodes experienced by people diagnosed with bipolar disorder. However, research shows that psychosocial and environmental stressors are more evident prior to the onset of the early episodes of this illness. The influence of these stressors seems to play little or no role after the first few episodes (Goodwin & Jamison, 1990). Clearly the etiology of these disorders is complex and cannot be explained simply as extreme sensitivity to stress.

The Stress/Vulnerability/Coping/Competence Model

The stress/vulnerability/coping/competence model was proposed by two individuals who are well known in the field of psychiatric rehabilitation, William A. Anthony and Robert Paul Liberman (1986). An elaboration of the diathesis stress model described earlier, the stress/vulnerability/coping/competence model provides both a theory about the cause of severe mental illness and an explanatory framework for the impact that psychiatric rehabilitation and treatment interventions can have on the symptoms and functional level of people who have psychiatric disabilities. The model proposes the following: Individuals inherit or otherwise acquire a vulnerability (sometimes referred to as diathesis) to major mental illnesses such as schizophrenia, major depression, or bipolar disorder. This vulnerability results in abnormal development of brain structures and processes or an unusual type of stress reaction.

Fortunately, a number of protective factors can either prevent the onset of an acute episode of illness or lessen the impact of symptoms. These factors include coping skills, supportive resources, competence in relevant life activities, and psychotropic medications. According to this model, the severity and outcome of these disorders have a lot to do with whether or not these protective factors are in place when a stressful event occurs. If an individual does not have adequate coping skills or does not acquire resources or supports that enhance coping, he or she remains very vulnerable to the influence of future stressors and more vulnerable to frequent or prolonged relapses. Conversely, a person with well-developed coping skills and a reliable support system is likely to experience fewer acute episodes of mental illness, as well as episodes that are less severe and shorter in duration. Consider the following vignette:

> *Cheryl has been coping with schizophrenia for 10 years. For the last 2 years she has been relatively stable, experiencing some negative symptoms, but very few positive symptoms. She sees a psychiatrist once a month who prescribes a relatively low dose of antipsychotic medication for her. Sometimes Cheryl forgets to take her medication, or chooses to skip her morning dose because it makes her drowsy. She used to attend a peer support group regularly, but has gradually lost touch with the group. Cheryl has a part-time clerical job that she likes. She is not particularly close to friends or family, and when not at her job she prefers to keep to herself. Cheryl was doing well at her job until her supervisor, whom she liked and trusted, left to take another position. About a week later she began to hear disturbing voices. She also had difficulty sleeping and could not concentrate on her filing duties at work. She missed some days*

at work and was occasionally late. Her new supervisor criticized her performance and questioned her recent tardiness and absenteeism. Unable to face an increasingly stressful work environment, Cheryl quit her job.

While Cheryl's job history suggests that she had some coping skills and a certain level of vocational competence, she lacked the problem-solving skills and support system she needed to help her cope with a major change at work. The fact that she was not taking her medication regularly at the time she was exposed to psychosocial stress may also have affected her vulnerability to psychosis and the distressing results.

An important role of psychiatric rehabilitation is to aid the individual in the development of coping skills and competence (Anthony & Liberman, 1986). By enhancing coping ability and competence in social and vocational environments, the vulnerability to stress is reduced. Psychotropic medications are also an important protective factor, and PsyR practitioners can play an important role in helping consumers obtain the information and skills they need to utilize medications appropriately. For individuals who have mastered coping skills, future stressors, which everyone faces, will be much less devastating.

Etiology Summary

Summarizing all available evidence on the etiology of schizophrenia, Walker et al. (2004) reached the conclusion that both genetic (inherited) and prenatal (before birth) factors can give rise to a vulnerability to schizophrenia. The subsequent processes, which affect the development of neurons in the brain, especially those that occur during adolescence and exposure to stressful events, can trigger the behavioral expression of this vulnerability. Walker and colleagues point out that the etiology of schizophrenia involves the interaction among vulnerabilities within the brain and environmental factors. The illness does not emerge from a single defect in a specific brain region but rather from the dysfunction of neuronal circuits in multiple brain regions. The brain's maturational processes play a critical role.

Obsolete Etiological Theories

The scientific community has made real progress in its understanding of the etiology of the major mental illnesses. At the same time, the public is still exposed to a number of discredited or obsolete theories about what causes major mental illness. Most of these obsolete theories center on early childhood psychological trauma or abusive family environments as causal factors. Harding and Zahniser (1994) describe the familial role in etiology as one of the great myths about schizophrenia. While a dysfunctional family environment is clearly unpleasant, often stressful, and may be associated with some psychiatric disorders, it apparently is not the primary cause of severe and persistent mental illness.

One discredited theory traced the cause of schizophrenia to "schizophrenegenic" mothers. Supposedly, these mothers caused schizophrenia in their children by giving them mixed messages, for example, simultaneously encouraging independence and engendering unnatural levels of maternal dependence (Lidz, 1992). Empirical research has provided no support for this theory and others that focus on parentally induced intrapsychic conflict, yet some professionals and members of the general public still subscribe to them.

These theories are not only erroneous, they are harmful. Adherents to these theories have blamed family members for the illness of their loved ones. This, in turn, fostered guilt and animosity among family members, making for tense, counterproductive relationships between family members and professionals (Torrey, 2001). This disservice to consumers and their families is also being perpetuated by some educators, who persist in training mental health professionals in these discredited theories, despite the lack of evidence for them (Harding et al., 1992; Lefley, 1989). Many individuals and family members still believe in primarily psychological causes for the illness (Holzinger et al., 2003).

The Myth of the Myth of Mental Illness

The views of Thomas Szasz (1976) were popular in the 1960s and 1970s. He proposed that rather than being an actual disease, mental illnesses, including schizophrenia, were artifacts or creations of psychiatry. In short, he believed that mental illness does not really exist. The extensive biological evidence that an active disease process exists has discredited this theory. Szasz built his theory on a single observation, which was undoubtedly true at the time, but reached a conclusion that was undoubtedly false. Szasz believed that all assertions about human behavior (including diagnoses) by psychiatrists and psychologists are subjective observations based on value judgments, not scientific judgments. In short, judgments, like diagnoses and competency, were solely matters of opinion rather than scientific facts. There is a body of research that supports this contention (Rosenhan, 1973). Szasz's position was simple: He believed that we should not define mental illness as a disease unless a "brain lesion" could be found.

Since that time, a variety of functional and structural problems have been found in the brains of people with schizophrenia; specific regions of the brain and neurotransmitters have been identified as described earlier in this chapter. In addition, the symptoms and functional deficits experienced by the millions of people who have schizophrenia are quite real and have a profound effect on their lives.

Other outdated theorists include the late British psychiatrist and author R. D. Laing who believed that psychosis was actually a healing process (Torrey, 2001). Laing believed that through psychosis the individual regresses to the developmental stage at the core of the problem. From this stage, it then becomes possible to bring about a cure. Based on that idea, Laing believed that the professionals' task was to encourage regression, or psychosis, rather than try to stop it. The helper would work with the individual in the psychotic state to help them mend themselves. To accomplish this for his patients, Laing created a clinic where they could experience their psychosis in a safe environment without interruption. Laing's approach was not only unhelpful, it was probably harmful. There is strong evidence that psychosis and regression are accompanied by sometimes irreversible brain tissue atrophy.

The beliefs of Loren Mosher (Mosher & Burti, 1989), formerly of the National Institute of Mental Health, are similar to Laing's. He believed people with schizophrenia should not be treated with medication because it deprives patients of "the experience" of their symptoms. His concern was that they would become out of touch with themselves. Given the growing evidence of the medical-biological nature of mental illness, such thinking is tantamount to saying that people suffering from heart disease should not be treated because it would interfere with their experience of angina (chest pain).

Summary

Individuals who are served in psychiatric rehabilitation programs have various psychiatric diagnoses including schizophrenia, schizoaffective disorder, bipolar disorder, and recurrent major depressive disorder. Generally speaking, within PsyR programs, the most common diagnoses are schizophrenic disorders, while in the general population, mood disorders are more common. Details of the criteria of these diagnoses are reported in the American Psychiatric Association's DSM-IV-TR manual (APA, 2000). These disorders are long term and characterized by episodes of acute illness followed by periods of residual symptoms and remission. In the acute phases of these disorders and occasionally at other times, the resulting symptoms have serious behavioral manifestations, and often come to preoccupy the sensory and cognitive experience of the individual.

Most people receiving PsyR services have experienced psychotic symptoms, such as hallucinations, delusions, and thought disorders, which are very severe and disruptive to daily life. The preponderance of evidence is that these major mental illnesses are biological, brain disorders. Studies of the structure of the brain through MRIs and CAT scans and studies of the functioning of the brain using PET scans and cerebral blood flow analysis confirm this hypothesis. Indeed, the National Alliance for the Mentally Ill has established a nationwide public relations campaign to replace the term *mental illness* with *brain disorder.*

Genetic studies, twin studies, and epidemiological investigations all suggest that the vulnerability to schizophrenia and other severe mental illnesses is inherited. Stresses, including biological/physical risk factors and psychosocial/environmental events, contribute to further harm in already vulnerable individuals. This combination of biological influences, environmental factors, and psychosocial stressors apparently changes the structure and functioning of the brain, which results in symptoms such as hallucinations, delusions, and other serious difficulties. These symptoms have severe cognitive (thinking), psychological, and social consequences for the individual.

Chapter 3 will focus on the persistence of these disorders, addressing their treatment, course, and outcome. It will discuss the positive impact of medication, rehabilitation, and other psychosocial interventions, as well as the varied outcomes for persons with these disorders.

Class Exercise

The experience of a severe and persistent mental illness raises many questions in the minds of people with the illness. These concerns are shared by loved ones. At times, mental health professionals have been less than forthcoming or honest in their responses to questions. This has often led to misunderstandings and a lack of trust. Sometimes, it has led to the development of very serious misconceptions and misinformation about mental illness. Consider how you might respond in the following circumstances.

Scenario 1

A member of the PsyR program you work in has approached you, telling you that he does not have schizophrenia, because he has only one personality. You say that multiple personalities is not what schizophrenia is all about and try to leave it at that. But he persists by asking you, "Then what is schizophrenia?" How do you respond?

Scenario 2

The mother of another member of the program you work for approaches you by asking why her daughter should take medication. She says, "After 20 years they have told me she has a *mental* disease, but they want her to take pills, I think to dope her up. Pills! They can only help if you have a problem with the body, but her problem is with her mind!" How would you help to clarify matters here?

Scenario 3

Another member of the program and his family believe that the reason he has mental illness is from a curse. They say, "An evil eye was put on him, a spell put upon him by an evil spirit." How can you address this issue?

Scenario 4

Another individual that you are working with has obvious symptoms of an active psychosis. He believes he shares responsibility for the assassination of President Kennedy in 1963, that he had indications it would happen and did not prevent it. He also thinks that coconspirators in the plot are now after him, have him under the surveillance, and send him cryptic e-mail with veiled threats. The man involved in the story was a child at the time and has no connection to the president's death. When someone tried to explain these ideas were delusions, he responded, "That's what they want you to think, that I'm paranoid crazy." He doesn't think he is ill and does not want treatment. How might you reach out to this individual?

References

Amador, X., & Johanson, A. L. (2000). *I am not sick: I don't need help.* Peconic, NY: Vida Press.

Amador, X. F., & Paul-Odouard, R. (2000). Defending the Unabomber: Anosognosia in schizophrenia. *Psychiatric Quarterly, 71,* 363–371.

American Psychiatric Association. (2000). *Diagnostic and statistical manual of mental disorders* (4th ed., text revision). Washington, DC: Author.

Anthony, W. A., & Liberman, R. P. (1986). The practice of psychiatric rehabilitation: Historical, conceptual, and research base. *Schizophrenia Bulletin, 12*(4), 542–559.

Arns, P. (1998, June). *Update on using the IAPSRS Toolkit for measuring psychosocial rehabilitation outcomes.* Paper presented at the International Association of Psychosocial Rehabilitation Services Conference, Orlando, FL.

Buchanan, R. W. & Carpenter, W.. (1997). The neuroanatomies of schizophrenia. *Schizophrenia Bulletin, 23*(3), 367–372.

Buchsbaum, M. S., & Haier, R. J. (1987). Functional and anatomical brain imaging: Impact on schizophrenia research. *Schizophrenia Bulletin, 13*(1) 115–132.

Cannon, M., Jones, P. B., & Murray, R. M. (2002). Obstetric complications and schizophrenia: Historical and meta-analytic review. *American Journal of Psychiatry, 159,* 1080–1092.

Conklin, H. M., & Iacono, W. G. (2002). Schizophrenia: A neurodevelopmental perspective. *Current Directions in Psychological Science, 11,* 33–37.

Cotter, D. R., & Pariante, C. M. (2002). Stress and the progression of the developmental hypothesis of schizophrenia. *British Journal of Psychiatry, 181,* 363–365.

Drake, R. E., McLaughlin, P., Pepper, B., & Minkoff, K. (1991). Dual diagnosis of major mental illness and substance disorder: An overview. *New Directions for Mental Health Services, 50,* 3–12.

Frith, C. D. (1997). Functional brain imaging and the neuropathology of schizophrenia. *Schizophrenia Bulletin, 23*(3), 403–422.

Goodwin, F. K., & Jamison, K. R. (1990). *Manic depressive illness.* New York: Oxford University Press.

Gur, R. E., & Pearlson, G. D. (1993). Neuroimaging in schizophrenia research. *Schizophrenia Bulletin, 19*(2), 163–181.

Harding, C. M., & Zahniser J. H. (1994). Empirical correction of seven myths about schizophrenia with implications for treatment. *Acta Psychiatrica Scandinavica, Supplementum, 384,* 140–146.

Harding, C. M., Zubin, J., & Strauss, J. S. (1992). Chronicity in schizophrenia: Revisited. *British Journal of Psychiatry, Supplement, 18,* 27–37.

Heckers, S. (1997). Neuropathology of schizophrenia: Cortex, thalamus, basal ganglia, and neurotransmitter projection systems. *Schizophrenia Bulletin, 23*(3),525–528.

Holzinger, A., Kilian, R., Lindenbach, I., Petscheleit, A., & Angermeyer, M. C. (2003). Patients' and their relatives' causal explanations of schizophrenia. *Social Psychiatry & Psychiatric Epidemiology, 38,* 155–162.

Kato C, Petronis A, Okazaki Y, Tochigi M, Umekage T, Sasaki T. (2002). Molecular genetic studies of schizophrenia: Challenges and insights. *Neuroscience Research, 43*(4):295–304

Kendler, K. S., & Deihl, S. R. (1993). The genetics of schizophrenia: A current genetic-epidemiologic perspective. *Schizophrenia Bulletin, 19*(2), 87–112.

Kurachi, M. (2003a). Pathogenesis of schizophrenia: Part I. Symptomatology, cognitive characteristics and brain morphology. *Psychiatry & Clinical Neurosciences, 57,* 3–8.

Kurachi, M. (2003b). Pathogenesis of schizophrenia: Part II. Temporo-frontal two-step hypothesis. *Psychiatry & Clinical Neurosciences, 57,* 9–15.

Lefley, H. P. (1989). Family burden and stigma in major mental illness. *American Psychologist, 44*(3), 556–560.

Lidz, T. (1992). *The relevance of the family to psychoanalytic theory.* Madison, CT: International Universities Press.

Luke, D. A., Mowbray, C. T., Klump, K., Herman, S. E., & Boots-Miller, B. (1996). Exploring the diversity of dual diagnosis: Utility of cluster analysis for program planning. *Journal of Mental Health Administration, 23*(3), 298–316.

Marcus, J., Hans, S. L., Nagler, S., Auerbach, J. G., Mirsky, A. F., & Aubrey, A. (1987). Review of the NIMH Israeli kibbutz-city study and the Jerusalem infant development study. *Schizophrenia Bulletin, 13*(3), 425–437.

Mauch, D. (1991). Separate paths to a common understanding: Treating the human condition of a disability. In *The community integration of persons labeled as dually diagnosed: Issues and models, selected conference proceedings* (pp. 1–14). Cincinnati, OH: University Affiliated Cincinnati Center for Developmental Disorders.

Mosher, L. R., & Burti, L. (1989). *Community mental health.* New York: W. W. Norton.

New Jersey Developmental Disabilities Council. (1997/1998). *Resources directory* (8th ed.). Trenton, NJ: Author.

Parsons, J. A., May, Jr., J. G., & Menolascino, F. J. (1984). The nature and incidence of mental illness in mentally retarded individuals. In F. J. Menolascino & J. A. Stark (Eds.), *Handbook of mental illness in the mentally retarded* (pp. 3–43). New York: Plenum Press.

Pitiladar, A. Gonul, A.S., Taneli, F. , & Akdeniz, F. (2004) Low serum levels of brain-derived neurotrophic factor in patients with schizophrenia do not elevate after anti-psychotic treatment. *Progress in Neuropsychopharmacology & Biological Psychiatry, 28*, 709–713

Raine, Adrian; Lencz, Todd; Yaralian, Pauline; Bihrle, Susan; LaCasse, Lori; Ventura, Joseph; Colletti, Patrick (2002). Prefrontal structural and functional deficits in schizotypal personality disorder. *Schizophrenia Bulletin. 28*(3), 501–513

Roberts, M. (Ed.). (1996). *Supported employment training: Competency-based instructional modules* (3rd ed.). Piscataway, NJ: University Affiliated Programs of New Jersey, University of Medicine and Dentistry of New Jersey.

Rosenhan, D. L. (1973). On being sane in insane places. *Science* (179), 250–258.

Schulze, K., McDonald, C., Frangou, S., Sham, P., Grech, A., Toulopoulou, T., et al. (2003). Hippocampal volume in familial and nonfamilial schizophrenic probands and their unaffected relatives. *Biological Psychiatry, 53*, 562–570.

Schwartz, D. B. (1992). *Crossing the river: Creating a conceptual revolution in community and disability.* Cambridge, MA: Brookline Books.

Sciacca, K., & Thompson, C. M. (1996). Program development and integrated treatment across systems for dual diagnosis: Mental illness, drug addiction, and alcoholism (MIDAA). *Journal of Mental Health Administration, 23*(3), 288–297.

Stark, J. A., McGee, J. J., Menolascino, F. J., Baker, D. H., & Menousek, P. E. (1984). Treatment strategies in the habilitation of severely mentally retarded—mentally ill adolescents and adults. In F. J. Menolascino & J. A. Stark (Eds.), *Handbook of mental illness in the mentally retarded* (pp. 189–218). New York: Plenum Press.

Szasz, T. (1976). *Schizophrenia: The sacred symbol of psychiatry.* New York: Basic Books.

Szymanski, L. S., King, B., Goldberg, B., Reid, A. H., Tonge, B. J., & Cain, N. (1998). Diagnosis of mental disorders in people with mental retardation. In S. Reiss & M. G. Aman (Eds.), *Psychotropic medication and developmental disabilities: The international consensus handbook* (pp. 3–17). Columbus: The Ohio State University Nisonger Center.

Torrey, W. C., (1993). Psychiatric care of adults with developmental disabilities and mental illness in the community. *Community Mental Health Journal, 29*(5), 461–473.

Torrey, E. F. (2001). *Surviving schizophrenia.* New York: Harper Perennial.

U.S. Department of Health and Human Services. (1995). *Assessment and treatment of patients with coexisting mental illness and alcohol and other drug abuse* (Treatment Improvement Protocol Series 9). Washington, DC: Substance Abuse and Mental Health Administration.

Walker, E., Kestler, L., Bollini, A., & Hochman, K. M. (2004). Schizophrenia: Etiology and course. *Annual Review of Psychology, 55*, 401–430.

Weiss, R. D., Mirin, S. M., & Frances, R. J. (1992). The myth of the typical dual diagnosis patient. *Hospital and Community Psychiatry, 43*, 107–108.

Chapter 3

Course, Treatment, and Outcome of Severe and Persistent Mental Illnesses

Introduction   70

Course   72

Short-Term Course of These Diseases   72

The Experience of Hospitalization   73

Long-Term Course of These Diseases   73

Course of Mood Disorders   77

Do Rehabilitation Services Matter?   78

Not Just New England   79

Treatment   79

Biological (Somatic) Treatments   79

Efficacy of Antipsychotic Medication   79

Atypical or Second-Generation Antipsychotic Medication   80

Reasons Medications Fail   81

Medication Side Effects   82

What Are the Best Antipsychotic Medications?   83

Do Traditional versus Second-Generation Antipsychotics Have Different Therapeutic Effects?   84

Pharmacological Treatment of Bipolar Disorder and Mania   85

Course of Bipolar Disorder When Taking Lithium   86

Pharmacological Treatment of Major Depressive Disorders   86

Does Antidepressant Medication Improve the Course and Outcome of Major Depression?   87

Future Possibilities   87

Medication Compliance   88

Role of Psychoeducation in Illness Self-Management   91

Staff Competencies Required for Effective IMR   92

Psychosocial Treatments   93

Psychosocial Treatments of Bipolar Disorder   95

Combined Treatment (Medication and Psychosocial) of Major Depression   95

Some Ineffective Treatments   95

Maria's Story   96

Understanding Course, Treatment, and Outcome: What the Staff and Consumers Don't Know Can Hurt Them!   97

Special Treatment Considerations with Dual Diagnoses   99

Service for Persons with Developmental Disabilities and Mental Illness   99

Summary   101

Class Exercise   102

References   102

An individual's experience of severe and persistent mental illness can be several months to many decades in length. The course of the illness is usually characterized by a significant risk of relapse and may include persistent symptoms. Psychiatric treatments, both pharmacological and psychosocial in nature, are intended to positively impact the course of mental illness by controlling, eliminating, and reducing symptoms and reducing the length, frequency, and severity of relapses. For schizophrenia and mood disorders, psychotropic medications are often the primary treatment. These medications, when properly prescribed and taken by the individual, often result in a less virulent course of the illness. Unfortunately, although many individuals experience a great deal of relief, the outcome is rarely a cure. Responsiveness to treatment may vary widely for individuals with the same diagnosis. There is also wide heterogeneity of outcomes among people with severe and persistent mental illness, ranging from those who deteriorate over time to individuals who have no symptoms at all and no relapses.

While these disorders require biological treatments, they also demand psychosocial interventions such as support and rehabilitation to promote the best possible outcomes. Longitudinal studies that tracked people with severe mental illness for more than 30 years have found that in the long run, most people who receive these services cope better, have decreasing symptoms, and function better in the community. Unfortunately, even those who are coping well may suffer occasional relapses. However, these relapses do not preclude other positive outcomes such as the attainment of living, learning, and working goals. Thus, in addition to the heterogeneity of outcomes between individuals, there is a multiplicity of outcomes for each individual. That is, over the course of many years of dealing with mental illness, one individual may experience numerous negative outcomes (e.g., persistence of symptoms, relapses) and positive outcomes (e.g., remission of symptoms and achievement of independent living goals).

This chapter will answer the following questions:

1. *Does the functioning of people with severe and persistent mental illness deteriorate or improve over the long term?*
2. *What are the probable short-term and long-term outcomes for persons diagnosed with schizophrenic disorders or mood disorders?*
3. *If these illnesses are caused by biological factors, why are psychosocial treatments effective?*
4. *Can support and rehabilitation impact the course of severe and persistent mental illness and bring about positive outcomes?*

Introduction

To understand the course, treatment, and outcome of severe and persistent mental illness, one must consider the interrelatedness of these three areas. The *course* of an illness is its natural history, that is, the sequence of events throughout the length of the illness. For persons experiencing severe and persistent mental illness, this course can be lifelong and marked by a risk of recurrence of severe symptoms. *Treatment* is defined as any action designed to cure a disease or reduce its symptoms. Treatments are intended to alter the course of these illnesses in a positive manner by reducing the intensity of symptoms and the frequency of *relapses*. If treatments succeed, they are said to have good outcomes. *Outcomes* can refer to specific results, the end of a specific course of treatment, or to the end result of the course of an entire illness. The term *outcome* can also refer to the long-term consequences of having a severe and persistent mental illness on the life of a person with the disorder.

In general, the course or natural history of severe mental illness is uncertain. It is clear, however, that the longer a psychosis goes untreated, the more difficult its course and the more negative are its long-term outcomes (Bottlender et al., 2003). As just mentioned, among the most prominent characteristics of severe and persistent mental illnesses is the risk of relapse, which is the recurrence of acute phases, after periods of remission or lack of symptoms. Concomitant with relapse are disruptions in functioning and independent living.

Relapse can lead to the loss of homes, jobs, the disruption of one's education, and familial discord. But the most serious harm a relapse presents may be to the individual's personal health. Each additional relapse may contribute to a further disordering of brain structure and functioning (Conklin & Iaconoa, 2002; Cotter & Pariante, 2002; Schulze et al., 2003; Torrey, 2001). The costs to the individual incurred from the chronic and recurrent course of severe and persistent mental illness is staggering. Keck and McElroy (1998) cite a U.S. Public Health Service study that projected the devastation of bipolar disorder on an individual's life. As an example, consider a woman who at the age of 25 has the onset of bipolar disorder. She can expect a 9-year reduction in life expectancy based on a 25% chance of attempting suicide and poorer overall health. In the remaining 40 or so years of her life, she can expect 12 years of overt or acute illness and 14 years of reduced productivity (vocationally, scholastically, and as a parent) (Keck & McElroy, 1998).

The personal damage of schizophrenia may be even more severe. Wiersma, Nienhuis, Slooff, and Giel (1998) conducted a *longitudinal study* of 82 people with schizophrenia living in the Netherlands. They periodically assessed these individuals over a 15-year period. Their findings revealed a pattern of chronicity and relapses consistent with other studies cited later in this chapter; 67% of the individuals had at least one relapse. An additional negative finding was that after each relapse, 16% of these subjects (11% of the entire cohort) did not fully recover from the episode. Even more disturbing, 10% of the individuals committed suicide during the 15-year period.

The Wiersma et al. (1998) study highlighted the increased risks associated with each additional relapse. That is, with each relapse the individual has a higher likelihood of suicide and of having persistent symptoms that do not remit. Nevertheless, while 21% of the people in this study had very negative outcomes, almost 80% did experience some significant form of recovery. Still, their findings demonstrate the need for an effective relapse prevention program as part of all psychiatric rehabilitation services.

In a subsequent study, Wiersma and colleagues (2000) examined the social disability (e.g., lack of relatedness, withdrawal) among 349 persons with schizophrenia in several European countries. At the 15-year follow-up, individuals with schizophrenia still had persistent social deficits. Nevertheless, the majority lived in normal settings with their family, a partner, or alone, as opposed to a residential program or hospital. Although, overall, the severity of social disability decreased during the follow-up period, the social disability of those in the hospital or in shelters and residences supervised by staff did not decrease. The severity of an individual's disability in social functioning at the beginning of the study was predictive of the level of social disability 15 years later.

Course

Short-Term Course of These Diseases

What is the probable short-term prognosis for someone suffering from a severe mental illness? For some, accurate diagnosis and effective treatment take place rapidly. But for others, this process can be difficult, making the time it takes to receive effective treatment extremely lengthy. Certainly, for most persons who develop schizophrenia the initial phase before effective treatment has begun can be the most devastating and the most frightening. As you will see, determining how to treat these diseases can be a very complicated process. In addition, during the initial stages of the disease the individual is often very unstable, making an accurate diagnosis even more difficult (Chen, Swann, & Johnson, 1998; Wiersma et al., 1998). For example, many people who are given a diagnosis of a mood disorder will later be diagnosed with schizophrenia. At the same time, those with a diagnosis of schizoaffective disorder are most likely to have their diagnosis changed at a subsequent psychiatric evaluation (Chen et al., 1998; Marneros, Tottig, Wenzel, & Brieger, 2004; Wiersma et al., 1998). Similarly, many people who receive a diagnosis of depression are later found to have bipolar disorder (Angst, 2004). In most cases effective treatment cannot be provided until an accurate diagnosis is made.

The short-term course of these diseases is stormy for several other reasons. Most persons are diagnosed with these conditions during their late teens or early twenties, a time of life when most people feel almost invulnerable to disease. For many of these young people, the most common response to a diagnosis of mental illness, especially if a remission of symptoms is obtained through medication, is denial (Fox, 2004). Active denial of a potentially lifelong, debilitating mental illness is, in some ways, a natural, expected, life-affirming response. Unfortunately, it often leads to noncompliance or nonadherence with medication regimens and severe relapse.

An alternative conceptualization to the phenomenon of denial is anosognosia discussed earlier in Chapter 2. This is the lack of awareness that the symptoms of the illness are in fact symptoms. Whatever the cause, for many persons, it takes many cycles of relapse, remission, denial, medication noncompliance, and relapse again before they accept the reality of their condition. This cycle is often an important contributor to the high relapse rate among newly diagnosed consumers. It is important for practitioners to be sensitive to the fact that denial or anosognosia, especially in the early stages of severe mental illness, is a normal, expected response. Practitioners should avoid interpreting related behavior, such as noncompliance with medication regimens, as abnormal or intentionally antagonistic.

The Experience of Hospitalization

For many of those with severe mental illness, their first significant treatment experience is hospitalization. There are important reasons why this is often the preferred treatment. In the hospital, the person can be observed to ensure that he or she is not a danger to self or others. The hospital is also the best environment to try out different medications in an attempt to reduce psychotic symptoms. Many medications have side effects that range from mildly annoying to highly dangerous; often these side effects can be very frightening or very uncomfortable. Side effects are often treated with medication changes or the addition of medicines designed to specifically treat their effects. Despite the fact that hospitalization is sometimes required to stabilize symptoms and determine the most effective medication regimen, from the patient's point of view it can be a frightening and dehumanizing experience. On the typical psychiatric ward, locked doors, limited visiting hours, and restricted use of telephones leave people feeling cut off from the outside world. Sometimes the experience of hospitalization is traumatic in itself, for example, when a person is physically restrained or is forced to spend time in a "quiet room." Inpatient hospital treatment will be discussed in greater detail in Chapter 14.

After being discharged from the hospital, what is the likelihood of rehospitalization? One of the most illustrative articles on this topic was published by Anthony, Cohen, and Vitalo (1978). By comparing the reported *recidivism* (rehospitalization) rates from the studies available at the time (see Table 3.1), the authors demonstrated that the probability of relapse in the short term (1 to 5 years) is very high. An examination of Table 3.1 reveals that as the follow-up period increases from 3 months to 5 and 10 years, the corresponding cumulative rate of recidivism also increases from 10% to 15% to as high as about 75%. Clearly, if you have been hospitalized because of a serious mental illness, the chance you will need rehospitalization at some point in time is very high. This high risk of relapse is true of schizophrenia, schizoaffective disorder, major depression, and bipolar disorder.

In recent years these figures have improved in terms of the proportion of individuals who relapse. For example, the 1-year relapse rates have decreased from a range of 20% to 40% to a range of 15% to 23% for individuals being treated with antipsychotic medication (Leucht et al., 2003). Klinkenberg and Calsyn (1996) reviewed research on predictors of recidivism among individuals with severe and persistent mental illnesses. They found that those individuals receiving aftercare (post-hospital care) and assertive community treatment (see Chapter 7) in addition to their medication experienced lower rates of rehospitalization.

Long-Term Course of These Diseases

Until recently, the long-term prognosis for a person with a severe mental illness such as schizophrenia was considered bleak. Even the American Psychiatric Association manual,

TABLE 3.1
Recidivism Rates by Follow-up Periods

Follow-up Period	Recidivism (%)	Authors
3 months	10	Ellsworth et al. (1971)
	15	Orlinsky and D'Elia (1964)
	16	Johnston and McNeal (1965)[c]
	11 to 22[b]	Moos, Shelton, and Petty (1973)
6 months	14	Angrist et al. (1961)[c]
	27	Johnston and McNeal (1965)
	30	Orlinsky and D'Elia (1964)
	33	Friedman, von Mering, and Hinko (1966)
	33	Miller and Willer (1976)
	35	Morgan (1966)[c]
	40	Fairweather et al. (1960)
9 months	29	Lorei (1964)[c]
6 to 13 months[a]	33	Franklin, Kittredge, and Thrasher (1975)
7 to 10 months[a]	39	Cumming and Markson (1975)
1 year	35	Pishkin and Bradshaw (1960)[c]
	36	Wolkon, Karmen, and Tanaka (1966)
	37	Johnston and McNeal (1965)
	37	Michaux et al. (1969)[c]
	37	Katkin et al. (1975)
	38	Williams and Walker (1961)
	38	Freeman and Simmons (1963)
	39	Lorei (1967)
	40	Miller (1966)
	40	Miller (1967)
	41	Schooler et al. (1967)[c]
	42	Bloom and Lang (1970)
	46	Orlinsky and D'Elia (1964)
	48	Savino and Schlamp (1968)
	50	Friedman, von Mering, and Hinko (1966)
1 to 2 years	20	Lewinsohn (1967)[c]
15 months	45	Wilder, Levin, and Zwerling (1966)
18 months	46	Wolkon, Karmen, and Tanaka (1971)
2 years	51	Johnston and McNeal (1965)
	55	Wolkon, Karmen, and Tanaka (1971)
	55	Katkin et al. (1975)
	75	Mendel (1966)[c]
2$^{1}/_{2}$ years	60	Wolkon, Karmen, and Tanaka (1971)
3 years	56	Johnston and McNeal (1965)
	64	Sherman et al. (1964)[c]
	65	Olshansky (1968)
5 years	67	Friedman, von Mering, and Hinko (1966)
	70	Freyhan (1964)
	70	Miller (1966)
	75	Miller (1967)
10 years	77	Gurel (1970)

[a] Length of follow-up period not the same for every patient in the study.
[b] Data were presented for individual hospital wards.
[c] Recidivism percentages for these studies were excerpted from a review by Clum (1975).

DSM-IIIR (APA, 1987), reported that in most cases the long-term course of schizophrenia worsened. This was partially due to the fact that for many persons struck with this disorder, the initial effects are catastrophic, reducing functioning and leading to marked disabilities. Besides the symptoms of the illness, stigmatizing public attitudes have a negative affect on quality of life and community adjustment.

Today the picture is much more optimistic. Recent studies have challenged the negative prognosis associated with this disease and given hope to many. Torrey (2001) has summed up the research on the long-term course of schizophrenia (e.g., Harding, Brooks, Ashikaga, Strauss, & Breier, 1987a, 1987b) by placing outcomes in five possible categories: (1) completely recovered, (2) much improved, (3) improved, (4) hospitalized, and (5) dead. By comparing Figures 3.1 and 3.2 at 10 and 30 years, respectively, we can see that the long-term prognosis for schizophrenia is generally positive and appears to improve slightly with time. At both 10 and 30 years, 75% of people stricken with schizophrenia are in a recovered, recovering, or improved category. It appears that between 10 and 30 years, an additional 10% improved to the point where they no longer required extensive support and became relatively independent. Thus, after 30 years, while more people have died (as would be expected by aging), fewer are hospitalized, fewer require extensive support networks, and a larger number are functioning more independently.

The Vermont study conducted by Harding and her colleagues (1987a, 1987b) focused directly on those individuals who might be expected to have the worst prognosis. This study examined a group of 269 patients who had been discharged, literally from the back wards of Vermont's State Psychiatric Hospital 32 years before. Vermont was one of the first states to begin deinstitutionalizing its psychiatric hospital population, starting in the

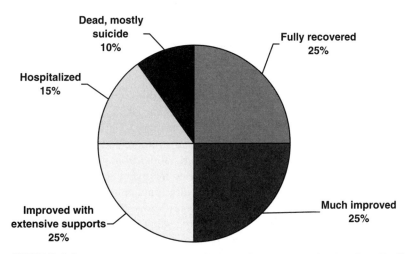

FIGURE 3.1 Outcomes 10 years after discharge from back wards. (Based on Harding et al., 1987a, 1987b.)

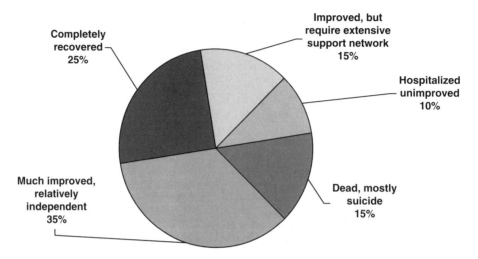

FIGURE 3.2 Outcomes 30 years after discharge from back wards. (Based on Harding et al., 1987a, 1987b.)

1950s. Researchers spent a good deal of time locating people as well as interviewing family members and others who knew the subjects. Their findings strongly contradicted the poor prognosis everyone had assumed for those most severely afflicted with schizophrenia.

At 10 years' postdischarge, 70% of the study participants were still out of the hospital, although many required treatment and social supports. At 30 years' postdischarge, 50% to 66% were recovered or improved. Table 3.2 provides additional detail on the functional level of the study's subjects. As you can see many of them attained valued social roles and utilized natural supports within the community.

Although the long-term outcome of schizophrenia is hopeful for many people, all people with schizophrenia still face a number of challenges including cognitive deficits. Cognitive processes include such functions as thinking and processing information. Deficits in these areas include problems sustaining attention, so-called executive functions (e.g., the ability to plan ahead), and verbal memory (Hoff & Kremen, 2003). These deficits are likely to be a function of the abnormal structure and function of specific areas of the brain including the hippocampus and parts of the frontal lobes as discussed in Chapter 2. Some of these cognitive deficits respond to treatment and improve, but others do not and can significantly interfere with community functioning. Dickinson and Coursey (2002) found that cognitive functions are strong predictors of how well people with schizophrenia cope with their illness. For example, "processing" speed and working memory are important cognitive functions. Slowed processing of information and poor working memory interfere with both social and vocational outcome.

TABLE 3.2
Results from the Strauss-Carpentar Levels of Function Scale for the 168 Subjects of the Vermont Study Who Were Alive and Interviewed[a]

Area of Functioning	N	%
Not in hospital in past year	140	83
Met with friends every week or two	111	66
Had one or more moderately to very close friends	128	76
Employed in past year[b]	79	47
Displayed slight or no symptoms	121	72
Able to meet basic needs	133	79
Led moderate to very full life	128	76
Slight or no impairment in overall function	92	55

[a] Reprinted with permission from C. M. Harding, G. W. Brooks, T. Ashikaga, et al. (1987a).
[b] Quality of work could not be rated; issues of confidentiality prevented visits to subjects' work sites.

Course of Mood Disorders

Although there is some evidence that the course of schizophrenia does not progressively worsen for the majority of individuals with that diagnosis, some studies suggest that the course of chronic or recurrent mood disorders may worsen over time (Kessing, 1998; Kessing, Andersen, Mortensen, & Bolwig, 1998). Outcomes studies of 2 to 5 years' duration have found that for individuals with bipolar disorder, recurrent episodes lead to deterioration in both social and vocational functioning (Keck & McElroy, 1998). This observation may seem unexpected to some mental health professionals. Generally speaking, between acute episodes of mood disorders, there is a greater remission of symptoms than is typically found in schizophrenic disorders (APA, 1994). That is, the person with a mood disorder is likely to be symptom free between acute episodes. Interestingly enough, this does not necessarily imply that the course of a mood disorder is less serious or less virulent. Kessing and his colleagues (1998) found that the number and frequency of episodes of increased symptomatology for persons with mood disorders increase with age. This is in contrast to schizophrenia, in which the number and frequency of episodes generally decrease with age.

In one study, Kessing and his colleagues followed all individuals admitted for psychiatric care in Denmark diagnosed with an affective disorder over a period of 20 years. During this time, more than 20,000 first-admission patients had been discharged with a diagnosis of major depression or bipolar disorder. The results indicated that the rate of recurrence increases with the number of previous episodes for people with these disorders. The natural history of severe depression and bipolar disorder seems to be progressively worse, regardless of gender, age, and type of disorder. This suggests that for some, the course of these disorders is progressive, or worsening despite treatment. In short, an increasing number of relapses predicts an acceleration of relapses for the future (Kessing, 1998; Kessing et al., 1998).

In a more recent study, Kennedy, Abbott, and Paykel (2003) followed 70 individuals to ascertain whether the course of depression had improved given more recent developments in pharmacological and psychosocial treatments. Individuals with a history of severe recurrent depression originally recruited in 1990–1992 were reassessed after 8 to 11 years. The great majority (92%) of the participants recovered during follow-up. Nevertheless, two-thirds suffered a recurrence of symptoms at some point. Unfortunately, one out of six (17%) suffered from an episode of chronic depression of at least 2 years' duration during the 8- to 11-year follow-up. Generally, social functioning at follow-up was good and there were high levels of participation in pharmacological and psychosocial treatments. Greater severity of illness was the most consistent predictor of poor outcome.

Do Rehabilitation Services Matter?

The results from the Vermont study (Harding et al., 1987a, 1987b), which looked at the long-term outcome of schizophrenia, have greatly encouraged the psychiatric rehabilitation community. Regardless of how symptomatic individuals are, there is hope that at some future date they will be able to function independently in the community with reduced symptoms and little or no supports. Is this positive prognosis a result of the disease process or is it due to the services that people receive? Some of the researchers from the Vermont study set out to answer this question.

When it began deinstitutionalization, Vermont had a comprehensive rehabilitation system, with elements comparable to today's supported employment and supported living initiatives (see Chapters 9 and 11, respectively, for details on these programs). A neighboring state, Maine, adopted a more traditional approach for the treatment of its deinstitutionalized population consisting of traditional inpatient treatment and aftercare. Using the same strategy that had been employed in the original Vermont study, DeSisto, Harding, McCormick, Ashikaga, and Brooks (1995a, 1995b) compared 180 deinstitutionalized patients from Vermont with 119 similar patients from Maine. The results were very clear. Individuals from Vermont were more productive, less symptomatic, and had better community adjustment and higher levels of functioning.

In both states, the symptomatology and functioning of persons with these illnesses improved over the very long term. However, in Maine, these improvements took much longer. Sometimes it took 10 years longer for people from Maine to achieve the same gains that the Vermonters had attained. Because of this time lag, people in Maine required more mental health services. The authors concluded that these differences were probably the result of Vermont's efforts at community psychiatric rehabilitation. In short, better services produce better outcomes for people with psychiatric disabilities. The comparison of the Maine to Vermont outcomes suggests that features of the service system can significantly influence outcomes.

Not Just New England

In addition to the studies conducted in Vermont and Maine, methodologically sound studies in both the United States and Europe, involving more than 1,300 individuals with schizophrenia, have found that 46% to 68% of these folks either improved or recovered significantly over periods of time ranging from 23 to 37 years (Harding, Zubin, & Strauss, 1992). Thus, one of the basic values of psychiatric rehabilitation, hopefulness, which is discussed in detail in Chapter 4, actually has a scientific basis.

Treatment

As defined in Chapter 1, treatment seeks to cure a disease or reduce its symptoms. Treatment for serious mental illnesses can be broken into two broad categories: biological (somatic) and psychosocial. The biological or somatic category usually refers to medications, but also electroconvulsive therapy. The psychosocial category refers to efforts to reduce symptoms and improve functioning by employing interventions that influence social or psychological factors.

Biological (Somatic) Treatments

One of the primary approaches in the treatment of severe and persistent mental illness is to use pharmacological agents to treat acute episodes of psychotic and/or mood symptoms (Lehman & Steinwachs, 1998; Leucht et al., 2003; Walker, Kestler, Bollini, & Hochman, 2004). In the treatment of schizophrenia, it is clear that antipsychotic or neuroleptic medications are required for any effective symptom reduction to take place (Lehman & Steinwachs, 1998; Mueser, Torrey, Lynde, Singer, & Drake, 2003). Thus for a disorder such as schizophrenia or another psychosis, antipsychotic medications, which are intended to reduce or eliminate psychotic symptoms, are often used as the first-line treatment (Lehman & Steinwachs, 1998).

For acute episodes of major depression, the current treatment of choice is antidepressant medications, such as Tofranil and Prozac. For bipolar disorder, the treatment of choice is a mood stabilizer, such as Lithobid (lithium) (Keck & McElroy, 1998).

Efficacy of Antipsychotic Medication

A large body of evidence supports the efficacy of antipsychotic medication in the treatment of schizophrenia, with more than 100 well-controlled studies showing that 50% to 85% of persons will improve significantly with reductions in hallucinations, delusions, thought disorders, and bizarre behavior (Lehman & Steinwachs, 1998).

Those who experience symptom relief with an antipsychotic medication typically will be prescribed this medication for at least 1 year after the acute symptoms have been reduced (Lehman & Steinwachs, 1998). The purpose of this long-term treatment is to reduce the risk of relapse or the worsening of positive symptoms. Medications are used in the *acute phases* of an illness such as schizophrenia, in the *residual phases* to keep symptoms from recurring, and also in the *prodromal phases* to avert relapse. In the case of most serious mental illnesses, medications are also used during periods of remission.

Summarizing studies that looked at the outcomes of more than 2,300 patients with schizophrenia, Hogarty (1993) found that medication alone could reduce the rate of relapse from 67% to 39% in the first year. After the first year, by continuing antipsychotic medication, relapse rates were reduced from a level of 65% annually to only 15% annually (Hogarty, 1993). This has been confirmed in more recent review articles. As mentioned earlier, more than 30 well-controlled studies have been conducted that show that the annual relapse rate can be reduced from a rate of 15% to 25% if antipsychotic medication is continued (Leucht et al., 2003).

At one time, it was noted that in many treatment studies about 40% of the people taking antipsychotic medication relapsed anyway in the first year after discharge from a hospital (Hogarty, 1993). This was often attributed to suspected medication noncompliance (Gray, Wykes, & Gournay, 2002). Many mental health professionals continue to attribute psychotic relapse to medication noncompliance (Gray et al., 2002). However, as Hogarty (1993) has pointed out, even patients whose compliance was known because they received long-acting *intramuscular injections* (also known as a "depot" medications) had approximately the same relatively high rate of relapse, reduced only slightly in comparison to those taking pills orally. Subsequent research has found the injectable medication is actually somewhat more effective at reducing symptoms than oral medications (Adams, Fenton, Quraishi, & David, 2001).

Atypical or Second-Generation Antipsychotic Medication

Clozapine, first introduced in the 1950s, but not widely used in the United States until the 1990s, and a number of other antipsychotics are a heterogeneous group of medications that are commonly referred to as the "atypical" antipsychotics. The "atypicals" differ significantly from one another in terms of the neurotransmitter receptors that they occupy, such as different types of dopamine receptor and serotonin receptors. However, they all act as dopamine antagonists to some extent (see Chapter 2). In addition to affecting other neurotransmitter systems, they have a reduced risk of both the early and late emerging movement disorders, which are among the many side effects of antipsychotic medications (Marder et al., 2002). In addition, clozapine has been shown to be highly effective for treatment-resistant schizophrenia. However, its use is generally confined to individuals whose psychotic symptoms have not responded to one or more antipsychotic medications, because of its potentially serious side effects, which include agranulocytosis, an immune system problem, and the requirement for frequent blood monitoring (Alphs & Anand, 1999; Naheed & Green, 2001). Clozaril has also been associated with loss of energy and fatigue.

With the exception of clozapine, the atypicals have now become the first line in the treatment of schizophrenia and other psychotic disorders (Walker et al., 2004). They are sometimes referred to as "second generation" or "new generation" antipsychotics, which is probably a more accurate description than "atypical." Commonly prescribed atypical antipsychotics include Risperdal (risperidone), Zyprexa (olanzapine), Solian amisulpride, Seroquel (quetiapine), and Geodon (ziprasidone). Still, questions are raised about the overall efficacy of these new drugs. A study by Lieberman and colleagues (2005) compared several of these new drugs with an older drug, perphenazine (brand name Trilafon). After 18 months the majority of persons receiving each of the prescribed drugs had discontinued treatment. The authors speculated that these dropout rates were mostly related to side effects and concluded that the newer drugs offered no advantage over the more traditional drug in the trial.

Leucht and colleagues (2003) did a meta-analysis (a study combing the effects of multiple smaller studies) that compared "atypical" antipsychotic medication to the older, conventional antipsychotics, usually Haldol (a traditional antipsychotic medication). This review examined overall relapses (the recurrence and aggravation of symptoms) and treatment failure (that is, the need to discontinue a medication because of side effects or increased symptoms). The studies with the strictest methodology have found lower rates of both treatment failure and relapse when second-generation antipsychotics are used (Leucht et al., 2003). In terms of annual relapse rates, individuals treated with Haldol have a relapse rate averaging 23%, whereas those who are treated with atypicals have a relapse rate of only 15% (Leucht et al., 2003). In terms of overall treatment failure, both groups of medications have fairly high rates on a given trial with a particular medication, the traditional antipsychotic medications failing 66% of the time and the atypicals 49%, a difference of practical significance. Treatment failure is usually followed by trying one or more other antipsychotics before a successful medication is found. This highlights the fact that different medications must be tried in order to find the one with the best treatment effect for a particular individual.

Reasons Medications Fail

Psychotropic medications must be tried for a sufficient length of time and under appropriate psychiatric supervision. However, traditional antipsychotic medications fail initially about two-thirds of the time, requiring a change in treatment strategy. A psychiatrist may determine that a particular medication is ineffective because symptoms do not improve, side effects are intolerable, or relapse occurs (Leucht et al., 2003). Initial medication failure decreases to about 50% of the time when atypical, second-generation medications are prescribed. According to Conley and Buchanan (1997), a systematic approach to the evaluation and characterization of treatment resistance is increasingly important. Since the introduction of many new drugs, consumers are more likely than ever to be prescribed a variety of psychotropic medications if the first one tried does not work well. The need for accurate evaluation will continue to increase as even more new medications are introduced. Psychiatrists facing the decision of when to change from one medication to another must clearly understand the appropriate length of a trial and what target symptoms respond to a particular medication in order to maximize the response in persons with treatment-resistant symptoms.

The medication challenges for both the physician and the individual usually revolve around a number of questions. First, which psychotropic medication will be most effective? Second, what dosage is needed to be effective, while at the same time not putting the person at unnecessary risk for side effects? Third, how does one cope with the long-term need to take pills regularly, possibly accompanied by frequent blood tests required for certain medications such as lithium (a mood stabilizer) and clozapine (an antipsychotic medication)? Further complicating matters, even if the right medication is prescribed, there is always some risk of symptom exacerbation and relapse.

Conley and Buchanan (1997) provided several additional reasons why people with schizophrenia have a poor response to various psychotropic medications:

- Partial compliance of person with the treatment regimen
- Inappropriate dosing or length of trial (most medications require 4 to 6 weeks to determine efficacy)
- True resistance of the disorder to the medication, simply using the wrong medication to try to bring about a therapeutic effect.

Medication Side Effects

Side effects of psychotropic medication are particularly important. They can be very severe and harmful to the individual. Some common side effects are increased appetite, hormonal difficulties (e.g., failing to menstruate), motor difficulties (e.g., shuffling gate), muscular problems (e.g., stiffness), dryness of mouth, blurred vision, impotence, low blood pressure, seizures, and immune system reactions.

The burden of side effects can be illustrated by looking at two common and very troubling side effects associated with antipsychotic medication: pseudo-parkinsonism and tardive dyskinesia. Antipsychotic medication, because it affects the functioning of the neurotransmitter, dopamine (discussed in Chapter 2), interferes significantly with motor functions. Some patients, regardless of age, develop the symptoms (but not the actual disease) of Parkinson's disease: resting tremors, poor control of their own movements, and shuffling movements. Another side effect that may occur from use of these medications is *tardive dyskinesia*, which involves an uncontrollable twisting or writhing movement of the mouth and limbs. Unlike some of the other side effects, tardive dyskinesia is usually not reversible once it appears. As if it were not enough to endure the symptoms and behaviors associated with psychosis, the involuntary movements of tardive dyskinesia can make someone appear bizarre to others, which increases stigma.

Some side effects are eminently treatable with changes in dosage or type of medication. Certain side effects can be treated with other medications, but of course, these medicines can have their own side effects as well. A common remark about these drugs is that if they were not therapeutic, they would be poison. Antipsychotic medications differ from each other in terms of side effect profiles. Movement abnormalities are the main side effect associated with the typical or older antipsychotics. There are both early and late emerging motor side effects (Sadock & Sadock, 2000). Early emerging "extrapyramidal" syndromes include pseudo-parkinsonism symptoms, dystonic reactions (sudden onset of sustained intense muscle contraction), and akathisia (restlessness). The most common late emerging syndrome is tardive dyskinesia. These side effects caused by the typical antipsychotics have led many psychiatrists to abandon them in favor of second-generation medications. Nonetheless, these medications contributed to our understanding of the neurochemistry of schizophrenia, and offered many patients the first opportunity to live outside an institution.

Atypical antipsychotic medications may produce fewer adverse effects, particularly less extrapyramidal motor dysfunction (Allison & Casey, 2001; Bradford, Stroup, & Lieberman, 2002) and tardive dyskinesia (Kane, 2003). However, for some people serious physical problems or conditions may result from the use of these medications. A problem for many consumers on psychotropic medications is *weight gain* and the newer atypical antipsychotics can cause this problem (Allison & Casey, 2001; Green, Patel, Goisman, Allison, & Blackburn, 2000). In fact, one study found that the mean weight gain for those treated with one of the atypical medications (such as clozapine, risperidone, amisulpride and zotepine) was significantly more than for those treated with the older antipsychotic medications (Wetterling & Muessigbrodt, 1999). Weight gain is not only unpleasant for the individual, but can also lead to medical consequences such as diabetes (Allison & Casey, 2001). Treatments such as behavior therapy can control weight gain in the short term and "lifestyle changes" can improve the issue long term (Green et al., 2000). It is hoped that using these techniques to maintain a healthy weight will lead to better compliance with medication. Another physical problem is that some individuals exhibit *abnormal EKG* patterns with the start of Clozaril; however, this may normalize with continued treatment (Kang et al., 2000).

What Are the Best Antipsychotic Medications?

The simple answer to the question is "The medicine that provides the individual with an optimal therapeutic response and the fewest possible side effects." It is difficult, at this point, to know in advance which medication meets those criteria for a given individual (Kane, 2003; Walker et al., 2004). Traditional antipsychotics, given at the appropriate dosage level, have established therapeutic efficacy, but have the drawback of many side effects, particularly in terms of movement. As discussed earlier, the second-generation antipsychotics fail less frequently and are associated with somewhat lower relapse rates (Leucht et al., 2003). These medications are superior in that they do not have the serious motor side effects. Unfortunately, they result in more weight gain and an increased risk for diabetes. Clozapine (Clozaril) is very effective in helping individuals whose symptoms have not responded to other antipsychotics, yet as discussed earlier it has the risk of a number of serious side effects.

Evidence-based Practice: Medication Management Approaches in Psychiatry (MedMAP):

Medication is the most powerful tool we have for controlling the symptoms of these diseases. Yet, as the Schizophrenia Patient Outcome Research Team (PORT) studies (Lehman & Steinwachs, 1998) suggest, the quality of psychiatric care provided to persons with severe mental illness has been very uneven. Medication management approaches in psychiatry (MedMAP) is an evidence-based practice designed to correct these problems (SAMHSA/CMHS, 2005). MedMAP was developed from a series of medication algorithm (series of standard procedures) studies.

Critical Ingredients of MedMAP

1. *Systematic approach*: Utilization of a systematic approach to medication management
2. *Measurement of outcomes*: Objective assessment of the symptoms that the medications are supposed to affect
3. *Documentation*: Clear, concise documentation of the treatments and their outcomes
4. *Consumer involvement*: Efforts to enhance medication adherence through consumer education and involvement in medication decisions

Service Outcomes of MedMAP

Effective application of MedMAP principles results in more uniform and effective application of medications and improved medication regimen adherence. While for many persons medication does not result in the total remission of symptoms, effective application of MedMAP principles will help to maximize the effects that can be gained.

Do Traditional versus Second-Generation Antipsychotics Have Different Therapeutic Effects?

Corrigan and his colleagues (2003) compared the effects of atypical second-generation antipsychotics to conventional antipsychotics. They reviewed 31 published studies on more than 12,000 individuals. The findings generally showed that atypical medications led to significant decreases in negative symptoms (see Chapter 2 for a list of these symptoms) compared to conventional antipsychotics. One study found that in addition to reducing negative symptoms, atypical antipsychotics also reduced cognitive problems, hostility, and excitement (Meyer, Bond, Tunis, & McCoy, 2002). Effects on psychosocial functioning and on the quality of life were mixed. Only half of the studies reported significant improvements in these areas. One medication (Olanzapine) yielded the best results on psychosocial functioning. Corrigan et al. (2003) concluded that some atypical antipsychotics may have more of a direct effect on some of the psychosocial disabilities that result from serious mental illness than do traditional antipsychotic medications.

Given different therapeutic profiles, do they have different effects on rehabilitation outcomes? It was found that the atypical antipsychotic medications compared to traditional antipsychotics were associated with better symptom control. However, no difference in work status was found based on type of medication (Meyer et al., 2002).

Bond and colleagues (2004) studied three groups of unemployed people receiving (1) olanzapine, an atypical second-generation antipsychotic; (2) risperidone, an atypical second-generation antipsychotic; or (3) a first-generation antipsychotic medication. On most vocational measures, subjects receiving second-generation agents (groups 1 and 2) did not differ from those receiving first-generation agents. However, at 9 months, the second-generation group had a significantly higher rate of participation in vocational training and began trending toward a higher rate of paid employment. All groups, regardless of type of medication, showed substantial improvement in employment outcomes after entering a vocational program. The hypothesis that second-generation antipsychotic medications promote better employment outcomes was not upheld (Bond et al., 2004).

Pharmacological Treatment of Bipolar Disorder and Mania

Lithium is a mood stabilizer that has been used as a treatment for bipolar disorder in the United States since 1970 and was being used in other countries even earlier. It is an effective medication for both the treatment of acute mania and the prevention of the recurrence of both manic and depressive symptoms in bipolar disorders (Keck & McElroy, 1998). Belmaker (2004) and Keck and McElroy (1998) reviewed numerous studies showing that lithium reduces the symptoms of acute mania. Like antipsychotic medications, mood stabilizers work by influencing neurotransmitter activity in the brain.

Numerous well-controlled studies involving hundreds of patients have demonstrated that lithium prevents recurrent affective episodes of both depressed and manic types (Belmaker, 2004; Keck & McElroy, 1998). At the same time, a significant number of individuals do *not* respond that well to lithium maintenance therapy. Poor medication compliance, in large part due to lithium's side effects, has interfered with its effective use. The prevention of future episodes, while an important goal in itself, has the additional benefit of perhaps reducing the likelihood of increased frequency of episodes and more rapid cycling, that is, an acceleration in the number and severity of acute episodes (Cusin, Serretti, Lattuada, Mandelli, & Smeraldi, 2000).

The effective treatment of mania needs to anticipate the future course of the illness (Licht, 1998). Lithium is still considered the best mood-stabilizing substance although it may be insufficient in mixed episodes and severe mania (Licht, 1998). For those who do not respond to lithium as an ongoing treatment, other medications are available including carbamazepine and valproate. Carbamazepine is an anticonvulsive medication that is also used to treat seizure disorders. Valproate is preferred for acute episodes, in particular, for mixed episodes. Because the mood stabilizers work slowly, antipsychotic medications are also sometimes used to treat severe mania, particularly during the acute phase, to decrease potentially dangerous behavior (Belmaker, 2004). However, in general, their use should not be prolonged into the maintenance phase. Antidepressants have also been used for the relief of depressive episodes (Keck & McElroy, 1998). Unfortunately, persons who also suffer manic episodes, can have a manic state induced by the use of antidepressants (Belmaker, 2004).

Freeman and Stoll (1998) report that polypharmacy, or the use of multiple medications, is common in the treatment of *refractory bipolar disorder*, a term used to describe conditions that do not respond readily to a single medication. Very few controlled studies on the use of combinations of mood stabilizers have been conducted. The interactions of such combinations can be useful, but can also be very complicated and are potentially dangerous. The safest and most efficacious mood stabilizer combinations appear to be the mixtures of anticonvulsants, particularly valproate, and lithium.

Course of Bipolar Disorder When Taking Lithium

What typically transpires when someone with bipolar disorder takes lithium? Compared to many of the clinical studies described earlier, the results from the field are mixed and disappointing. Lithium does not seem to consistently reduce the risk of recurrence of manic episodes as often as might be expected. Silverstone, McPherson, Hunt, and Romans (1998) examined the effectiveness of lithium in preventing recurrent episodes of bipolar disorder over a 2-year period following hospital discharge. Results showed that overall, 67% had a relapse. While a major reason for this may have been poor compliance by study participants, some even discontinuing the lithium, it is clear that this drug is not effective in many cases.

Maj, Pirozzi, Magliano, and Bartoli (1998) collected information on 402 people started on lithium as a maintenance treatment in order to prevent relapse. Five years after starting treatment, 38% were still taking lithium and had experienced at least one recurrence of the disorder. Conversely, 23% were still taking lithium and had experienced no recurrent episodes. Those who had discontinued their lithium at follow-up had poorer outcomes than those still taking lithium.

Pharmacological Treatment of Major Depressive Disorders

For depressive disorders, controversy remains regarding whether medication or psychosocial interventions are more effective in bringing symptom relief (Craighead, Milkowitz, Vajk, & Frank, 1998a; Friedman et al., 2004; Nemeroff & Schatzberg, 1998). Nevertheless, there is little question that those treated with antidepressants will have a more favorable course than those who do not take these medications (Angst, 1998).

The treatments of choice for the relief of major depressive disorders are the drugs known as *selective serotonin reuptake inhibitors*, such as Prozac (Nemeroff & Schatzberg, 1998). This class of drugs is named for the nature of the effect they have on the neurotransmitter serotonin. Next, most commonly used are the tricyclic antidepressants such as Tofranil (imipramine), which are named for their chemical structure of three molecular circles. A third group of drugs, monoamine oxidase (MAO) inhibitors, although effective, is rarely used. Typically, it takes at least 3 to 6 weeks to determine whether an antidepressant is being effective. Tricyclic antidepressants, at full dose, have been found to be effective in reducing the recurrence of major depressive symptoms or episodes (Frank, Kupfer, & Perel, 1990, 1993).

Viguera, Baldessarinand Friedberg (1998) note that the benefits of long-term antidepressant treatment in major depression and the risks of discontinuing medication are now well established. Reviewing 27 studies, with more than 3,000 patients with depressive symptoms, they compared the course and outcome of the illness between patients whose antidepressants were discontinued and those with continued treatment. Those who had continued treatment showed much lower relapse rates (2% versus 6% per month) and a lower 12-month relapse risk (20% versus 45%). Contrary to prediction, gradual discontinuation (dose-tapering or use of long-acting agents) did not yield lower relapse rates. As mentioned earlier, the number of previous depressive episodes—particularly three or more prior episodes, which was considered a chronic course—was strongly associated with higher relapse risk after discontinuation of antidepressants. Nevertheless, a chronic course did not negatively affect responsiveness to continued treatment. That is, even those with multiple episodes were likely to respond well to medication.

Does Antidepressant Medication Improve the Course and Outcome of Major Depression?

Can antidepressant medication be used to improve the long-term course and outcome of major depression? The use of antidepressants appears to have a positive effect on relapse rates. In the first year, those not receiving antidepressants had a 45% chance of relapse, while those who did receive these medications had a relapse rate of 20%. Among the groups without antidepressants, at the 14-month follow-up, 50% had relapsed. Among those being treated with antidepressants, the 50% relapse rate was not reached until 48 months. More previous episodes were associated with higher relapse. However, more previous episodes did not predict responsiveness to treatment. Although these findings highlight the efficacy of antidepressants, they also point out, once again, that, like the other severe mental illnesses, major depression relapses are a matter of time, even when medication is taken (Viguera et al., 1998).

Future Possibilities

Many of the studies mentioned in preceding sections demonstrate that while medication helps many people cope with severe and persistent mental illness, prescription guidelines are hardly an exact science. Many people suffer for years without finding an effective medication regimen that has tolerable side effects. With a better understanding of the human genome (the entire human genetic profile), the potential exists to tailor medication to an individual's genetic profile. The emerging fields of pharmacogenomics and pharmacogenetics are seeking to uncover the genetic basis of differences in medication

TABLE 3.3
Medication Treatment Summary

Broad Diagnostic Categories	Category of Commonly Prescribed Medications	Examples
Schizophrenic disorders	Traditional antipsychotics (oral) Traditional (injectable) Atypical antipsychotics	Haldol, Mellaril, Prolixin, Thorazine Haldol, Prolixin Risperdal (risperidone), Zyprexa (olanzapine), Seroquel (quetiapine), and Solian (amisulpride) Geodon (ziprasidone) Clozaril (clozapine)
Mood disorder: Depressive disorders	Selective serotonin uptake inhibitors Tricyclics MAO inhibitors	Prozac, Zoloft Tofranil
Bipolar disorder or mania (manic phases only)	Mood stabilizers Anticonvulsant (with mood- stabilizing properties	Lithium carbonate Lithobid Valproate Carbamazepine

therapeutic response and side effects (Walker et al., 2004). The field of pharmacogenomics looks at the determinants of drug response at the level of the entire human genome using DNA analysis. The goal is to eventually individualize therapy based on a person's genetic makeup (Basile, Masellis, Potkin, & Kennedy, 2002).

Table 3.3 is meant to provide an overview of some of the commonly used medications. It is by no means exhaustive, nor does it serve as guide to prescribing medications. It is included solely to share information that mental health consumers and the staff that serve them must know.

Today, it is rare that a person with severe and persistent mental illness would go completely untreated with medication, although there are still individuals who receive no care at all. Unfortunately, it remains a very typical situation that a large number of individuals receive inadequate care, and there is only a small number who are served well (Lehman & Steinwachs, 1998; President's New Freedom Commission, 2003; Satcher, 2000).

Medication Compliance

The term *compliance* has the connotation of "giving in," going along with, or submitting to a more powerful authority. Medication compliance refers to adhering to the prescribed schedule of time, dosage, and amounts of medication. Many individuals, indeed most individuals with long-term disorders, struggle with complying or adhering to their medication regimens. Unfortunately, *noncompliance* rates are about 50% (Gray et al., 2002). Although this percentage sounds high, it may be no higher than the rates of noncompliance for all disorders and all medical conditions (Gray et al., 2002). Noncompliance is also potentially a preventable cause of the serious consequences of relapse (Gray et al., 2002).

Injectable medications, also known as depot antipsychotics, are sometimes used for individuals who do not want to take pills or cannot remember to take them regularly. As mentioned earlier, individuals taking depot antipsychotics experience greater symptom reduction and relapse less often, suggesting better medication compliance (Adams et al., 2001). Clearly, for some people, taking an intramuscular injection at an interval somewhere between once a week and once a month is less troublesome than taking pills daily.

An inability to remember, an unwillingness to be reminded repeatedly of one's illness, serious side effects, or insufficient therapeutic effects may all be contributing to medication noncompliance. Feeling better or improving is also a cause of noncompliance, because in the face of improved or eliminated symptoms, stopping the medication seems a logical step (Fox, 2004). Some experts, to avoid the connotation of submission and disempowerment, refer to the issue as medication "adherence," sticking to a prescribed schedule and dose.

Another factor consistently associated with decreased medication compliance is substance abuse (Heyscue, Levin, & Merrick, 1998). Some individuals discontinue medication when drinking alcohol or abusing substances. Some of these individuals also take to "self-medicating" with both legal prescription drugs and illicit drugs on a dosage and schedule they choose. This is discussed in more detail in Chapter 8, which addresses dual diagnoses.

Because of their awareness of the relationship between medication nonadherence to the aggravation of symptoms and the advent of relapses, many PsyR staff understandably feel compelled to promote medication compliance. Indeed for some it becomes a preoccupation and, occasionally, staff fall into the trap of blaming individuals for their own relapses, assuming medication noncompliance was necessarily involved.

The issue of medication compliance is a sensitive and emotional one. Many consumers have had the experience of medications being misused as "chemical restraints." In other words, they were given high dosages of medication to obtain a sedative effect intended to control psychotic symptoms very quickly. Many others have had the experience of troubling side effects that indeed are not only very distressing, but also potentially harmful, as they can cause serious health problems.

People taking psychotropic medications are often reluctant to discuss these matters with their doctors. They may not have the confidence to confront, disagree, or even question a physician or other professionals. They may not even know they are "allowed to," or have no experience working collaboratively with a psychiatrist. Sometimes, in one's role as a patient, it is just easier to say "I'm fine" and not bring up troubling concerns. Some may even lie about what might be going on to avoid hospitalization.

How then can the right medication be prescribed at the right dosage in a manner that maximizes therapeutic effects, reduces side effects, and informs consumers about the choices they actually have? Can communication about these issues be improved, so that consumers can exercise informed choice and self-determination over their medication? Would not better communication regarding symptoms and side effects empower doctors as well, by helping them to be better informed on these issues?

Kim Mueser and colleagues (2003) discuss two related solutions to these problems called *collaborative psychopharmacology* and *illness management and recovery* services. Both are based on the same premise as a chain store's advertisement slogan, "An educated consumer is our best customer."

Collaborative Psychopharmacology

Collaboration means laboring or working together. Collaborative psychopharmacology involves consumers working with their psychiatrists and other professionals to determine the right medications to use according to up-to-date guidelines. Although medications are clearly effective, research has also found that many psychiatrists do not follow the appropriate dosage ranges nor take into account the time course for therapeutic response and dosage adjustment, also known as *titration* (Lehman & Steinwachs, 1998). Similarly, guidelines on the identification and management of side effects, and methods for the treatment of refractory symptoms are frequently not followed by psychiatrists (Lehman & Steinwachs, 1998).

Because of the complexity of pharmacological treatment for severe mental illness, as well as the rapid evolution in the field as new medications are developed, a recent trend has been to establish *algorithms* for prescribing medications based on research (SAMHSA-CMHS, 2005). Algorithms are step-by-step instructions to proceed with certain actions based on specific conditions and responses to previous steps. Many of these recommendations require adding expert clinical consensus to the scientific evidence. Implementation procedures for collaborative pharmacological treatment have been developed that include a standard approach to documenting and monitoring symptoms and side effects, guidelines for systematically making decisions about medications, and attempts to engage consumers in decision making about medication-related decisions.

Illness Management and Recovery

Integral to collaborative psychopharmacology is the fact that individuals with mental illness need to be educated and informed in order to make sound decisions regarding their medication. Illness management and recovery (IMR) training is an evidence-based practice intended to help consumers acquire the knowledge and skills to work effectively with professionals in their treatment and rehabilitation in order to minimize the effects of the mental illness on their lives and pursue personally meaningful goals. A variety of methods are aimed at helping consumers deal more effectively with their disorder, including the following:

1. *Psychoeducation*: knowing the factual information about mental illness and its treatment.
2. *Medication management education*: teaching strategies that promote effective use of medication.
3. *Relapse prevention skills*: identifying symptoms and precursors for relapses, as well as planning ahead for crises. This may include assisting consumers in establishing *advance directives*, which are legal documents that empower consumers to make decisions about their treatment prior to becoming too ill to do so themselves.

4. Cognitive behavioral approaches, strategies for thinking about and understanding problems and symptoms.

Role of Psychoeducation in Illness Self Management

Psychoeducation is an important ingredient in most approaches to IMR training. Psychoeducation involves providing consumers with basic information about diagnoses, symptoms, medications, medication side effects, treatment options, the role that stress can play, and prodromal symptoms that signal a relapse. Psychoeducation is often provided in groups, although it can be provided in a one-to-one format. Typically psychiatric rehabilitation programs run time-limited psychoeducation groups that last approximately 6 to 12 sessions. To maximize the effectiveness of a psychoeducation intervention, practitioners should do the following:

- Provide it to consumers who are asking for information about their illness.
- Tailor the content so that consumers clearly understand the information.
- Enhance didactic presentations with handouts, articles, videos, and structured small-group discussions.
- Avoid overloading consumers with too much information in a single session.
- Show consumers how the information is relevant to their goals.

The research that has been done on psychoeducation for consumers shows that this approach increases consumers' knowledge, but has little or no impact on consumers' behavior. For example, it has *not* been shown to be an effective way to increase medication compliance. Therefore, according to the studies that have been conducted thus far, consumer psychoeducation groups—when used alone—are not a particularly effective intervention in terms of helping consumers to manage their illness and achieve desired outcomes such as reduced symptoms, fewer hospitalizations, and improved quality of life (Mueser et al., 2002). However, if psychoeducation is combined with or incorporated into other illness self-management strategies, such as the cognitive behavioral interventions described later, other positive outcomes can be realized.

Consumers are probably capable of participating in the *delivery* of illness management interventions. Kim Mueser et al. (2002) commented:

> Research on illness management has thus far focused on programs developed and run by professionals. This research provides support for illness management programs and guidance on their effective components. Similar research on peer-based illness self-management programs may inform professional-based services and lead to *collaborative* efforts. (p. 1282)

Mueser suggests that consumers implementing this evidence-based practice will actually inform the practice of nonconsumer professionals, and lead to a new, more effective collaboration between consumers and professionals in the provision of illness management services. For more on consumer-run services, see Chapter 12.

Reviewing dozens of studies, Mueser and colleagues (2002) reported that psychoeducational methods were effective at improving consumers' knowledge of mental illness, but tended not to affect other outcomes. Second, medication education strategies were effective at helping consumers choose to take medication and incorporate it into their daily routines. Third, they found that relapse prevention and cognitive-behavioral approaches helped consumers to learn how to identify and respond to the early warning signs of relapse, thereby preventing relapses and rehospitalizations. Fourth, cognitive-behavioral approaches were successful in helping consumers develop more effective strategies for coping with symptoms, leading to decreases in symptom severity and distress.

Cognitive-behavioral interventions for symptom management consist of strategies designed to help the individual gain insight regarding his or her symptoms through the application of learning theory. These techniques, for example, encourage the individuals to evaluate the real-world evidence supporting delusional beliefs, literally test out their beliefs, and when the test results are inconsistent with their beliefs to develop new understanding. Cognitive interventions have been found to be effective at reducing the severity of psychotic symptoms as well as relieving distress (Mueser et al., 2002, 2003).

Staff Competencies Required for Effective IMR

The staff competencies necessary to provide effective IMR training go well beyond what would be considered the typical level of training for psychiatric rehabilitation staff. To provide effective IMR training, a staff member should have a fair knowledge of mental illness, have good coping skills, and be proficient at motivational interviewing and cognitive behavioral techniques. In addition to being good educators/trainers, staff members need to understand the IMR training strategy, recovery, and effective goal setting. Given this wide array of knowledge and skills, IMR training is often more effectively provided by a staff team rather than an individual staff member.

Evidence-based Practice: Illness Management and Recovery

Illness management and recovery (IMR) training is a multifaceted evidence-based practice (EBP) built around skill training and acquisition. The goal of IMR is to give the individual the knowledge and skills he or she needs to effectively cope with aspects of the illness. These knowledge and skills include (1) understanding the illness, including symptoms, possible course, and probable long- and short-term outcomes; (2) understanding the prescribed medications and the possible side effects that may occur; (3) developing strategies to help ensure medication compliance; (4) learning how to identify relapse early warning signs and how to respond to these; (5) developing effective coping skills to effectively deal with persistent symptoms; and (6) developing social support systems. These goals are accomplished using four different strategies that have been found effective in clinical trials: psychoeducation, behavioral tailoring, relapse prevention training, and coping skills training.

Critical Ingredients of Illness Management and Recovery

1. Psychoeducation about illness, medications, and so forth
2. Behavioral tailoring for medication regimen compliance
3. Relapse prevention training including warning sign recognition
4. Teaching coping strategies for persistent symptoms
5. Building social support systems.

Service Outcomes of Illness Management and Recovery

1. Increased knowledge of mental illness
2. Increased knowledge of medications and side effects
3. Reduced relapse rates and reduced severity of relapses
4. Fewer hospitalizations and hospital utilization.

Psychosocial Treatments

In addition to pharmacological treatments, the other broad category of treatment for severe and persistent mental illnesses is psychosocial treatment. *Psychosocial treatments* are approaches that attempt to effect change through the manipulation of social or psychological factors. Psychosocial interventions have been found to be very important in the care of persons with these disorders and are discussed throughout this text. Specific models that employ psychosocial strategies include some types of day programs, assertive community treatment, supported employment, and family psychoeducation. (These approaches are all described in detail in subsequent chapters of this book.) Also the various forms of psychotherapies are psychosocial interventions.

Many experts, such as Craighead and colleagues (1998a, 1998b), Harding and colleagues (1992), and Hogarty (1993), believe the most effective impact on the course of severe and persistent mental illness is achieved through a combination of biological and psychosocial interventions. Based on the available evidence, Hogarty (1993) concluded that the right combination of these two categories of treatments resulted in the lowest possible relapse rates. It is the conventional wisdom that pharmacological interventions are a necessary prerequisite for any psychosocial interventions to be effective. While some experts consider this to be an established fact, others such as Harding and her colleagues consider this to be a myth. They believe that psychosocial interventions can be effective regardless of the use of psychotropic medication (Harding & Zahniser, 1994).

CONTROVERSIAL ISSUE
Psychotropic Medications versus Alternative Treatments

Should PsyR practitioners always take a strong pro-medication stance, prioritizing medication compliance because it is the surest route to stabilization and good community adjustment? Are there situations in which a professional should support a consumer's choice to refuse psychotropic medications in favor of alternative treatments?

As discussed earlier, there is strong evidence that medications are the most effective way to treat the symptoms of severe mental illness. PsyR practitioners should share this knowledge with their clients, assist consumers in accessing good psychiatric treatment, and assist consumers in acquiring the skills and resources needed to take medication as prescribed and communicate effectively with their psychiatrist when problems arise. However, these interventions may fail when individuals refuse to take, or stop taking their medications.

How should PsyR practitioners react when an individual is not taking prescribed medication? In some programs, particularly those that adhere in part to the medical model or employ medical personnel, staff may view medication compliance as a primary goal even if the consumer is resistant to the idea of taking medication. In such programs interventions utilized to increase compliance are sometimes coercive in nature (Diamond & Wikler, 1985), for example, withholding privileges or monetary resources if a client has not taken medication. As you will see in Chapter 4, which covers the goals, values, and principles of PsyR, both coercive interventions and identification of treatment goals that are not client chosen are inconsistent with PsyR philosophy.

As addressed earlier, there are many reasons for medication noncompliance, including denial of the illness and discomfort due to side effects. Assisting a consumer in coming to terms with his or her mental illness and eventually accepting psychiatric treatment, or working with the consumer and his or her psychiatrist to develop a strategy to reduce side effects, are appropriate responses to these issues. Psychoeducational approaches can also be effective in terms of increasing adherence to a medication regimen.

Some consumers object to taking medications because of concern about the long-term use of psychotropic medication, or because they are opposed to the ingestion of chemical substances for philosophical or religious reasons. Such individuals may explore alternative treatments. Nutritional supplements and special dietary regimens have been used since the 1950s, but thus far there is no solid scientific support for this approach (Torrey, 2001). Others try homeopathic remedies, or relaxation techniques. Patricia Deegan, a consumer advocate, has written a manual on nonmedical strategies for reducing and coping with symptoms called *Coping with Voices: Self Help Strategies for People Who Hear Voices That Are Distressing* (1995). For example, when experiencing aversive auditory hallucinations, some consumers may obtain relief by listening to soothing music with headphones. (For more information on Dr. Deegan, see the biography in Chapter 12.) The exploration and use of alternative treatments for a variety of physical illnesses is currently widespread in the United States. Some of these approaches have even begun to attain respectability in medical and scientific circles. It is important for practitioners, including those who may be dubious about alternative medicine, to recognize consumers' rights to explore other approaches to treatment, just as many nonconsumers might when faced with a chronic disease. Unfortunately, because they have a mental illness, consumers' judgments of alternative approaches are often considered to be suspect. Instead, such individuals are more likely considered to be in a state of denial regarding their illness.

The questions that this issue raises are numerous. How far should PsyR practitioners go in supporting a client who chooses to utilize an alternative treatment? Should they help consumers gain access to alternative treatment resources? How should they handle a situation in which it seems obvious that a consumer is not benefiting from an alternative treatment approach? Should practitioners continue to counsel clients to reconsider medications, even when a client has expressed resistance to the idea for a number of years? It is important for PsyR practitioners to be thoughtful, to consider ethical implications, and to have an open dialogue with consumers and other professionals when struggling with such questions.

Psychosocial Treatments of Bipolar Disorder

Colom, Vieta, Martinez, Jorquera, and Gasto (1998) review and critique the different types of psychotherapy employed in the treatment of bipolar disorder. To date, none have established efficacy in controlled clinical trials regarding outcomes such as hospitalization, relapses, or suicidal behavior. This is in contrast to the numerous controlled studies highlighting the effectiveness of medication. Instead, a psychoeducational approach, either individually or in a group, seems to be the most promising.

Combined Treatment (Medication and Psychosocial) of Major Depression

Depression can often be a chronic disorder with a high risk of relapse that requires active treatment, often with a combination of medication and psychotherapy. Identifying which individuals would particularly benefit from psychosocial as compared to pharmacological approaches and developing an understanding of the mechanisms of action of these therapies remain major challenges (Scott & Watkins, 2004). In the treatment of major depression, behavioral therapy, cognitive-behavioral therapy, marital therapy, and interpersonal therapy have all been found to reduce depressive symptoms (Craighead et al., 1998a). A complete discussion of these treatments is outside the scope of this book.

Depressive disorders that are treated definitely have a better course than depressions that remain untreated (Angst, 1998). Interventions using behavior therapy, cognitive-behavioral therapy, and interpersonal therapy have all brought about significant reductions in depressive symptoms. In 12 out of 15 studies, cognitive-behavioral therapy significantly lowered the relapse or recurrence rate for depression (de Almeida & Neto, 2003). These treatments have also been found to be successful in the sense that the gains of the therapy are maintained. Arnow and Constantino (2003) reviewed the controlled research on the effectiveness of treatments for dysthymic disorder (relatively mild, nonepisodic but fairly constant chronic depression) and for long-term major depression. In trials conducted with persons with dysthymic disorder, medication has been superior to psychotherapy, with limited evidence that combined treatment has advantages over medication or psychotherapy alone. However, with long-term major depression, combined treatment has demonstrated superiority over medication or psychotherapy alone (Arnow & Constantino, 2003). Similarly, reviewing the literature, Friedman et al. (2004) found that combined treatment is associated with improvements over medication alone. Adding psychotherapy to antidepressant medication may be particularly effective among severely depressed patients. Further, adding cognitive-behavioral therapy to medication may be particularly important in preventing relapse, particularly among individuals discontinuing their medication (Friedman et al., 2004).

Some Ineffective Treatments

In the past, some treatments deservedly received a bad name for their ineffectiveness or actual harm in helping people with serious and persistent mental illness. There were efforts to treat people with schizophrenia without antipsychotic medication (available since the 1950s) and with only psychotherapies, such as traditional insight-oriented individual and group therapy. These resulted in very poor outcomes for the treatment recipients (Hogarty, 1993; Lehman & Steinwachs, 1998).

Insight-oriented, psychodynamic therapies can be defined as those that use interpretation of unconscious material and focus on therapeutic transference. In the treatment of serious mental illnesses of all types, this form of psychotherapy has been found to be generally ineffective. Actually, some studies have found psychodynamic treatments to be harmful. The consensus is that these therapies should no longer be used to treat schizophrenia (Lehman & Steinwachs, 1998), bipolar disorder (Keck & McElroy, 1998), or major depression (Craighead et al., 1998a). There is, however, a role for providing support through individual counseling identified in the research of Hogarty (1993). Effective individual counseling with people who have severe mental illness generally focuses on support, the person's present life situation (rather than past experiences), and problem solving.

Psychodynamic therapy is not the only treatment approach that may have a negative impact. Therapeutic settings that seem very positive might actually promote relapse in some individuals with schizophrenia, especially if they are very high in intensity and expectations (Hogarty, 1993). For example, as will be addressed in Chapter 6, programs that combine intensive group therapy with a short length of stay are associated with more hospitalization and longer relapses (Linn, Caffey, Klett, Hogarty, & Lamb, 1979).

Maria's Story

Maria is a new PsyR worker just learning "the ropes." As you read about what happens to Maria and the consumer she is working with, think about how the situation might have been avoided. Also, consider who was really responsible for the problem. (*Hint:* There was more than one way to avoid this problem and more than one person responsible.)

Maria always knew that she wanted to work with people. During high school she volunteered at a geriatric home on weekends, reading to some of the residents or helping them with activities such as shopping for personal items or just keeping them company. She majored in psychology at the small Midwestern college she attended. Most of the courses she took covered basic psychological theory, research methods, and statistics. Her dream was, someday, to get her Ph.D. and do private therapy. During college she volunteered at a private psychiatric hospital working with the activity therapist. She liked working with the patients. Maria could relate well because many of the patients were her age. She found it very interesting to talk with them about their symptoms.

During her senior year, she applied to several doctoral programs in clinical psychology. One of her psychology professors told her that it was harder to get into a clinical psychology program than to get into medical school. She wasn't even contacted for an interview. After graduation Maria went home and searched for a job where she could use her psychology degree. After looking all summer she ended up working as a clerk in a local bookstore. One day a friend of her mother told Maria about a program for people with severe mental illnesses that was looking for people with B.A. degrees to provide services. Maria applied, and on the strength of her previous experience and education, she got her first psychiatric rehabilitation job. She was really excited.

After a week-long orientation to the program she was assigned to work with Mark. Mark had a master's degree in rehabilitation counseling and more than 4 years of experience working in the program. Mark and Maria were responsible for a caseload of 11 clients. Maria quickly got to know the clients and the tasks she had to perform as a case manager. After only a few months, she and Mark decided that she would be the primary case manager for John and Helen, two clients with whom she had developed a close relationship. Maria felt that she was really starting to grow as a professional.

When it came to her role as case manager, Maria made sure that she covered all the bases. She genuinely liked John and Helen and she also wanted to prove to Mark that she could do a good job. She reviewed their treatment plans with them and established regular goals for them to achieve. Best of all, they were achieving these goals, and sometimes faster than scheduled. One day Helen was absent on a day when she had an important meeting. That afternoon, Maria called her boarding home, but they said Helen was out; they thought she had gone to the program. The next day Helen was absent again. Maria called the boarding home right away and they said that she had left that morning at her regularly scheduled time; they assumed she had gone to the program. Maria became very worried and went to tell Mark what was happening. The police brought in Helen that afternoon. They had found her acting strangely in the park and when they had asked if she needed any help she had started screaming and run away. Helen was hospitalized that evening.

When Helen returned to the program, Maria asked her what had happened. Why had she stopped going to the program when she was doing so well? Helen said she knew that she was making real progress with Maria's help. One day she began hearing voices and she became unable to sleep at night. She remembered that Maria had said that if she took her medication and worked on her treatment plan she would get better, but at the same time she knew she was getting sick. She knew how much effort Maria put into helping her and what a caring person she was. She felt like she was letting Maria down. Maybe Maria would be very disappointed in her or even very angry. When she got too sick to control her symptoms, she would go to the park rather than let Maria see her that way after all the work she had done.

Understanding Course, Treatment, and Outcome: What the Staff and Consumers Don't Know Can Hurt Them!

The bewildering and sometimes confusing array of information regarding course, treatment, and outcome highlights the need for consumers and their families, as well as staff, to be informed about medications, symptom relief, and so forth. Illness self-management and recovery strategies such as those mentioned earlier make up an important aspect of the PsyR process. Consider the issue of continuing medication after someone is symptom free. We know that continuing medication during time periods of remission significantly reduces the likelihood of relapse for people with schizophrenia as well as bipolar disorder, and recurrent major depression (Keck & McElroy, 1998; Nemeroff & Schatzberg, 1998). Still, the need to take medication on a long-term basis presents a major challenge for consumers, their loved ones, PsyR staff, and psychiatrists. Because it may take weeks or months for the effects of the medication to weaken and leave the body completely, the connection between discontinuing medication and a relapse is sometimes difficult for both the individual and the family to recognize. Conveying the knowledge of the importance of continuing medication is imperative. These truths highlight the necessity for collaborative psychopharmacology, illness management and recovery training (discussed earlier) and family psychoeducation (see Chapter 13).

Knowledge of the facts of the course and outcome of severe and persistent mental illnesses is essential for effective psychiatric rehabilitation services. Practitioners who are unfamiliar with the findings regarding the probability of relapses, especially that relapse is still likely even with treatment compliance, may set inordinately high expectations for consumers and themselves. At the same time, ignorance of the numerous positive outcomes that are possible, indeed likely, also can lead to undue feelings of helplessness, inordinately low expectations, and the self-fulfilling prophecy of pessimistic expectations leading to negative outcomes. A realistic understanding of the limited efficacy of treatment, the "rocky" or stormy course of the illness, and the variety of potential outcomes is more likely to result in high-quality services and better rehabilitation outcomes.

Consider the following: Many well-meaning, enthusiastic staff lack education specific to the severe mental illnesses. As illustrated in Maria's story, some of these individuals inform consumers that strict adherence to their treatment plan, taking their medication as prescribed, and so forth, will result in the prevention of relapse. When, despite following a treatment plan, relapse occurs, both the consumer and the staff may feel that they have failed. That is, the relapse is their fault rather than the disease itself. For consumers, this might result in hiding, denying symptoms, or dropping out of treatment because they are so disenchanted with being misled. For the staff person, this can produce frustration, a sense of failure, and eventually "burnout." Consumers and staff need to know that these illnesses do flare up, requiring medication changes, more intense treatment, support, and sometimes hospitalization. Indeed, most consumers are well aware of this, but do not necessarily attribute relapse to the illness itself.

When periodic relapse is seen as a function of the type of illness rather than a personal failure, the chances of a timely intervention are greatly increased. Prompt intervention can sometimes avert severe relapse and help ensure that the consumer is less debilitated. Probably the most important benefit of this knowledge is that relapse is no longer seen as a failure on the part of the consumer or the staff.

Similarly, inordinately low expectations—believing, for example, that the probability of relapse precludes other positive outcomes—may be just as harmful to both staff and consumers. Deegan (1992) described a vicious cycle of disempowerment. She observed that staff expectations of inevitable consumer incompetence lead to learned helplessness on the part of the consumer. In other words, low or negative expectations on the part of staff promote feelings of powerlessness among mental health consumers. Feeling they are unable to affect their own lives, some consumers have learned to become helpless and inadvertently fulfill the staff's expectation of incompetence. Thus, inordinately low expectations for positive outcomes result in the staff not supporting consumers in their educational aspirations, vocational goals, or independent living goals.

Believing that positive outcomes are possible often results in the successful pursuit of a higher quality of life. There is evidence also that successful psychiatric rehabilitation may positively impact the symptomatology. For example, it was found that successful vocational rehabilitation actually resulted in lower symptomatology, suggesting that rehabilitation itself may positively affect the course of the illness (DeSisto et al. 1995a, 1995b; Bond et al., 2001; Lysaker & Bell, 1995). Other examples of the positive impact of psychiatric rehabilitation interventions on the course of mental illness appear throughout this text.

Special Treatment Considerations with Dual Diagnoses

Dual diagnosis, the presence of two disorders within one individual, is a common situation. Two of the most prevalent and relevant to severe and persistent mental illness are (1) mental illness and addictive disorders (substance abuse or chemical abuse) and (2) mental illness and developmental disability.

Drug abuse is a significant complicating factor, associated with medication noncompliance, among other issues. *Substance abuse* also contributes to relapses, homelessness, medical problems, disruption in employment, and many more problems (Krystal, D'Souza, Madonick, & Petrakis, 1999). The issue of combined mental illness and substance abuse will be dealt with extensively in Chapter 8.

Developmental disabilities include conditions that are present prior to adulthood and are associated with intellectual, social, or physical impairments that continue into adulthood, such as autism and mental retardation. Because the issue of the dual diagnosis of mental illness and developmental disabilities is not covered thoroughly elsewhere in the book, an introduction to this special issue is presented next.

Service for Persons with Developmental Disabilities and Mental Illness

Historically, medications have been used to sedate individuals or control undesired behavior even when no mental illness had been diagnosed. Kalachnik and his colleagues (Kalachnik et al. 1991) cite a survey done by Lipman in 1967, which revealed that more than 50% of individuals with developmental disabilities in institutions were prescribed psychotropic medication, especially thioridazine (Mellaril) and chlorpromazine (Thorazine). These authors allude to an order from a U.S. district court judge handed down in 1972 that stated:

> Medication shall not be used as punishment, for the convenience of staff, as a substitute for a habilitative program, or in quantities that interfere with the resident's habilitation program. (p. 47)

To examine the efficacy of using antipsychotic medication to treat people with a dual diagnosis of intellectual disability and schizophrenia, Duggan and Brylewski (1999) reviewed the literature and found only one relevant randomized clinical trial (Foote, 1958). This study included four people with a dual diagnosis of schizophrenia and intellectual disability, but results were only available for two people. The reviewers found no evidence to guide the use of antipsychotic medication for those with both intellectual disability and schizophrenia. Until the urgent need for randomized controlled trials is met, clinical practice will continue to be guided by evidence from trials involving people with schizophrenia but without intellectual disability.

In 1980, in response to the overuse and misuse of psychotropic medications for people with developmental disabilities, the Accreditation Council for Services for Mentally Retarded and Other Developmentally Disabled Persons (ACMRDD) recommended the use of interdisciplinary teams for planning and oversight (Davis et al., 1998). These teams would include consumers, family members, and direct service staff, as well as physicians and other specialists. The team would do more than just monitor medication use. They would provide information to improve the data available for making a diagnosis, help to identify and access needed services, promote self-determination, encourage consumer choice, and aid in decision making.

Recognizing that services for people with developmental disabilities are moving from institutions to community settings, Davis and her colleagues (1998) articulated a list of attitudes, skills, and behaviors that should guide interdisciplinary teams. Among other things, these include (1) accessing adequate training on the needs of people with developmental disabilities as well as the use, abuse, and misuse of medications; (2) ensuring the inclusion of consumers and family members in decision making; and (3) focusing on community inclusion of consumers.

Stark, McGee, Menolascino, Baker, and Menousek (1984) attempted to describe quality services for people with this dual diagnosis. They identified seven necessary characteristics of effective alternatives to traditional services. These characteristics, described next, are consistent with many of the principles and values of PsyR. As you read these, see if you can identify which PsyR principles are related:

1. *Comprehensive community programs:* All learning should take place in real-life community-based situations.
2. *Functional, individualized approach:* Interventions focus on the individual in a specific environment developing the skills needed by the individual to be successful there.
3. *Training rather than testing:* Observing individuals in their environments helps to assess skills and deficits and informs the training process. Testing merely provides a description of the person's performance at that particular moment on tasks that often were designed for people with greater cognitive abilities.
4. *Unconditional positive regard:* The individual is given the respect, concern, courtesy, attention, and affection that would be afforded any human being. It also means that the person is not blamed for his or her disability or the resulting lack of experiences or skills.
5. *Understanding behavior as communication:* Behavior is a means of communication. This is particularly true for people with little or no ability in expressive language. Behavior therefore is viewed as such and rather than being punished is used to understand the person and inform services.

6. *Ecological behaviorism:* Behavior is seen as a complex interrelated system that is influenced by the environment rather than a simple example of stimulus-response.

7. *Balanced approach:* Both psychotropic medication and behavioral programming are useful tools to assist an individual to achieve independence.

Summary

Psychiatric symptoms can dominate the individual's experience, at times controlling a person's thoughts and feelings as presented in some of the vignettes in Chapter 2. These symptoms can be harmful to the self-esteem and hopefulness of the individual and may put the person at risk for suicide. Functional deficits are associated with these illnesses, specifically in self-care, employment, home making, educational achievements, and independent living. Because of these illnesses, individuals sometimes do not acquire important life skills or are unable to practice the skills they mastered previously.

There is no uniform outcome for each of these disorders. Instead, there are a variety of outcomes. For example, many people with depression, bipolar disorder, and some people with schizophrenia will have only one or two episodes and never relapse again. Alternatively, most people with a chronic or recurrent depression, bipolar disorder, or schizophrenia will have a variety of positive and negative outcomes over the course of their lifetime. Knowledge of this information is essential for consumers, their families, and their staff. Communication about these issues is critical. To avoid burnout and pessimism on the part of the staff, alienation and learned helplessness on the part of consumers, both need to be informed in order to develop expectations that are appropriate and realistic.

Individuals with these disorders are often prone to relapse, the risk of which is reduced, but not eliminated, by medication. All of these conditions are treated with powerful psychotropic medications that in addition to their therapeutic effects have numerous side effects. Because of side effects, the limited efficacy of these medicines, and many other reasons, many consumers find it difficult to comply with their medication regimens. The issue of compliance with medication, informed choice, and clear communication between the consumer and his or her psychiatrist is an important issue with all of these disorders.

In addition to biological or somatic treatments such as medications, psychosocial interventions are also needed. The symptoms of depression seem to be particularly helped by approaches such as cognitive and behavioral therapies. The symptoms of schizophrenia and bipolar disorders are not helped by insight-oriented psychotherapy; however, cognitive-behavioral techniques may help individuals cope with symptoms. Nevertheless, supportive counseling is useful, as are psychoeducation and illness management strategies such as the evidence-based IMR training.

The deficits or impairments in functioning caused by these illnesses are best addressed by psychiatric rehabilitation. Psychiatric rehabilitation can eliminate or reduce the impairment the person experiences in his or her living, learning, working, or social environments.

In addition, it can help the individual pursue his or her personal goals, achieve these goals, and maintain these gains.

Class Exercise

Misconception, Truth, or a Little of Both?

The word *myth* is often taken to mean misconception. Yet, many myths besides being fictions have a grain of truth. There are numerous myths about severe and persistent mental illness.

1. Consider the list of statements that follows these questions.
2. Do you consider each of them to be myths? Are they complete misconceptions?
3. Do they have any grains of truth?

Decide how to answer these questions based on the scientific evidence presented and cited in your text during the last three chapters.

> *"Once a person with schizophrenia, always a person with schizophrenia."*
> *"All people with schizophrenia are alike."*
> *"Rehabilitation can only happen when someone is completely stable."*
> *"Psychotherapy is a waste of time for people with severe and persistent mental illness."*
> *"All people with severe and persistent mental illness must be on medication for the rest of their lives."*
> *"People with mental illness can only do low-level jobs."* (You may want to peek at Chapter 9 before guessing on this one.)
> *"Families cause mental illness."* (See Chapters 2 and 13.)

References

Adams, C. E., Fenton, M. K., Quraishi, S., & David, A.S. (2001). Systematic meta-review of depot antipsychotic drugs for people with schizophrenia. *British Journal of Psychiatry, 179*(4), 290–299.

Allison, D. B., & Casey, D. E. (2001) Antipsychotic-induced weight gain: A review of the literature. *Journal of Clinical Psychiatry, 62*(Suppl 7), 22–31.

Alphs, L. D., & Anand, R. (1999). Clozapine: The commitment to patient safety. *Journal of Clinical Psychiatry, 60*(Suppl. 122), 39–42.

American Psychiatric Association. (1987). *Diagnostic and statistical manual of mental disorders.* (3rd ed.) Washington, DC: Author.

American Psychiatric Association. (1994). *Diagnostic and statistical manual of mental disorders.* (4th ed.) Washington, DC: Author.

Angst, J. (1998) Treated versus untreated major depressive episodes. *Psychopathology, 31*(1), 37–44.

Angst, J. (2004). Bipolar disorder: A seriously underestimated health burden. *European Archives of Psychiatry and Clinical Neuroscience, 254,* 59–60.

Anthony, W. A., Cohen, M. R., & Vitalo, R. (1978). The measurement of rehabilitation outcome. *Schizophrenia Bulletin, 4,* 365–383.

Anthony, W. A., & Jansen, M. A. (1984). Predicting the vocational capacity of the chronically mentally ill: Research and policy implications. *American Psychologist, 39*(5), 537–544.

Arnow, B. A., & Constantino, M. J. (2003). Effectiveness of psychotherapy and combination treatment for chronic depression. *Journal of Clinical Psychology, 59*(8), 893–905.

Basile, V. S., Masellis, M., Potkin, S. G., & Kennedy, J. L. (2002). Pharmacogenomics in schizophrenia: The quest for individualized therapy. *Human Molecular Genetics, 11*(20), 2517–2530.

Belmaker, R. H. (2004). Medical progress: Bipolar disorder. *New England Journal of Medicine, 351*(5), 476–486.

Bond, G.R., Resnick, S. G., Drake, R. E., Xie, H., McHugo, G. J. & Bebout, R. R. (2001). Does competitive employment improve nonvocational outcomes for people with severe mental illness? *Journal of Consulting and Clinical Psychology, 69*(3), 489–501.

Bond, G. R., Kim, H.-W., Meyer, P. S., Gibson, P., Tunis, S., Evans, J. D., et al. (2004). Response to vocational rehabilitation during treatment with first- or second-generation antipsychotics. *Psychiatric Services, 55*(1), 59–66.

Bottlender, R., Sato, T., Jaeger, M., Wegener, U., Wittmann, J., Strauss, A., et al. (2003). The impact of the duration of untreated psychosis prior to first psychiatric admission on the 15-year outcome in schizophrenia. *Schizophrenia Research, 62,* 37–44.

Bradford, D.; Stroup, S.; Lieberman, J. (2002) Pharmacological treatments for schizophrenia, in Nathan, P. E.; Gorman, J. M. (Ed). A guide to treatments that work (2nd ed.). London, England: Oxford University Press., pp. 161–169.

Chen, Y. R., Swann, A. C., & Johnson, B. A. (1998). Stability of diagnosis in bipolar disorder. *Journal of Nervous and Mental Disease, 186*(1), 17–23.

Colom, F., Vieta, E., Martinez, A., Jorquera, A., & Gasto, C. (1998). What is the role of psychotherapy in the treatment of bipolar disorder? *Psychotherapy and Psychosomatics, 67*(1), 3–9.

Conley, R. R., & Buchanan, R. W. (1997). Evaluation of treatment-resistant schizophrenia. *Schizophrenia Bulletin, 23*(4), 663–674.

Conklin, H. M. & Iacono, W. G. (2002). Schizophrenia: A neurodevelopmental perspective. *Current Directions in Psychological Science, 11,* 33–37.

Corrigan, P.W., Reinke, R.R., Landsberger, S.A., Charate, A., & Toombs, G. A. (2003) The effect of atypical anti-psychotics medication on psychosocial outcomes. *Schizopnrenia Research, 63,* 97–101.

Cotter, D. R. & Pariante, C. M. (2002). Stress and the progression of the developmental hypothesis of schizophrenia. *British Journal of Psychiatry, 181,* 363–365.

Craighead, W. E., Craighead, L. W., & Ilardi, S. S. (1998a). Psychosocial treatments for major depression. In P. E. Nathan & J. M. Gorman (Eds.), *A guide to treatments that work* (pp. 226–239). New York: Oxford University Press.

Craighead, W. E., Milkowitz, D. J., Vajk, F. C., & Frank, E. (1998b). Psychosocial treatment for bipolar disorders. In P. E. Nathan & J. M. Gorman (Eds.), *A guide to treatments that work* (pp. 240–248). New York: Oxford University Press.

Cusin, C., Serretti, A., Lattuada, E., Mandelli, L., & Smeraldi, E. (2000). Impact of clinical variables on illness time course in mood disorders. *Psychiatry Research, 97*(2–3), 217–227.

Davis, S., Wehmeyer, M. L., Board, J. P., Jr., Fox, S., Maher, F., & Roberts, B. (1998). Interdisciplinary teams. In S. Reiss & M. G. Aman (Eds.), *Psychotropic medication and developmental disabilities: The international consensus handbook* (pp. 73–83). Columbus, OH: Nisonger Center for Mental Retardation and Developmental Disabilities.

de Almeida, A. M., & Neto, F. L. (2003). Cognitive-behavioral therapy in prevention of depression relapses and recurrences: A review. *Revista Brasileira de Psiquiatria, 25*(4), 239–244.

Deegan, P. E. (1992). The independent living movement and people with psychiatric disabilities: Taking back control over our own lives. *Psychosocial Rehabilitation Journal, 15*(3), 3–19.

Deegan, P. E. (1995). *Coping with voices: Self help strategies for people who hear voices that are distressing.* Lawrence, MA: National Empowerment Center.

DeSisto, M. J., Harding, C. M., McCormick, R. V., Ashikaga, T., & Brooks, G. W. (1995a). The Maine and Vermont three-decade studies of serious mental illness. I. Matched comparison of cross-sectional outcome. *British Journal of Psychiatry, 167*(3), 331–338.

DeSisto, M. J., Harding, C. M., McCormick, R. V., Ashikaga, T., & Brooks, G. W. (1995b). The Maine and Vermont three-decade studies of serious mental illness. II. Longitudinal course comparisons. *British Journal of Psychiatry, 167*(3), 338–342.

Diamond, R. J., & Wikler, D. I. (1985). Ethical problems in community treatment of the chronically mentally ill. *New Directions for Mental Health Services, 26*, 85–93.

Dickinson, D., & Coursey, R. D. (2002). Independence and overlap among neurocognitive correlates of community functioning in schizophrenia. *Schizophrenia Research, 56*(1–2), 161–170.

Duggan, L., & Brylewski, J. (1999) Effectiveness of antipsychotic medication in people with intellectual disability and schizophrenia: A systematic review. *Journal of Intellectual Disability Research, 43*(2), 94–104.

Foote, E. S. (1958). Combined chlorpromazine and reserpine in the treatment of chronic psychotics. *Journal of Mental Science, 104*, 201–205.

Fox, V. (2004). Cresting. *Psychiatric Services, 55*(6), 641–642.

Frank, E., Kupfer, D. J., & Perel, J. M. (1990). Three-year outcome for maintenance therapies in recurrent depression. *Archives of General Psychiatry, 47*, 1093–1099.

Frank, E., Kupfer, D. J., & Perel, J. M. (1993). Comparison of full-dose versus half-dose pharmacotherapy in the maintenance treatment of recurrent depression. *Journal of Affective Disorders, 27*, 139–145.

Freeman, M. P., & Stoll, A. L. (1998). Mood stabilizer combinations—A review of safety and efficacy. *American Journal of Psychiatry, 155*(1), 12–21.

Friedman, M. A., Detweiler-Bedell, J. B., Leventhal, H. E., Horne, R., Keitner, G. I., & Miller, I. W. (2004). Combined psychotherapy and pharmacotherapy for the treatment of major depressive disorder. *Clinical Psychology: Science & Practice, 11*(1), 47–68.

Gray, R., Wykes, T., & Gournay, K. (2002). From compliance to concordance: A review of the literature on interventions to enhance compliance with antipsychotic medication. *Journal of Psychiatric & Mental Health Nursing, 9*(3), 277–284.

Green, A. I., Patel, J. K., Goisman, R. M., Allison, D. B., & Blackburn, G. (2000) Weight gain from novel antipsychotic drugs: Need for action. *General Hospital Psychiatry, 22*(4), 224–235.

Harding, C. M., Brooks, G. W., Ashikaga, T., Strauss, J. S., & Breier, A. (1987a). The Vermont longitudinal study of persons with severe mental illness, I: Methodology, study sample, and overall status 32 years later. *American Journal of Psychiatry,* (6), 718–726.

Harding, C. M., Brooks, G. W., Ashikaga, T., Strauss, J. S., & Breier, A. (1987b). The Vermont longitudinal study of persons with severe mental illness, II: Long-term outcome of subjects who retrospectively met DSM-III criteria for schizophrenia. *American Journal of Psychiatry, 144*(6), 727–735.

Harding, C. M., & Zahniser, J. H. (1994). Empirical correction of seven myths about schizophrenia with implications for treatment. *Acta Psychiatrica Scandinavica, Supplementum, 384*, 140–146.

Harding, C. M., Zubin, J., & Strauss, J. S. (1992). Chronicity in schizophrenia: Revisited. *British Journal of Psychiatry—Supplement, 18*, 27–37.

Heyscue, B. E., Levin, G. M., & Merrick, J. P. (1998). Compliance with depot antipsychotic medication by patients attending outpatient clinics. *Psychiatric Services, 49*, 1232–1234.

Hogarty, G. E. (1993). Prevention of relapse in chronic schizophrenic patients. *The Journal of Clinical Psychiatry, 54*(3), 18–23.

Hoff, A. L. & Kremen, W. S. (2003) Neuropsychology in schizophrenia: an update, *Current Opinion in Psychiatry, 16*, 149–155.

Kalachnik, J. E., Leventhal, B. L., James, D. H., Sovner, R., Kastner, T. A., Walsh, K., et al. (1991). Guidelines for the use of psychotropic medication. In S. Reiss & M. G. Aman (Eds.), *Psychotropic medication and developmental disabilities: The international consensus handbook* (pp. 45–72). Columbus, OH: Nisonger Center for Mental Retardation and Developmental Disabilities.

Kane, J. M. (2003). Long-term treatment of schizophrenia: Moving from relapse-prevention model to a recovery model. *Journal of Clinical Psychiatry, 64*(11), 1384–1385.

Kang, U. G., Kwon, J. S., Ahn, Y. M., Chung, S. J., Ha, J. H., Koo, Y. J., & Kim, Y. S. Electrocardiographic abnormalities in patients treated with clozapine. *Journal of Clinical Psychiatry.* Vol 61(6) Jun 2000, 441–446.

Keck, P. E., & McElroy, S. A. (1998). Pharmacological treatment of bipolar disorders. In P. E. Nathan & J. M. Gorman (Eds.), *A guide to treatments that work* (pp. 249–269). New York: Oxford University Press.

Kennedy, N., Abbott, R., & Paykel, E. S. (2003). Remission and recurrence of depression in the maintenance era: Long-term outcome in a Cambridge cohort. *Psychological Medicine, 33*(5), 827–838.

Kessing, L. V. (1998). Recurrence in affective disorder: II. Effect of age and gender. *British Journal of Psychiatry, 172,* 29–34.

Kessing, L. V., Andersen, P. K., Mortensen, P. B., & Bolwig, T. G. (1998) Recurrence in affective disorder: I. Case register study. *British Journal of Psychiatry, 172,* 23–28.

Klinkenberg, W., & Calsyn, R. J. (1996). Predictors of receipt of aftercare and recidivism among persons with severe mental illness: A review. *Psychiatric Services, 47*(5), 487–496.

Krystal, J. H., D'Souza, D. C., Madonick, S., & Petrakis, I. (1999). Toward a rational pharmacotherapy of comorbid substance abuse in schizophrenic patients. *Schizophrenia Research, 35*(Suppl), 35–49.

Lehman, A. F., & Steinwachs, D. M. (1998). At issue: Translating research into practice: The Schizophrenia Patient Outcomes Research Team (PORT) treatment recommendations. *Schizophrenia Bulletin, 24*(1), 1–10.

Leucht, S., Barnes, T. R. E., Kissling, W., Engel, R. R. Correll, C., & Kane, J. M. (2003). Relapse prevention in schizophrenia with new-generation antipsychotics: A systematic review and exploratory meta-analysis of randomized, controlled trials. *American Journal of Psychiatry, 160*(7), 1209–1222.

Licht, R. W. (1998). Drug treatment of mania—A critical review. *Acta Psychiatrica Scandinavica, 97*(6), 387–397.

Lieberman, J. A., Stroup, T. S., McEvoy, J. P. Swartz, M. S., et al. (2005). Effectiveness of antipsychotic drugs in patients with chronic schizophrenia. *The New England Journal of Medicine, 353*(12), 1209–1223.

Linn, M. W., Caffey, E. M., Klett, C. J., Hogarty, G. E., & Lamb, H. R. (1979). Day treatment and psychotropic drugs in the aftercare of schizophrenic patients. *Archives of General Psychiatry, 36,* 1055–1066.

Lysaker, P., & Bell, M. (1995). Work rehabilitation and improvements in insight in schizophrenia. *Journal of Nervous & Mental Disease, 183*(2), 103–106.

Maj, M., Pirozzi, R., Magliano, L., & Bartoli, L. (1998). Long-term outcome of lithium prophylaxis in bipolar disorder: A 5-year prospective study of 402 patients at a lithium clinic. *American Journal of Psychiatry, 155*(1), 30–35.

Marder, S. R., Essock, S. M., Miller, A. L., Buchanan, R. W., Davis, J. M., et al. (2002). The Mount Sinai conference on the pharmacotherapy of schizophrenia. *Schizophrenia Bulletin, 28,* 5–16.

Marneros, A., Tottig, S., Wenzel, A. R., & Brieger, P. (2004). Affective and schizoaffective mixed states. *European Archives of Psychiatry and Clinical Neuroscience, 254,* 76–81.

Meyer, P. S., Bond, G. R., Tunis, S. L., & McCoy, M. L. (2002). Comparison between the effects of atypical and traditional antipsychotics on work status for clients in a psychiatric rehabilitation program. *Journal of Clinical Psychiatry, 63*(2), 108–116.

Mueser, K. T., Drake, R. E., & Bond G. R. (1997). Recent advances in psychiatric rehabilitation for patients with severe mental illness. *Harvard Review of Psychiatry, 5*(3), 123–137.

Mueser, K. T., Torrey, W. C., Lynde, D., Singer, P., & Drake, R.E. (2003). Implementing evidence-based practices for people with severe mental illness. *Behavior Modification, 27*(3), 387–411.

Naheed, M., & Green, B. (2001). Focus on clozapine. *Current Medical Research Opinion, 17*(3), 223–229.

Nemeroff, C. B., & Schatzberg, A. F. (1998). Pharmacological treatment of unipolar depression. In P. E. Nathan & J. M. Gorman (Eds.), *A guide to treatments that work* (pp. 212–225). New York: Oxford University Press.

President's New Freedom Commission. (2003). *Achieving the promise: Transforming mental health care in America.* Available online at http://www.mentalhealthcommission.gov

Sadock, B.J., & Sadock, V. A. (Eds.). (2000). *Kaplan and Sadock's comprehensive textbook of psychiatry.* Baltimore, MD: Williams & Wilkins.

Satcher, D. (2000). Mental health: A report of the Surgeon General Executive Summary. *Professional Psychology—Research and Practice, 31*(1), 5–13.

Scott, J., & Watkins, E. (2004). Brief psychotherapies for depression: Current status. *Current Opinion in Psychiatry, 17*(1), 3–7.

Schulze, K., McDonald, C., Frangou, S., Sham, P., Grech, A., Toulopoulou, T., Walshe, M., Sharma, T., Sigmundsson, T., Taylor, M. & Murray, R. M. (2003). Hippocampal volume in familial and nonfamilial schizophrenic probands and their unaffected relatives. *Biological Psychiatry, 53*, 562–570.

Silverstone, T., McPherson, H., Hunt, N., & Romans, S. (1998). How effective is lithium in the prevention of relapse in bipolar disorder? A prospective naturalistic follow-up study. *Australian & New Zealand Journal of Psychiatry, 32*(1), 61–66.

Stark, J. A., McGee, J. J., Menolascino, F. J., Baker, D. H., & Menousek, P. E. (1984). Treatment strategies in the habilitation of severely mentally retarded–mentally ill adolescents and adults. In F. J. Menolascino & J. A. Stark (Eds.), *Handbook of mental illness in the mentally retarded* (pp. 189–218). New York, Plenum Press.

Substance Abuse Mental Health Services Administration-Center for Mental Health Services (2005). *Evidence-Based Practice Implementation Toolkits* accessed at http://www.samhsa.gov.

Torrey, E. F. (2001). *Surviving schizophrenia*. New York: Harper Perennial.

Viguera, A. C., Baldessarini, R. J., & Friedberg, J. (1998). Discontinuing antidepressant treatment in major depression. *Harvard Review of Psychiatry, 5*, 293–306.

Walker, E., Kestler, L., Bollini, A., & Hochman, K. M. (2004). Schizophrenia: Etiology and course. *Annual Review of Psychology, 55*, 401–430.

Wetterling, T., & Muessigbrodt, H. E. (1999). Weight gain: Side effect of atypical neuroleptics? *Journal of Clinical Psychopharmacology, 19*(4), 316–321.

Wiersma, D., Nienhuis, F. J., Slooff, C. J., & Giel, R. (1998). Natural course of schizophrenic disorders: A 15-year follow-up of a Dutch incidence cohort. *Schizophrenia Bulletin, 24*(1), 75–85.

Wiersma, D., Wanderling, J., Dragomirecka, E., Ganev, K., Harrison, G., An Der Heiden, W., et al. (2000). Social disability in schizophrenia: Its development and prediction over 15 years in incidence cohorts in six European centres. *Psychological Medicine, 30*(5), 1155–1167.

Part II

Psychiatric Rehabilitation Principles and Methodology

Chapter 4

Goals, Values, and Guiding Principles of Psychiatric Rehabilitation

Introduction   110
   Physical Rehabilitation as a Model for Psychiatric Rehabilitation   110
The Concept of Recovery   111
Goals, Values, and Guiding Principles   112
   The Goals of Psychiatric Rehabilitation   113
   The Values of Psychiatric Rehabilitation   115
Guiding Principles of Psychiatric Rehabilitation   119

A Proposed Integrated-Structural Model of Psychiatric Rehabilitation   125
Psychiatric Rehabilitation Ethics   126
   Researching the Principles of Psychosocial Rehabilitation   130
   Researching and Promoting Recovery   132
The Future of Psychiatric Rehabilitation Thought and Practice   133
Summary   134
Class Exercise   134
References   135

This chapter reviews the goals, values, and guiding principles of psychiatric rehabilitation (PsyR). Like any new and evolving discipline, the strategies and methods used in PsyR constantly undergo adjustment and change as the field matures and the methods become more refined. These differences are reflected by the wide scope of PsyR practice currently in use. Despite the diversity of practice, you will see that there is a great deal of agreement about the core elements that make up the belief system; that is, the goals and values of PsyR. This agreement is clearly demonstrated by the similarity among the many formulations of PsyR principles that have been suggested by different groups and authors.

This chapter will answer the following questions:

1. How does the concept of recovery inform the goals, values, and philosophy of psychiatric rehabilitation?

    2. *What are the goals of psychiatric rehabilitation?*

    3. *What are the defining values held by psychiatric rehabilitation professionals?*

    4. *What are the guiding principles that inform state-of-the-art PsyR practice today?*

    5. *What are the ethics of PsyR?*

Introduction

This chapter deals with the shared ideas and philosophy of psychiatric rehabilitation professionals as reflected in the services they provide. These concepts contribute to making PsyR a unique discipline. A relatively young field, PsyR is actively defining itself by amending its principles as its techniques and skills become more refined. PsyR is one specialty in the broader field of rehabilitation, to which it owes much of its philosophical base.

Physical Rehabilitation as a Model for Psychiatric Rehabilitation

Several authors have suggested that the rehabilitation of persons with physical disabilities provides an apt and instructive model or analogy for understanding the rehabilitation of persons with psychiatric disabilities (e.g., Anthony, Cohen, & Farkas, 2002; Deegan, 1988). An obvious benefit of this comparison is that rehabilitation from physical injury or disease is a relatively common and acceptable phenomenon in modern society. Sports figures recovering from injuries sustained on the playing field and aging public figures recovering from heart attacks or strokes are frequent subjects of media coverage. In addition, as medicine improves, life expectancy increases, making it more likely that a family member, friend, or acquaintance will develop a physical handicap.

The individual who has a disability due to a severe mental illness may experience difficulty with aspects of everyday life that require assistance, increased time and effort, or environmental modifications. As with the individual with a physical disability, one of the first steps in the rehabilitation process is acceptance of the disability and a willingness to work to overcome it. Unlike the individual with a physical disability, however, the reason for a person's disability due to mental illness may be less apparent to others.

Sadly, it is still true for many people that signs of a physical handicap (e.g., wheelchair) cause less negative stereotyping than indicators of a mental, cognitive, or emotional *handicap* (e.g., talking to oneself). These cues, which can be signals for stigma, may trigger stereotypic responses and discrimination (Corrigan, 2002). On the positive side, as our understanding of the brain and nervous system increased in the latter part of this century, so has our understanding of mental illness. Initially, the idea was that as public knowledge increased, the stigma associated with mental illness would be reduced. Recent studies suggest that as public understanding of mental illness increases, stigma about these diseases changes (Link, Phelan, Bresnhan, Stueve, & Pescosolido, 1999; Phelan, Cruz-Rojas, & Reiff, 2002). For example, as the public becomes more aware that severe mental illness has a genetic component, less blame is assigned to the ill individual. However, this new understanding suggests that other family members may be more likely to become ill

(Phelan et al., 2002). Still, as knowledge increases and medications and services improve, there is good reason to assume that stigma will decrease.

The Concept of Recovery

An exciting recent addition to PsyR thinking has been the development of a concept of *recovery*. The idea of recovery represents optimism about the future. Because the conditions associated with a severe mental illness are often lifelong, it was necessary to adopt a new conception of recovery that could coexist with the illness and its symptoms. Today, the concept of recovery from severe mental illness, with its promise of hope for the future, is becoming widely accepted.

Based on models of rehabilitation and recovery from physically handicapping conditions, a number of researchers and scholars have helped to develop a concept of recovery for severe mental illness (Anthony, 1993; Davidson & Strauss, 1992; Deegan, 1988; Jacobson, 2001; Onken, Ridgway, Dornan, & Ralph, 2002; Ridgway, 2001; Smith, 2000). For many conditions, recovery refers to a cure. In the context of a lifelong mental illness, recovery refers to a reformulation of one's life aspirations and an eventual adaptation to the disease. Nationally known consumer advocate, Patricia Deegan, Ph.D., and William Anthony, Ph.D., the director of the Center for Psychiatric Rehabilitation at Boston University, have both spent considerable time and energy spreading the concept of recovery throughout the PsyR community. Both Deegan and Anthony believe that the first step a person must go through in the recovery or rehabilitation process is acceptance of the handicap or disability. For a person with a cyclical mental illness, this step alone may take years. Deegan (1988) believes that to achieve an effective recovery the individual has to develop a new world view that incorporates one's mental illness as part of his or her reality. Dreams and aspirations may have to be modified to include the mental illness. Deegan points out that helping someone achieve this kind of fundamental change in self-concept is an important aspect of the PsyR practitioner's task.

This fundamental change in self-concept implies awareness of several other important aspects of the recovery process. Deegan (1988) stresses that one of the most important new ideas is that recovery and rehabilitation are not linear processes. People going through these types of changes naturally experience setbacks and temporary failures. When doing better, it is very tempting to forget or ignore the idea that one has a severe mental illness (Fox & Geller, 2004). Real recovery is a journey that requires exploring new ideas and new self-concepts and that means being open to failure, disappointment, and possible relapse. By this logic, PsyR services that do not make realistic allowances for failure do a disservice to people in recovery.

Another corollary of the recovery concept is that each person's road to recovery is unique. Because recovery is based on developing a new self-image, we might assume that there may be as many roads to recovery as there are people. The uniqueness of each person's rehabilitation has a direct bearing on PsyR services. Effective programs respect diversity and provide many individualized services for their *service recipients*. "One size fits all" services may be easier and more efficient to operate but, especially in the long run, they are inherently less effective at helping persons recover.

Because the core task that the recovering person needs to accomplish is the development of a new and positive sense of self or self-image that incorporates his or her mental illness, other consumers also have an important role to play in the recovery process. Consumers who have achieved a positive self-image despite their illness serve as role models and they provide evidence that it can be done. Role modeling is a fundamental PsyR strategy. An aspect of Bandura's social learning theory (1977), which is covered in more depth in Chapter 5, role modeling is the principle way individuals learn to behave in different settings or environments. At the core of many PsyR approaches, role modeling is a powerful tool for providing both hope and specific strategies to achieve goals. The staff members of effective PsyR services, for example, act as role models for their service recipients. This is one reason why many PsyR professionals strive to reduce the barriers between themselves and their clients as much as possible. For example, staff members may dress less formally and share in everyday functions and chores as a means of emphasizing their similarities with the individuals they are serving.

The concept of recovery is bolstered by the increasing progress being made in psychiatry and psychiatric rehabilitation. This progress is seen in a number of different developments:

- The results of landmark longitudinal studies on the outcome of schizophrenia (e.g., Harding, Brooks, Ashikaga, Strauss, & Breier, 1987; described in Chapter 3)
- The introduction of improved medications that have better results in terms of decreasing both symptomatology and side effects for many consumers (described in Chapter 3)
- The identification of evidence-based practices that reliably produce positive outcomes for consumers. Supported employment may be the best example of this (see Chapter 9).
- The debunking of many of the myths about schizophrenia and mental illness that support continued stigma against people with mental illness (e.g., Harding & Zahniser, 1994).

The concept of recovery embodies the optimism and hope that underlie the entire PsyR enterprise. The goal of recovery for every individual with mental illness is an important element in the definition of the PsyR profession.

Goals, Values, and Guiding Principles

This chapter discusses the goals, values, and guiding principles of PsyR. *Values* are deeply held beliefs that may inform specific behaviors, attitudes, and ideas. An individual's values tend to be stable over time. Because they are deeply held, a person may not articulate or question his or her own values. For example, individuals who value the free expression of ideas may not even be aware of that value until they find themselves coming to the defense of someone who is prevented from expressing their opinion at a meeting or gathering.

Even then, they may not consider why they felt so strongly about what had just taken place.

Goals represent desired states or objectives to strive for and achieve. Goals are usually identified based on their relationship or presumed relationship with values. Again, if we value free expression we might work hard to achieve the goal of defeating a bill that we believe would stifle free speech on the Internet. Goals are more specific than values. Goals can usually be arrived at by different paths. For example, the goal of an improved quality of life might be achieved in a different manner for each person.

Principles, in contrast to goals, are more specific statements specifically designed to promulgate values and goals by providing guidelines for addressing specific situations or behaviors as they arise. As an example, consider the community mental health principle of least restrictive treatment environment. This widely held principle states that an individual should always receive treatment in the most autonomous (least restrictive) setting or environment that is possible but still effective. This means, for example, that no one should be treated in a psychiatric hospital if there is a community-based program available where he or she can receive equally effective treatment. We can see that this principle is designed to promote the goals of community integration and quality of life, as well as foster the value of respect for the dignity of each human being.

Table 4.1 provides a preview of the goals, values, and guiding principles of PsyR that are discussed in the following sections.

The Goals of Psychiatric Rehabilitation

As we stated above, the goals of PsyR represent the objectives of PsyR services. These are what all PsyR services strive to achieve for their clients. In that sense, goals are guidelines for service and go hand in hand with PsyR values. The combination of goals and values helps determine the guiding principles. Our review of several efforts to identify these ideas (Anthony et al., 2002; Anthony & Nemec, 1983; Cnaan, Blankertz, Messinger, & Gardner, 1988, 1989, 1990; International Association of Psychosocial Rehabilitation Services [IAPSRS], 1996) suggests that there is near universal agreement on three goals of PsyR, as discussed next.

1. PsyR Services Are Designed to Help Persons with Severe Mental Illness Achieve Recovery

The goal of recovery illustrates both the hope and the difficulty of the PsyR enterprise. Recovery, which we discussed earlier, is the defining goal of PsyR. Because recovery is unique for each person, guidelines for achieving this goal may vary. You will see that some of the values and guiding principles we outline are designed to promote the idea that each individual must follow his or her own path to recovery. Because recovery is really an abstract idea defined by each individual, it is something that each person must achieve for himself or herself rather than something that we can do for or to someone. Achieving this goal presents the PsyR worker with an important challenge. The worker

TABLE 4.1
The Goals, Values, and Guiding Principles of PsyR

Goals (3)
1. Recovery
2. Community integration
3. Quality of life

Values (5)
1. Self-determination
2. Dignity and worth of every individual
3. Optimism
4. Capacity of every individual to learn and grow
5. Cultural sensitivity

Guiding Principles (13)
1. Individualization of all services
2. Maximum client involvement, preference, and choice
3. Partnership between service provider and service recipient
4. Normalized and community-based services
5. Strengths focus
6. Situational assessments
7. Treatment/rehabilitation integration, holistic approach
8. Ongoing, accessible, coordinated services
9. Vocational focus
10. Skills training
11. Environmental modifications and supports
12. Partnership with the family
13. Evaluative, assessment, outcome oriented focus

has to help and encourage the individual to do something that the individual has to accomplish on his or her own.

2. PsyR Services Are Designed to Help Persons with Severe Mental Illness Achieve Maximum Community Integration

This goal, for the individual to be able to live with a degree of independence in the community of his or her choice, is the most consistently stated goal of PsyR services both nationally and worldwide (e.g., Cnaan et al., 1988, 1989; IAPSRS, 1996). In a very real sense, this was the starting point on which all the other goals and values emerged. Residing in the community, instead of in an institution, offers the opportunity for self-direction, rehabilitation, and recovery.

How this goal can be best achieved is still a matter of some contention. A good deal of criticism has been directed at some PsyR services accused of keeping consumers segregated by creating small institutions in the community rather than working toward community integration. Some housing advocates feel strongly that housing facilities should be integrated (a percentage of residences open to the public at large) rather than designated specifically for persons with severe mental illness (e.g., Carling, 1995). Ultimately, many advocates believe that there should be no housing designated for people with psychiatric disabilities at all. Instead, people with disabilities should live in regular community residences (e.g., homes, apartments) of their own choosing.

Some PsyR models, such as the Fairweather Lodges (Fairweather, 1980), continue to embrace sheltered support for some individuals as an appropriate strategy given the level of stigma that still exists in the community. Regardless of these differences, the maximum degree of community integration feasible continues to be a goal of the PsyR enterprise.

3. PsyR Services Are Designed to Help Persons with Severe Mental Illness Achieve the Highest Possible Quality of Life

The PsyR practitioner believes in the importance of achieving the highest quality of life possible for every individual regardless of the stage of his or her illness or the severity of his or her symptoms. The concept of *quality of life* refers to both the individual's subjective sense of life, for example, how the individual feels about his or her living arrangement, and to the objective, for example, yearly income. Much of this research is based on the Lehman (1983, 1988) quality-of-life interview, which takes aspects such as symptom level into account. This goal goes hand in hand with optimism about recovery and community integration, despite the presence of a handicapping condition. The presence of symptoms should not detract from the importance of those things that help ensure a reasonable quality of life such as social support, companionship, employment, recreation, food, shelter, clothing, and an active sex life. For the PsyR worker, quality of life is an important goal regardless of what stage of the illness the person is experiencing. For the individual, symptom reduction can be a quality of life issue as much as a treatment issue.

The Values of Psychiatric Rehabilitation

The values that underlie most, if not all, PsyR services relate directly to the goals that PsyR tries to achieve. Values are general attitudes that influence the professional's behavior in many ways. In fact, PsyR practitioners may hold these values without articulating them since they are embedded in the designs of the programs they work in and the service strategies they carry out. As you review the following five PsyR values, consider how they relate to the goals of PsyR.

1. Everyone Has the Right of Self-Determination, Including Participation in All Decisions That Affect Their Lives

In PsyR facilities this value is often referred to as empowerment. While this term's usage is nearly universal, because it encompasses so much, there is still no generally agreed-on definition of empowerment. Community psychologist Julian Rappaport (1987) characterized the term empowerment as conveying ". . . both a psychological sense of personal control or influence and a concern with actual social influence, political power, and legal rights" (p. 121).

Consumer involvement and empowerment directly relate to the importance of the recovery process. As Deegan (1988) pointed out, the essence of recovery is the individual's reestablishment of a self-concept that takes the mental illness into account. This is in contrast to the notion that the services provided constitute the rehabilitation itself. Instead, the services help make the rehabilitation process available, attractive, and possible for the individual with a disability who must do the very real work of self-change. As Deegan (1988) put it:

> "... persons with a disability do not "get rehabilitated" in the sense that cars "get" tuned up or televisions "get" repaired. They are not passive recipients of rehabilitation services. Rather, they experience themselves as recovering a new sense of self and of purpose within and beyond the limits of the disability. (p. 12)

How are these involvement and empowerment goals achieved for persons with severe mental illness? Many varied and innovative service delivery strategies are designed, developed, and refined in an effort to accomplish these goals.

One important aspect of involvement and empowerment concerns consumers' knowledge about their condition and their treatment. A study by Warner, Taylor, Powers, and Hyman (1989) examined the effect of labeling consumers as mentally ill. The authors had hypothesized that consumers who were accepting of their mental illness diagnosis would have lower levels of functioning. In fact, they found the opposite was true and concluded that empowerment, in the form of shared knowledge, may help reduce psychiatric disability.

Pratt and Gill (Pratt & Gill, 1990; Gill & Pratt, 1993) developed empowerment and involvement strategies for day treatment services that included sharing knowledge, power, and economic resources with consumers. From these starting points consumers were encouraged to extend their prerogatives to other aspects of their programs. These strategies produced greater consumer involvement with their program, increased acceptance and awareness of mental illness, and improved outcomes.

Another important aspect of self-determination or empowerment is ensuring that people with psychiatric disabilities are allowed to make decisions about their own lives—even if the decision could lead to a negative outcome. Another way of expressing this idea is that all people should have the right to take risks in their lives. Many well-intentioned practitioners struggle with consistently applying this value. They encourage consumers to make decisions, but also want them to play it safe and avoid any actions that could lead to a failure or setback. While it is important to be sure that people understand the potential consequences or their decisions and behaviors, it is ultimately the consumer's choice. For example, a person may feel ready to take on a full-time job, while staff members believe the person should take a less stressful part-time position. Sometimes, options that seem risky work out better than expected, whereas at other times the setback predicted by staff does occur. In either case, people should be empowered to direct their own lives and have experiences that will help them learn about their potential as well as their limitations.

While everyone uses the term there is still a good deal of debate about how to exactly define *empowerment*. One way of defining something is to formulate a working definition of it so that it can be measured. With input from several consumer groups around the country, Rogers, Chamberlin, Ellison, and Crean (1997) have begun development of a scale designed to measure empowerment. They suggest that empowerment is made up of three parts. The first element of empowerment is self-esteem/self-efficacy. This can be thought of as optimism and a sense of control over the future. The second element involves possessing actual power. The final element of empowerment, they suggest, is made up of righteous anger and community activism. It is important to recognize that these elements of empowerment describe characteristics of empowered people. Similar to the concept of recovery, empowerment is something that must come from within the individual, rather than something done *to* or *for* an individual.

2. PsyR Interventions Respect and Preserve the Dignity and Worth of Every Human Being, Regardless of the Degree of Impairment, Disability, or Handicap

This core value underlies every aspect of PsyR practice. People are in no way lessened as human beings by their illness. If asked, most service providers and consumers would personally endorse this position. Despite these socially correct declarations, the persistent stigma against people with mental illness suggests that in reality this is not a widely held value.

A lack of dignity or worth is conveyed in various ways, many of which are very subtle. Consider a setting where the service recipients are addressed by their first names but the staff members are only addressed by their titles or surnames. The message in such behavior is very clear; the service recipients have low status while the staff members have high status. This same message may be conveyed in other ways as well. For example, when different rules apply to program staff and service recipients regarding use of program areas (conference rooms where only staff are allowed to congregate, separate bathrooms for service recipients and staff, etc.). While individual situations like these are subtle, each sends a message that service recipients have low status and reduces their dignity.

If numerous such situations exist together in an insensitive environment, it conveys a clear message that persons with severe mental illness who require services have less worth than the persons who staff the program. Most of these situations, when they exist, are unintentional. The concept of staff bathrooms and lunchrooms is relatively common in many settings and does not carry a negative message. Most people address their own physician by the title "doctor." Nevertheless, for persons with mental illness an accumulation of these situations combined with societal stigma conveys a strong message that they are less valued by society. Wolf Wolfensberger's (1983) efforts to develop surveys and scales to identify these dignity-reducing situations are important simply because they are often subtle, unintended, and may be essentially invisible to the staff.

3. Optimism Regarding the Improvement and Eventual Recovery of Persons with Severe Mental Illness Is a Critical Element of All Services

Every person, regardless of his or her symptoms or handicaps, has the capacity to benefit from services. Real optimism on the part of service providers generalizes to the service recipients. Of course, the ultimate optimistic stance is represented by the concept of recovery described earlier in the chapter.

At the same time, providers who lack optimism regarding the potential of consumers may be hard pressed to maintain the requisite level of motivation to effectively carry out their functions. Worse, even the most symptomatic individuals are aware of when a practitioner believes that they will not achieve their goals.

The practical effects of a lack of optimism were often exemplified by the inadequate and inappropriate treatment provided for persons with severe mental illness by the traditionally trained staff of many community mental health centers (Torrey, 2001). Based on their training, these staff were often pessimistic about the long-term prognosis of persons who lacked appropriate ego functioning and the insight to benefit from treatment. Because of the pervasive belief that these persons could not improve, treatment resources were often allocated to programs providing services for persons with less severe conditions who could benefit from more psychodynamically oriented treatments. Persons experiencing severe and persistent mental illness, labeled "chronics," were often treated by the least trained staff, given minimal psychiatric time, and given minimal levels of supplies, space, and support staff.

4. Everyone Has the Capacity to Learn and Grow

This value is clearly a corollary of the value of optimism. The core message of this value is that all people, regardless of their level of disability, can benefit from modalities such as skill training and education. The presence of a mental illness does not preclude someone's ability to learn and grow.

Consider what happened to a consumer named William who had been in a PsyR day program for 5 years after spending the previous 13 years in a psychiatric hospital. William, who was always neat and well groomed, was almost entirely noncommunicative. One thing that he did communicate was a desire to work. Previous attempts at getting William to be more outgoing had all ended in failure. While he did not communicate, William did seem to like to be around people. Reviewing past failures, a new case worker hit on an idea. If William could learn to use a few phrases and operate the equipment, he could work as an elevator operator, a job for which some openings existed. William responded very positively to this idea. He learned to greet people and ask them what floor they wanted. He also learned to operate the elevator, paying particular attention to the doors and to whether it stopped evenly with the floor at each level. The staff were amazed that William could learn these things after years of being almost a recluse. William held that job for many years, rarely saying more than "Good morning!," "What floor?," and "Watch your step!"

5. PsyR Services Are Sensitive to and Respectful of the Individual, Cultural, and Ethnic Differences of Each Consumer

Severe mental illness knows no cultural or ethnic boundaries. Providers of PsyR services must be prepared to aid any individual experiencing these conditions. Sensitivity to cultural and ethnic differences is necessary when we consider that the task of PsyR is essentially reintegration with the consumer's community of choice. To successfully accomplish this goal, it is the responsibility of the practitioner to be sensitive to the particular beliefs, mores, and customs of the community in question. In short, the practitioner must become culturally competent and ensure that the services provided are also culturally competent. Tales abound of the kinds of social faux pas that occur when professionals make incorrect judgments about the consumers they serve because of a lack of knowledge of their culture. For example, when a person in the United States does not look at another person directly they might be suspected of having something to hide. However, looking at someone directly is considered rude or aggressive in some cultures.

This is an especially sensitive area for PsyR practitioners because they must constantly deal with the issue of societal stigma toward the consumers they serve. The constant problem of stigma helps to keep the practitioner aware of the importance of respectful communication and behavior. In one sense, having a severe mental illness constitutes a unique cultural identity in itself. The struggle to help consumers free themselves from the role of "mental patient" may be aided by increased respect and awareness for the consumer's ethnic and cultural background.

Guiding Principles of Psychiatric Rehabilitation

The guiding principles of psychiatric rehabilitation comprise a set of rules that can be applied to specific situations in order to achieve the goals and reflect the values of the field. In a sense, they constitute "rules of thumb" that PsyR practitioners can refer to when faced with important decisions. The principles are important tools for providing day-to-day guidance in clinical situations and for systematizing the practice of PsyR.

Although the higher order values and goals are widely shared by PsyR practitioners, there are still some questions about the application of specific principles. These differences are reflected in the formulations of PsyR principles that have been put forward in the discipline's short history (Anthony et al., 2002; Anthony & Nemec, 1983; Cnaan et al., 1988, 1989, 1990; IAPSRS, 1996). Rather than outright disagreement on these principles, professionals in different settings often prioritize principles differently. This reprioritization is often a response to real differences that exist between settings or unique situations. For example, in order to justify billing criteria, in some treatment settings staff are required to focus on the consumers' symptoms and deficits when writing clinical notes, rather than on their strengths. As you will see, this emphasis on symptoms and deficits violates the principle of focusing on an individual's strengths. Regardless, for these practitioners a refusal to comply with billing requirements might jeopardize the existence of PsyR services in general. In this paradoxical case, the best response might be to avoid emphasizing strengths when writing chart notes, but still emphasize strengths in actual practice.

As you review the 13 guiding PsyR principles discussed next, consider how they relate to the goals and values of PsyR.

1. Individualization of All Services

This principle means that rehabilitation goal formulation, assessment, and service provision respond to the individual needs and desires of the client. Because it allows each person to develop in the way he or she desires, individualization of services is a very important element of the recovery process. Because many PsyR services are carried out in groups, strict adherence to this principle is very important. Notice how the following supported employment (SE) program is designed to ensure individualization of services and how the curriculum is adjusted depending on the needs of members:

> *The SE program at Shore House offers a 6-week Vocational Exploration group. The curriculum for this group includes a review of each member's past experiences, including identification of their occupational values, skills, interests, and preferences. The final step for each group member is the development of a vocational goal. A new member, Arthur, wants to get a job and believes he will need the support of the job coach to secure and maintain employment. After several meetings, the job coach is satisfied that Arthur knows what kind of job he wants. Rather than spend 6 weeks in the group to gain information he already has, Arthur will begin working with the job coach immediately on job development.*

2. Maximum Client Involvement, Preference, and Choice

This principle is related to the very personal nature of recovery and rehabilitation. Each person has a unique set of preferences, values, and aspirations. Goals or services that are selected for the consumer by the practitioner or anyone else for that matter are meaningless. Consider the following situation that confronted Sharon. How would you feel in her shoes? Or, how would you feel if you were her counselor?

> *Sharon and her counselor Ann have completed work on her rehabilitation plan. Sharon's rehabilitation goal is to get a job doing clerical work. All of the interventions described in the plan are related to job acquisition (contacting employers, practicing interviewing, etc.). At her team meeting, Ann shares Sharon's plan with other staff. Some members of the team believe that before Sharon works on getting a job she needs to become more outgoing. Ann reminds them that there are many clerical jobs in quiet offices where workers are not expected to be outgoing, but the team thinks it would be good for her and Ann is pressured to change the plan. When Ann and Sharon meet to review and sign the plan, Ann explains that the team agreed that Sharon should volunteer to run the community meeting three times a week for the next 3-month period, and then, if she's more comfortable socializing, she should resume her work goal. Ann decides not to tell Sharon that she is very much against this plan. Despite feeling that she is not respecting Sharon's choice, she rationalizes this by thinking that running the community meeting may actually help Sharon.*

3. Partnership between Service Provider and Service Recipient

To assist a person with the rehabilitation and recovery process, the PsyR practitioner first needs to establish a positive connection with the person that is characterized by mutual respect and trust (Fox, 2000, 2004a, 2004b). It may take considerable time and effort to build such a working relationship. Once established, the relationships between PsyR practitioners and the people they serve are true partnerships (Fox, 2000, 2004a, 2004b). In other words, both parties—the consumer and the provider—work together to develop effective rehabilitation strategies. The perspectives of both of these participants are viewed as valuable and essential to the work. Practitioners bring specialized knowledge, skills, and techniques to the relationship; and consumers bring their experiences and a unique understanding of their own needs and preferences.

> *Larry, who has been a consumer of mental health services for many years, has had some negative experiences in his past relationship with staff members. He doesn't feel that they always understand his point of view and has sometimes felt that they pressure him to sign treatment plans and attend groups that don't pertain to his needs. He is skeptical when he meets Nicole, who introduces herself as his new counselor. What could this young woman possibly know about his life and his dreams? Nicole takes the time to get to know Larry. She encourages him to talk about himself and his interests. She puts in considerable time and effort to help him resolve an ongoing problem he has been having with his landlord. After several months Larry begins to think that Nicole really is concerned about him. When they begin discussing his rehabilitation plan, he is pleased that she encourages him to do most of the talking about his goals. She does offer helpful suggestions, but never tries to talk him into doing something that he's not interested in.*

4. Normalized and Community-Based Services

Wolf Wolfensberger, whose work was primarily with people who had developmental disabilities, coined the term *normalization*. Wolfensberger (1983) describes normalization as the promotion of valued social roles. Worker, student, parent, and neighbor are positive social roles that are valued in our society. Psychiatric patient and group home resident are examples of social roles that are devalued. PsyR services are designed to assist people in taking on and succeeding in valued social roles.

Normalized services are appropriate to the person's age, sex, culture, and so forth. For example, in a PsyR program you would not speak to the adults served as if they were children, or ask them to do finger paintings and then display their work on the wall. In normalized residential settings, consumers live in decent, safe neighborhoods; have access to transportation, shopping, and other community resources; interact with neighbors; and participate in community activities. In contrast, institutional settings and group homes in socially isolated locations would not assist consumers in developing valued social roles and would thus be inconsistent with this guiding principle.

5. Strengths Focus

PsyR services and practitioners recognize and build on an individual's strengths rather than focusing on his or her weaknesses or deficits. This can be a difficult task for both consumer and practitioner. Consumers who have a long history of psychiatric hospitalizations are accustomed to professionals focusing on their symptoms and problems. When asked "What are your strengths?" they are often at a loss. Initially, practitioners may also have difficulty seeing past psychotic symptoms and social deficits such as extreme withdrawal. However, PsyR programs typically allow consumers and practitioners to develop relationships around work and recreational activities. These experiences encourage practitioners to relate to consumers as they would to a colleague or friend, and to focus on what a consumer can do and likes to do. Perhaps this principle is best illustrated by the following professional descriptions of the same individual:

> *Joan is a psychiatric nurse who sees Peter once a month for medication maintenance group. In a chart note she describes Peter as appearing depressed and withdrawn with poor eye contact and constricted affect. Phil is a vocational rehabilitation counselor who is working with Peter in a supported employment program. His chart note, written on the same day as Joan's, describes Peter as a diligent worker who completes assigned tasks and communicates effectively with his supervisor. Both descriptions may be accurate and are appropriate to the professional's function. Joan's note may assist the psychiatrist in making a helpful medication adjustment, whereas Phil's PsyR assessment helps him determine that Peter's vocational rehabilitation goals are being achieved.*

This emphasis on consumer strengths has been championed by the work of Charles Rapp and his colleagues at the University of Kansas (Rapp, 1998).

6. Situational Assessments

Doing *situational assessments* rather than overall assessments means that the rehabilitation process focuses on the skills and modifications necessary for the client to function successfully in the environments (i.e., situations) of his or her choice. This is in contrast to doing a *global assessment* unrelated to specific client goals. For example, consumers attending a vocational readiness group may have markedly different employment goals. Sarah wants to get a job as a retail salesperson, while Tony would like to pursue work as a laboratory technician. Doing a general assessment of work readiness skills (e.g., ability to follow directions and complete assigned tasks) is not the best way to predict what they will need to succeed in their chosen jobs. The best way to assess their ability to meet the requirements of their chosen career is to observe them completing relevant tasks in these very different environments. It is likely that focusing on interpersonal skills will be crucial for success for Sarah. The ability to carry out precise measurements and record results will be important for Tony's chosen line of work.

7. Treatment/Rehabilitation Integration, Holistic Approach

This means that PsyR services and practitioners do not separate the treatment and rehabilitation processes. Rather, the client is viewed as a complex individual, taking into account all the aspects of his or her life impacted by these processes. The term *treatment* usually refers to symptom relief, while rehabilitation usually refers to overcoming barriers and the pursuit of goals. A modern understanding of PsyR views these as complementary endeavors, although historically medical and rehabilitation professionals have not always seen them as such.

Consider the issue of an essential component of the treatment of severe and persistent mental illness, compliance with psychotropic medication. A regimen of psychotropic medication is prescribed by a physician for relief (treatment) of psychotic symptoms. What is the role of rehabilitation in this intervention? On the face of it, one might say it is a simple issue of patient compliance or noncompliance with physician recommendations. However, consumers need knowledge and skills to comply with a medication regimen. In addition, they need to monitor their symptoms and side effects in order to communicate this information to their doctor. This is where rehabilitation can be of assistance to treatment. An individual's ability to monitor and share appropriate information about symptoms, medications, side effects, and so on, can be improved through psychoeducation (Pratt & Gill, 1990). Explicit training can be implemented to teach or increase these skills, such as instructional curricula developed by various groups, most notably Liberman and his colleagues (1993) at UCLA.

Another important point to consider is that rehabilitation goals may be hampered if treatment efforts are unsuccessful. Conversely, successful treatment should promote rehabilitation goals. Thus, treatment and rehabilitation are complementary and interdependent efforts.

8. Ongoing, Accessible, Coordinated Services

PsyR services should be unlimited with respect to time (e.g., there should not be a prescribed time length for services). They should be easily accessible and be coordinated to ensure availability and avoid duplication. As discussed in Chapter 2 and elsewhere in this book, not everyone experiences mental illness in the same way. Nor do the resulting service and support needs remain consistent over time. PsyR programs must be designed to accommodate the varied and changing needs of individuals who may require different levels of services during different phases of their illness. A clubhouse member may benefit from ongoing involvement with the program even after returning to full-time employment. Such involvement may take the form of a "graduate" group gathering one evening a week or occasional attendance at clubhouse-sponsored recreational activities on the weekends. For many consumers, continuous access to a PsyR program, and practitioners and peers whom they trust, is an essential ingredient for recovery.

Ruth Hughes, formerly executive director of IAPSRS, points out that for many consumers the issue is not membership for life but access for life. This means that "Just as we need to increase services, we also need to facilitate decreasing services and helping people move on when they no longer need us as much" (personal communication, August 31, 1998). Consumers who know that, if needed, they will always be welcome to return will have more courage to explore new opportunities.

Coordination of services is also a crucial aspect of successful community integration. Consumers may be involved with several different PsyR or mental health agencies at the same time, or may need to be referred to different service providers as their needs change over time. Case management services (see Chapter 7) are one effective strategy for accomplishing this coordination. Consider the problem of service coordination described in the following example:

> *Laura is a quiet and somewhat passive young woman who seeks to please both her family and the various practitioners who work with her. She sees a psychiatrist once*

*a month at a community mental health center where she and her family are also
involved in a family psychoeducation and support group. Currently, the group
facilitator is encouraging Laura and her family to work toward their stated goal of
Laura returning to college. Meanwhile, the free-standing clubhouse program that
Laura attends three times a week is in the process of placing her in a full-time position through their supported employment program. Laura is ambivalent about her
future and becoming increasingly anxious about working toward conflicting goals.*

Clearly the lack of service coordination described above can interfere with successful
rehabilitation. Even more important, more work needs to be done to help Laura clearly
determine what she wants. Such situations can result in both a waste of professional
resources and can set up consumers for failure.

9. Vocational Focus

Work is an important aspect of life and should be available to everyone who wants it.
Joe Marrone, a nationally known vocational services advocate believes that not working
is not really a viable choice, "I Think You Should Work, That's What I Think" is the title
of one of his regular talks; he points out the true drawbacks of not working including
poverty and isolation (Marrone & Golowka, 2000). In other words, all adults, with or
without disabilities, should work. PsyR practitioners do not question the ability of someone
to work, but rather assist the individual to acquire the skills, resources, and supports necessary for success. PsyR practitioners know that it is the absence of skills rather than the
presence of mental illness that create barriers to successful living.

A good example of this principle is the case study in Chapter 9 covering vocational
rehabilitation. Even though Carl had failed repeatedly at his attempts to work, the program
continued to support him in pursuing his goal. Rather than focusing on the failures, the
job coach focused on his strengths, skills, and interests and explored the supports that
might help him to succeed. Maintaining a consistent focus on the vocational goal eventually leads to vocational success.

10. Skills Training

PsyR services and providers should be capable of helping people in recovery acquire
the skills necessary to function successfully in the environments of their choice.

Skills training often encompasses much more than the specific skills one needs to work
on a job. We are often unaware of the skills we employ to negotiate everyday situations.
Consider the set of skills that need to be mastered just to get through a job interview. The
effective PsyR practitioner identifies the skills his client needs to succeed and then helps
him or her acquire them. Role playing the interview might reveal that the client speaks
too softly and does not make eye contact. The practitioner might role-play these skills for
the client, teach the skills, and then provide opportunities for practice until the practitioner
and the client feel the skill has been mastered.

11. Environmental Modifications and Supports

PsyR services and providers help people with disabilities access or negotiate the environmental modifications and supports necessary to function successfully in the environments of their choice. Environmental modifications and supports can take many forms.

For someone in a wheelchair, providing a ramp into a building is an important modification. For someone with mental illness, a change in working hours to accommodate a public transportation schedule might be a very important modification.

12. *Partnership with the Family*

Families are, in many cases, the most important and stable support system for persons with severe mental illness. State-of-the-art psychiatric rehabilitation includes family members as partners whenever possible if it is acceptable to the consumer. Thus, the best PsyR programs will have family members, together with consumers, on advisory and governing boards of directors. At the same time, consumer involvement is promoted among any services offered to families. Today, family psychoeducation in the form of ongoing multiple family groups with the consumer present is recognized as an evidence-based practice.

This strategy, which is described in more depth in Chapter 13, achieves important outcomes for the consumer as well as the family. PsyR professionals and agencies promote communication with interested family members, with the consent of consumers. For example, family members who inquire about their family member who is receiving PsyR service are often denied information for reasons of confidentiality and lack of a signed release. Best practice in this case means having an appropriate release of information or consent signed prior to a family member asking for information. Given that numerous consumers live with their families, it is critical that family members become engaged as partners in the processes of rehabilitation and recovery. For more information about the role of the family in PsyR, see Chapter 13.

13. *Evaluative, Assessment, Outcome-Oriented Focus*

To ensure that services are effective, providers must continuously evaluate and assess the outcomes they achieve and the quality of their services on both an individual and a system-wide level. Continued evaluation and assessment are very important, for instance, to identify changes in the needs of the population that programs are designed to serve. These population changes are much more common than might be imagined. Consider the apparent increase in the number of persons with a severe mental illness and a substance abuse problem. Since few of the newly deinstitutionalized persons had substance abuse problems in the 1960s, there was little need for substance abuse services. Long periods of hospitalization may have reduced the possibility of substance abuse for many of these people. After deinstitutionalization, when most persons with severe mental illness entered the community, professionals became aware of increasing numbers of consumers with substance abuse problems (Caton, 1981; Drake & Wallach, 2000; Pepper, Ryglewicz, & Kirshner, 1981). Facilities that employed program evaluation strategies and regularly monitored their outcomes were the first to identify this new need in their treatment population and begin to devise specifically designed services for them.

A Proposed Integrated-Structural Model of Psychiatric Rehabilitation

Corrigan (2003) has proposed a structural model of psychiatric rehabilitation that integrates a variety of models and approaches that have been implemented during the last few decades. His conceptualization includes (1) goals, (2) strategies, (3) settings, and (4) roles. Corrigan identifies goals as the overall mission and vision of PsyR. He identifies these goals as *inclusion*, *recovery*, and *quality of life*, similar to the conceptualization outlined in Table 4.1 near the beginning of this chapter. He also adds additional goals; *promoting opportunities, independence,* and *empowerment* of people with psychiatric disabilities. Corrigan makes a clear distinction between goals and tangible (measurable) benchmarks that indicate progress toward achieving goals. These benchmarks include reduced symptoms, improved social and coping skills, increased support, and better resources. A wide range of strategies or approaches are used in pursuit of the goals outlined earlier. Examples include instrumental support (assistance with problem solving), social support, goal setting, skills training, skills transfer training, cognitive rehabilitation, and family education and support.

The pursuit of these goals by means of various strategies can be implemented in three broad categories of settings: residential, vocational, and day/activity recreation. Residential can include hospitals, halfway houses, group homes, and, of course, a person's own home (see Chapter 11). Vocational settings include educational settings and competitive and supported employment (Chapters 9 and 10), and day activity/recreational settings (Chapter 6).

Corrigan (2003) emphasizes that different categories of individuals play important roles in the pursuit of the goals of PsyR. They play different "parts" in the PsyR process and are essential to the various settings. Clearly, the consumer or person with a disability is the most important participant. Practitioners who have different educational and skill levels are also critical to PsyR and, of course, most of the contents of this book are devoted to their role. Corrigan highlights other important roles such as the consumer's significant others, particularly family members (Chapter 13). In addition, he mentions a special group, consumers who are in professional helping roles with other consumers, sometimes known as "prosumers" (Manos, 1993), a word combining "professional" and "consumer." This is also discussed in Chapter 12.

Psychiatric Rehabilitation Ethics

A code of ethics is an intellectual framework that is consistent with the principles and values of a profession. It helps us analyze and make decisions when faced with moral choices. All professions (e.g., medicine, law, psychology) have a specific code of ethics. An important step in the evolution of PsyR from a service provision approach to a distinct profession was the development and adoption in 1996 of a Code of Ethics for Psychiatric Rehabilitation Practitioners by IAPSRS (now called USPRA). The USPRA code has five sections, each of which addresses a different aspect of professional practice: conduct and comportment, ethical responsibility to people receiving services, ethical responsibility to colleagues, ethical responsibility to the profession, and ethical responsibility to society.

The USPRA Code of Ethics addresses issues that often arise in day-to-day practice such as confidentiality, dual relationships with consumers, and consumers' right to make decisions about the services they receive, including the right to refuse services. What a code cannot do, however, is provide definitive answers for all situations that have ethical implications. Sometimes the guidelines are very clear; the USPRA code clearly states that it is unethical for a practitioner to have a sexual relationship with a client. It also cautions practitioners not to otherwise exploit their relationships with consumers. So it would be inappropriate for a practitioner who had a side business selling health care products to solicit sales to consumers.

BOX 4.1

USPRA, the Knowledge and Skills of Psychiatric Rehabilitation

As a first step toward professional certification and licensing, in 1996 the International Association of Psychosocial Rehabilitation Services, now the United States Psychiatric Rehabilitation Association (USPRA), established the national Registry for Psychiatric Rehabilitation Professionals. In 2001, the registry was replaced with a test-based certification program, establishing a new credential, the Certified Psychiatric Rehabilitation Practitioner (CPRP) administered by the Commission on the Certification of Psychiatric Rehabilitation (http://www.uspra.org/certification).

This exam is based on input from more than 500 subject matter experts—psychiatric rehabilitation practitioners from the United States and Canada. They defined the role of the psychiatric rehabilitation practitioner, identifying the knowledge and skills that are most important and most frequently used to deliver competent services. More than 90 tasks were identified, which were grouped into seven domains (IAPSRS, 2001):

1. *Interpersonal competencies:* Interpersonal communication that is both respectful and effective is integral to delivering effective PsyR services. Being a good listener, paraphrasing effectively, and communicating respect are essential to working with service recipients, their families, and others.
2. *Interventions of PsyR:* Interventions are actions taken by staff in collaboration with consumers. Many interventions are employed in PsyR, which we discuss in most of the chapters of this book including the evidence-based practices mentioned in this chapter, as well as promising practices such as recovery-oriented interventions, clubhouses, group interventions, and crisis interventions.
3. *Assessment, planning, and outcomes:* Rehabilitation or treatment planning is critical to the field and is discussed in detail in Chapter 5. Helping consumers define and refine their goals and developing the plans to achieve these is critical. Identifying personal strengths, personal interests, and assessing readiness for rehabilitation, as well as conducting specialized functional and environmental assessments are included.
4. *Community resources:* Knowing and accessing the resources and services the community offers that can promote the recovery and quality of life of those served by PsyR service recipients is essential.
5. *Systems:* Understanding large government systems, nonprofit, and community-based services is helpful to the work of the PsyR practitioner.
6. *Diversity:* PsyR practitioners serve persons of diverse cultural, racial, ethnic, and economic backgrounds; sensitivity to these factors and issues is important.
7. *Professionalism:* Knowledge of the Code of Ethics (IAPSRS, 2001), dedication to one's consumers, and respect for colleagues and the profession are also important. Also included is the desire to seek more knowledge and learn new practices thorough continuing education and other initiatives.

Source: From IAPSRS, 2001.

CONTROVERSIAL ISSUE
Self-Determination versus Quality of Life

Today, for all practical purposes, deinstitutionaliza-tion is an established fact. In addition, in many areas it is relatively rare for any persons with a severe and persistent mental illness to be hospitalized for any length of time. The era of long periods of treat-ment in psychiatric institutions is clearly at an end and a period of community treatment is well under way. Nearly all providers of community treatment are in agreement with the goals of deinstitutional-ization. The principle of least restrictive treatment environment is also widely supported. Through the courts in the United States and other countries, the right of persons not to be hospitalized against their own will has been greatly strengthened during the last four decades. Self-determination, consumer rights, and consumer empowerment are on the increase as is acceptance of the contribution of consumer providers. These changes appear to support the values, goals and principles of PsyR we have presented.

In *Out of the Shadows: Confronting America's Mental Illness Crisis*, E. Fuller Torrey (1997) makes a strong argument for both maintaining beds in psy-chiatric hospitals and liberalizing involuntary com-mitment for both outpatients and inpatients (the ability to hospitalize or treat someone with severe mental illness against his or her wishes). He starts with the fact that persons with severe mental illness frequently need hospitalization, if only for a short time, as part of their treatment. Torrey is not alone in this position. In his book, *I Am Not Sick: I Don't Need Help,* Amador (Amador & Johanson, 2000) focuses on the fact that some persons with severe mental illness are unaware they are ill. Hence, involuntary medication or hospitalization may be required. Indeed some consumers themselves have written of the utility and necessity of involuntary treatment in helping them begin to recover (e.g., Fox, 2000, 2004a, 2004b).

The goal of deinstitutionalization, Torrey goes on to argue, tends toward the reduction of too many hospital beds through hospital closings and reduced funding, which in turn encourages keeping people in the community when they should be in the hospital. In addition, he believes that the legal profession has gone too far in their campaign to liberate (sic) psychiatric patients. This effort has resulted in legal policies which dictate that persons can only be hospitalized against their will if they are a clear danger to themselves or others and the right of hospital patients to refuse medication. Torrey points out that some courts have ruled that living on the street and eating your own feces does not constitute a threat to the individual or others. He quotes a psychiatrist, Donald Trefert, commenting on a case where a judge found that a man was within his rights to refuse psychiatric treatment:

> The liberty to be naked in a padded cell in a county jail, hallucinating and tormented, without treatment that ought to be given is not liberty, it is another form of imprison-ment—imprisonment for the crime of being ill. (Torrey, 1997, p. 143)

It would be difficult for anyone to make an argu-ment that, whether right or wrong, Torrey does not have the best interests of persons with severe mental illness in mind. He has dedicated his profes-sional life to their cause, taking many difficult and unpopular stands along the way.

Another Viewpoint

Some advocates for the rights of people with severe mental illness have firsthand experience as psychi-atric inpatients. As such, they have been victims of (or witnesses of) atrocities carried out in the name of involuntary psychiatric treatment. Patricia Deegan (1990), a psychologist and activist diag-nosed with schizophrenia, describes watching a fellow inpatient suffer:

> Quietly I slipped past the mental health worker and looked inside the seclusion room. An old man, probably about 60 or so, with white hair and very thin, was strapped down

on a green rubber mattress. Heavy leather cuffs lashed his wrists and ankles to the cold steel of the metal bed frame. He was stripped naked except for his underwear. When I saw that mental health worker sitting in casual comfort outside of the room in which the man was restrained, humiliated and crying out for help, I froze in terror and disbelief. For a moment I could not move. I felt numb. Then I felt a tearing inside my heart. (p. 304)

Deegan has helped to form a campaign advocating against the use of both seclusion and restraint in psychiatric hospitals. Her fellow advocates include people who witnessed similar experiences with involuntary treatment and some who, "talked of being stripped naked and being left in their own urine and feces" (Stevens, 1991, p. 20). It is hard to imagine such individuals as being better off than those described above by Dr. Torrey.

A basic premise of activists in the ex-patient movement (also called the ex-psychiatric inmate movement or psychiatric survivor movement) is that service recipients experience much of what the mental health system calls treatment as unwanted control over their lives and in some cases as abuse. Individuals who are suffering from physical illnesses are rarely forced to take medication or remain in a hospital against their will, even despite the fact that a decision not to follow a doctor's order can have serious consequences. Consider the case below:

Jack is a 59-year-old man (with no apparent mental illness) who has been suffering from adult-onset diabetes for more than 10 years. One symptom of his disorder is ulcers on his hands and feet, which take many months to heal. His doctor warns him that if he does not take his medication regularly, alter his dietary habits, and keep regular medical appointments for ongoing wound care, he runs the risk of a gangrenous infection that could result in amputation or death. Jack does not heed his doctor's advice. His wife is extremely concerned and consults the doctor. They both come to the conclusion that

there isn't much that can be done, because Jack is an extremely stubborn man who mistrusts the medical profession. Forced treatment, such as commitment to a medical facility, is never considered as an option because Jack has a legal right to refuse treatment. It is very unlikely that a court would assume the parens patriae (parental) role and order medical treatment in the case of an adult not assumed to have a mental illness. A few months later Jack develops a severe enough infection to require amputation of both his legs.

Although involuntary treatment was never considered in Jack's case, people diagnosed with mental disorders are committed by the courts to psychiatric hospitals on a regular basis. According to ex-patient movement activist Judi Chamberlin (1990) this constitutes discrimination. She and other advocates maintain that:

The basic principle of the [ex-patient] movement is that all laws and practices which induce discrimination toward individuals who have been labeled as mentally ill need to be changed, so that a psychiatric diagnosis has no more impact on a person's citizenship rights and responsibilities than does a diagnosis of diabetes or heart disease. To that end, all commitment laws, forced treatment laws, insanity defenses, and other similar practices should be abolished" (p. 329).

Although we may wish that there were some way to force both an acutely psychotic individual who is living in squalor and "Jack" to accept treatment, there are some real issues we must grapple with before accepting Dr. Torrey's recommendations. One concern is raised by persons who question the effectiveness of psychiatric inpatient treatment, particularly as it is provided in large state institutions. Another issue is whether the individual's basic civil rights are violated with the loss of their freedom.

Who is right? Has deinstitutionalization and the movement for patients rights gone too far, as Torrey suggests? Or, are individual civil rights paramount in all cases?

Otherwise, there is a great deal of controversy in the PsyR field about what are the appropriate limits of relationships between practitioners and consumers. Sometimes practitioners are faced with difficult ethical dilemmas. For example, relationship boundaries between consumers and PsyR practitioners can be difficult to determine. While practice guidelines (IAPSRS, 1996) call for reduced professional boundaries and staff members are generally encouraged to develop friendly and informal relationships with consumers, some agencies have strict policies forbidding staff to socialize with consumers outside of the program environment. Other PsyR programs do not discourage the development of outside friendships with consumers, as long as the relationship is in the best interest of the consumer. Thus, in certain social situations PsyR providers have to make difficult decisions. Is it appropriate to take a consumer out to lunch to celebrate a birthday or achievement of a goal? Should one accept a Christmas gift from a client? Is it acceptable to attend a consumer's wedding reception?

Practitioners need to be aware of possible ethical dilemmas in their everyday activities. Familiarity with the USPRA Code of Ethics (see Box 4.2) is a good starting point. First of all, it can help practitioners recognize when they are grappling with an issue that has ethical implications. Secondly, it assists them in determining whether or not a considered solution is consistent with PsyR standards for ethical behavior. Practitioners also need to be aware of specific agency policies, and state laws that may apply to practice issues such as client confidentiality. Finally, good practitioners who recognize that they are on the horns of an ethical dilemma seek out supervision and/or team discussion of the situation in order to reach the best possible solution.

Researching the Principles of Psychosocial Rehabilitation

In an important set of studies, Cnaan and his colleagues (1988, 1989, 1990) addressed the lack of clarity around the definition of psychosocial rehabilitation (PSR). (*Note:* PSR and PsyR are different terms for the same set of practices.) They believed that the lack of agreement on the definition of PSR causes several problems. Lack of a clear definition tends to render any term, such as psychosocial rehabilitation, meaningless, since anything might be termed or labeled PSR. This all-inclusiveness also hinders the development of an agreed-on body of knowledge that represents PSR. Finally, because there is little agreement as to what constitutes PSR there is no way to evaluate a program regarding how well it is carrying out PSR. In response to these issues, Cnaan et al. attempted to identify, clarify, and confirm some of the definitional issues surrounding PSR.

In two initial studies (Cnaan et al., 1988, 1989), they identified 15 principles derived from the PSR and PsyR literature. Then, in a third study (Cnaan et al., 1990), the research team translated each principle into two or three specific PSR activities or practices. The presence of these practices indicated that the corresponding principle was adhered to. In other words, if an activity was deemed important in a particular PSR setting, they assumed that the principle that the activity represented was supported.

From this work, a survey instrument composed of activities and practices representing the 15 principles was created. Next, using a *Delphi* method (i.e., asking the experts for their opinions), the researchers identified a large group of PsyR experts from (1) authors

BOX 4.2
USPRA Code of Ethics

The following is taken from the Code of Ethics adopted by IAPSRS (now USPRA) in 1996 and updated in 2001.

Major Ethical Principles

The following principles should guide Psychiatric Rehabilitation Practitioners in their various professional roles, relationships and levels of responsibility in which they function professionally.

Conduct and Comportment

A. Practitioners maintain high standards of personal conduct in their role as a Psychiatric Rehabilitation Practitioner.
B. Practitioners strive to be proficient in Psychiatric Rehabilitation and in the delivery of services.
C. Practitioners regard as primary the obligation to help individuals achieve their needs and self-determined goals.
D. Practitioners promote multi-cultural competence in all places and relationships in the practice of Psychiatric Rehabilitation.

Ethical Responsibility to People Receiving Services

A. The primary responsibility of Practitioners is to persons receiving Psychiatric Rehabilitation Services.
B. Practitioners refrain from entering into dual relationships with persons receiving their services.

C. Practitioners act with integrity in their relationships with colleagues, families, significant others, other organizations, agencies, institutions, referral sources, and other professionals in order to maximize benefits for persons receiving services.
D. Practitioners make every effort to support the maximum self-determination of each person served.
E. Practitioners respect the privacy of consumers and hold in confidence all information obtained in the course of professional service.

Ethical Responsibility to Colleagues

A. Practitioners treat colleagues with respect, courtesy, fairness and good faith.

Ethical Responsibility to the Profession

A. Practitioners uphold and advance the mission, ethics and principles of Psychiatric Rehabilitation.
B. Practitioners assist the profession by promoting the field of Psychiatric Rehabilitation.
C. Practitioners take responsibility for identifying and developing experienced based psychiatric rehabilitation knowledge.

Ethical Responsibility to Society

A. Psychiatric Rehabilitation Practitioners promote the general welfare of society by opposing discrimination and increasing understanding of psychiatric disability and recovery.

of PsyR research literature, (2) the board of directors of IAPSRS (now USPRA), and (3) recent presenters at IAPSRS conferences. Seventy-two of these experts responded to the survey consisting of items about the importance of different activities PSR practitioners perform (that were presumed to relate to the 15 principles). Results from a factor analysis revealed support for 13 of the original 15 principles.

In another recent effort, also based on an extensive literature review, Cook and Hoffschmidt (1993) reviewed models (treatment strategies) of psychosocial rehabilitation. Their review identified 11 principles of PSR that are found, in different degrees, in nearly every PSR service. Both of these lists contributed to the goals, values, and guiding principles presented earlier in this chapter.

Researching and Promoting Recovery

Many consumers and service providers accept the general conception of recovery expressed by Deegan (1988), Leete (1989), and Anthony (1993, 2000). The idea of creating a recovery vision for the mental health system was introduced by Anthony (1993, 2000). He based his thesis on the experiences and writings of people living with a psychiatric disability. He described how persons in recovery have noted that it is a deeply personal and unique process involving the individual with a psychiatric disability changing his or her life goals, attitudes, and feelings. The individual develops hope and is able to go on with life despite the limitations of the illness. Several components of recovery have been identified in the writings of people living with a psychiatric disability. These include recovery factors internal to the individual such as gaining insight into their illness, empowerment, developing self-care strategies; and external factors such as relationships and supports. Still, how this process works, how recovery can be encouraged, helped, or enhanced, and a host of other questions remain unanswered.

Davidson and Strauss (1992) asked 66 participants who had been hospitalized and then followed for 2 to 3 years after discharge to describe their recovery process. Participants discussed the evolving sense of self as an important part of recovery. In another study, Davidson (1992) asked 46 people with psychiatric disabilities to identify the elements that helped them with recovery. Acceptance of the illness, feeling in control, and support from others were identified as three important elements.

Studies have focused on examining the published literature written by people with psychiatric disabilities. Jacobson (2001) reviewed 30 published recovery narratives and found that important recovery themes were focusing on the role of the self, support from others, the influence of the mental health system, and how the individual views the origin of the illness. Ridgway (2001) reviewed four published narratives and found the components of recovery to consist of experiencing a reawakening, having hope, accepting the illness, and the importance of support from others. Another project completed by Smith (2000) obtained 10 narratives from people who have psychiatric illnesses and attended a mental health consumer run program. Important parts of the recovery process appear to include medication management, needing to be in control of the illness, support from others, and having meaningful activities.

Despite the lack of understanding still surrounding the recovery concept, several initiatives have been developed to assist recovery. Spaniol, Kohler, and Hutchinson (1994) developed a workbook to help people with psychiatric disabilities learn about their own recovery. Part of the recovery process they describe encourages people with psychiatric disabilities to discuss their own experiences with mental illnesses. Another tool to help people with their recovery, the Wellness Recovery Action Plan (WRAP), was developed by Copeland (1997). This self-management strategy provides consumers with a tool to identify strengths and copings strategies that can be used to monitor triggers or early warning signs of symptom exacerbation and to develop a personal crisis plan to help them prevent relapses and foster personal wellness.

Onken and colleagues (2002) organized focus groups of mental health consumer leaders to examine recovery. They developed a definition of recovery that included the following elements: having hope, understanding and acceptance of the illness, developing a new sense of self, and the value of supports. They found that individuals attributed recovery to a diverse range of factors influencing their own journeys.

The Future of Psychiatric Rehabilitation Thought and Practice

It should be clear that some values, goals, and principles were derived from humanistic ideals that seemed "right" to practitioners at the time. Other ideas were borrowed from more established fields such as psychiatry, psychology, rehabilitation, and social work. Regardless of the source of these values, goals, and principles, their continued use will be based on their (1) utility as guides to effective rehabilitation and (2) ability to withstand testing through empirical research and evaluation.

No one should be surprised if some of the concepts put forth in this chapter are modified or even discarded over time. Consider, for example, how attitudes about hospitalization have evolved over time. During the period before deinstitutionalization, a person diagnosed with a major mental illness who experienced continuous psychotic symptoms had a very good chance of spending most of his or her life in a psychiatric institution. With deinstitutionalization the goal was to get people out of the institutions and into the community. Some practitioners embraced this policy with such fervor that one might have suspected that the community itself was a therapeutic agent. Once in the community the primary goal changed to the prevention of rehospitalization. Many services considered any client who did not require rehospitalization a success. Today, as our understanding of these illnesses has matured, we have adopted the goals of recovery, community integration, and quality of life. In this new conception, hospitalization, if it is necessary, is seen as a manifestation of the disease and treated as a minor setback.

Will our attitude toward hospitalization change again? We should not be surprised if it does. Each of these changes should reflect a better understanding of persons with mental illness and the conditions themselves. These changes usually represent progress.

Summary

Psychiatric rehabilitation shares many similarities with physical rehabilitation. The most important development in PsyR has been the development of a concept of recovery. Recovery in PsyR means that the individual establishes a new self-image that incorporates the fact that he or she has a mental illness, not absence of disease. The primary goals of PsyR are to achieve recovery, maximum community integration, and the highest possible quality of life. These goals are supported by values including self-determination, respect for human dignity, optimism, and the belief that all people have the capacity for growth. PsyR goals and values are actualized in practice by following specific guiding principles. USPRA, the national professional organization, has established practice guidelines and ethical principles to help guide the field. These goals, values, and guidelines may change as the field advances and new knowledge is created.

Class Exercise

Ethical Dilemma

The following vignette describes a situation that has ethical implications. Carefully read the vignette and then consider the questions that follow.

> Eric is a 29-year-old man with a history of many psychiatric hospitalizations. He has been referred to a number of PsyR programs in the past, but has been difficult to engage. Eric's symptoms typically include restlessness, confusion, and paranoia, and while he seems to respond well to antipsychotic medications, he frequently refuses to take them. Following a hospital discharge, Eric returns home to live with his mother and is assigned to an assertive community treatment program in which a team of staff provides services for Eric at his home. Eric is reluctant to talk with the team members when they visit and more often than not, despite pleas from his mother, refuses to take medication. The team decides to implement the following plan: Eric's mother, who is the payee for his monthly disability check, will give him a weekly allowance of spending money if he complies with the following conditions: (1) taking his medication as prescribed twice a day, and (2) talking with the team members when they visit. Each time Eric refuses to take a dosage or talk to the staff, he will be docked a specific amount of money. The staff's rationale is that coercion is necessary to both prevent exacerbation of symptoms and to establish a relationship with Eric. Eric resents the plan, but needs money for cigarettes so he goes along with it.

Questions
1. From the team's point of view, how can their plan help Eric achieve the PsyR goals of recovery, community integration, and a better quality of life?
2. From Eric's point of view, what are the negative implications of the team's plan? Can the plan interfere with the achievement of the PsyR goals mentioned above?
3. Is the plan consistent with PsyR values such as self-determination?

4. If the answer to Question 3 is no, can you think of a plan that would be helpful to Eric and be more consistent with PsyR values?

References

Amador, X., & Johanson, A. L. (2000). *I am not sick: I don't need help.* Peconic, NY: Vida Press.

Anthony, W. A. (1993). Recovery from mental illness: The guiding vision of the mental health service system in the 1990's. *Psychosocial Rehabilitation Journal, 16*(4), 11–23.

Anthony, W. A. (2000). A recovery-oriented service system: Setting some system level standards. *Psychosocial Rehabilitation Journal, 24*(3), 11–23.

Anthony, W. A., Cohen, M. R., & Farkas, M. D. (2002). *Psychiatric rehabilitation.* Boston: Center for Psychiatric Rehabilitation, Boston University.

Anthony, W. A., & Nemec, P. B. (1983). Psychiatric rehabilitation. In A. S. Bellack (Ed.), *The treatment and care of schizophrenia.* New York: Grune & Stratton.

Bandura, A. (1977). *Social learning theory.* Englewood Cliffs, NJ: Prentice Hall.

Carling, P. (1995). *Return to community.* New York, Guilford Press.

Caton, C. L. M. (1981). The new chronic patient and the system of community care. *Hospital and Community Psychiatry, 32,* 475–478.

Chamberlin, J. (1990). The ex-patient movement: Where we've been and where we're going. *Journal of Mind and Behavior, 11,* 323–336.

Cnaan, R. A., Blankertz, L., Messinger, K. W., & Gardner, J. R. (1988). Psychosocial rehabilitation: Towards a definition. *Psychosocial Rehabilitation Journal, 11*(4), 61–77.

Cnaan, R. A., Blankertz, L., Messinger, K. W., & Gardner, J. R. (1989). Psychosocial rehabilitation: Towards a theoretical base. *Psychosocial Rehabilitation Journal, 13*(1), 33–55.

Cnaan, R. A., Blankertz, L., Messinger, K. W., & Gardner, J. R. (1990). Experts assessment of psychosocial rehabilitation principles. *Psychosocial Rehabilitation Journal, 13*(3), 59–73.

Cook, J. A., & Hoffschmidt, S. J. (1993). Comprehensive models of psychosocial rehabilitation. In R. W. Flexer & P. A. Solomon (Eds.), *Psychiatric rehabilitation in practice* (pp. 81–97). Boston: Andover Medical Publishers.

Copeland, M. E. (1997). *Wellness recovery action plan.* West Dummerston, Vermont; Peach Press.

Corrigan, P. W. (2002). Testing cognitive models of mental illness stigma: The Prairie State stigma studies. *Psychiatric Rehabilitation Skills, 6*(2), 232–254.

Corrigan, P. W. (2003) Towards an integrated, structural model of psychiatric rehabilitation. *Psychiatric Rehabilitation Journal, 26,* 346–358.

Davidson, L. (1992). Developing an empirical-phenomenological approach to schizophrenia research. *Journal of Phenomenological Psychology, 23*(1), 3–15.

Davidson, L., & Strauss, J. S. (1992). Sense of self in recovery from severe mental illness. *British Journal of Medical Psychology, 65,* 131–145.

Deegan, P. E. (1988). Recovery: The lived experience of rehabilitation. *Psychosocial Rehabilitation Journal, 11*(4), 11–19.

Deegan, P. E. (1990). Spirit breaking: When the helping professions hurt. *The Humanistic Psychologist, 18*(3), 301–313.

Drake, R. E., & Wallach, M. A. (2000). Dual diagnosis: 15 years of progress. *Psychiatric Services, 51*(9), 1126–1129.

Fairweather, G. W. (Ed.). (1980). *The Fairweather Lodge: A twenty-five year retrospective* (New Directions for Mental Health Services No. 7). San Francisco: Jossey-Bass.

Fox, V. (2000). Empathy: The wonder quality of mental health treatment. *Psychiatric Rehabilitation Journal, 23*(3), 292–293.

Fox, V. (2002). First person account: A glimpse of schizophrenia. *Schizophrenia Bulletin, 28*(2), 363–365.

Fox, V. (2004a). First person account: Schizophrenia and motherhood. *Schizophrenia Bulletin, 30*(4), 763–765.

Fox, V. (2004b). Medication. *Psychiatric Rehabilitation Journal, 27*(3), 287–289.

Fox, V., & Geller, J. L. (2004). Cresting. *Psychiatric Services, 55*(6), 641–642.

Gill, K. J., & Pratt, C. W. (1993). Profit sharing in psychiatric rehabilitation: A five-year evaluation. *Psychosocial Rehabilitation Journal, 17*(2), 33–41.

Harding, C. M., Brooks, G. W., Ashikaga, T., Strauss, J. S., & Breier, A. (1987). The Vermont longitudinal study of persons with severe mental illness, II: Long-term outcome of subjects who retrospectively met DSM-III criteria for schizophrenia. *American Journal of Psychiatry, 144*(6), 727–35.

Harding, C. M., & Zahniser, J. H. (1994). Empirical correction of seven myths about schizophrenia with implications for treatment. *Acta Psychiatrica Scandanavica, 90*(Suppl 384), 140–146.

International Association of Psychosocial Rehabilitation Services. (1996). *Core principles of psychiatric rehabilitation*. Columbia, MD: Author.

International Association of Psychosocial Rehabilitation Services. (2001). *Role delineation study of psychiatric rehabilitation practitioner*. Morrisville, NC: Columbia Assessment Services.

Jacobson, N. (2001). Experiencing recovery: A dimensional analysis of recovery narratives. *Psychiatric Rehabilitation Journal, 24*(3), 248–256.

Leete, E. (1989). How I perceive and manage my illness. *Schizophrenia Bulletin, 15*, 197–200.

Lehman, A. F. (1983). The well-being of chronic mental patients: Assessing their quality of life. *Archives of General Psychiatry, 40*, 369–373.

Lehman, A. F. (1988). A quality of life interview for the chronically mentally ill. *Evaluation and Program Planning, 11*(1), 51–62.

Liberman, R. P., Wallace, C. J., Blackwell, G., Eckman, T. A., Vaccaro, J. V., & Kuehnel, T. G. (1993). Innovations in skill training for people with serious mental illness: The UCLA social and independent living skills modules. *Innovations & Research, 2*(2), 46–59.

Link, B. G., Phelan, J. C., Bresnahan, M., Stueve, A., & Pescosolido, B. A. (1999). Public conceptions of mental illness: Labels, causes, dangerousness, and social distance. *American Journal of Public Health, 89*, 1328–1333.

Manos, E. (1993). Prosumers. *Psychosocial Rehabilitation Journal, 16*(4), 117–120.

Marrone, J., & Golowka, E. (2000). If you think work is bad for people with mental illness, then try poverty, unemployment, and social isolation. *Psychiatric Rehabilitation Journal, 23*(2), 187–193.

Onken, S. J., Ridgway, P., Dornan, D. H., & Ralph, R. O. (2002). *Mental health recovery: What helps and what hinders?* Washington, DC: National Technical Assistance Center for State Mental Health Planning.

Pepper, B., Ryglewicz, H., & Kirshner, M. C., (1981). The young adult chronic patient: Overview of a population. *Hospital and Community Psychiatry, 32*, 463–469.

Phelan, J. C., Cruz-Rojas, R., & Reiff, M. (2002). Genes and stigma: The connection between perceived genetic etiology and attitudes and beliefs about mental illness. *Psychiatric Rehabilitation Skills, 6*(2), 159–183.

Pratt, C. W., & Gill, K. J. (1990). Sharing research knowledge to empower people who are chronically mentally ill. *Psychosocial Rehabilitation Journal, 13*(3), 75–79.

Rapp, C. (1998). *The strengths model.* New York: Oxford University Press.

Rappaport, J. (1987). Terms of empowerment/exemplars of prevention: Toward a theory for community psychology. *American Journal of Community Psychology, 15*(2), 121–144.

Ridgway, P. (2001). ReStorying psychiatric disability: Learning from first person recovery narratives. *Psychiatric Rehabilitation Journal, 24*(4), 335–343.

Rogers, E. S., Chamberlin, J., Ellison, M. L., & Crean, T. (1997). A consumer-constructed scale to measure empowerment among users of mental health services. *Psychiatric Services, 48*, 1042–1047.

Smith, M. K. (2000). Recovery from a severe psychiatric disability: Findings of a qualitative study. *Psychiatric Rehabilitation Journal, 24*(2), 149–158.

Spaniol, L., Kohler, M., & Hutchinson, D. (1994). *The recovery workbook: Practical strategies for people with psychiatric disability.* Boston: Center for Psychiatric Rehabilitation, Sargent College of Allied Health Professions, Boston University.

Stevens, K. (1991, November). The mental health liberation movement. *Sojourner: The Women's Forum*, pp. 20–21.

Torrey, E. F. (1997). *Out of the shadows: Confronting America's mental illness crisis.* New York: John Wiley & Sons.

Torrey, E. F. (2001). *Surviving schizophrenia.* New York: Harper Collins.

Warner, R., Taylor, D., Powers, M., & Hyman, J. (1989). Acceptance of the mental illness label by psychotic patients: Effects on functioning. *American Journal of Orthopsychiatry, 59*(3), 398–409.

Wolfensberger, W. (1983). Social role valorization: A proposed new term for the principle of normalization. *Mental Retardation, 21*(6), 235–239.

Chapter 5

Psychiatric Rehabilitation Methods

Introduction 140
Consumer Choice 141
  Environments of Choice 142
Psychiatric Rehabilitation
  Readiness 142
  Readiness Assessment 143
Rehabilitation Diagnosis 144
  Functional Assessment 146
  Resource Assessment 146
Rehabilitation Plan 147
Rehabilitation Interventions 147
The Story of Paul (Continued from
  Chapter 1) 147
Skill Acquisition and Development 149
  Skills Training and Direct Skills
    Teaching 149

Modeling 151
A Consumer-Centered Approach 151
Behavioral Strategies 152
Establishing a Rationale 153
Skill Generalization and Skill
  Maintenance 153
Principles of Skill Development 154
Resource Development 155
  Environmental Modifications 155
Evaluating Rehabilitation Progress 156
Summary 158
Class Exercise 159
References 160

This chapter will outline the basic strategies involved in the rehabilitation of persons with severe mental illness. Many of these ideas had their origin in the efforts to rehabilitate persons with physical disabilities. The inability to effect a cure and, in some cases, to arrest the symptoms of mental illnesses has been a barrier. The constant presence of the illness for many individuals and the subsequent emphasis on symptom reduction often relegated the rehabilitation process to a lower priority in the eyes of professionals and even some consumers. Today, as evidenced by the concept of recovery championed by Deegan, Anthony, and many others, there is general agreement that rehabilitation should begin as soon as possible. There is encouraging evidence of the numerous social, vocational, emotional, and psychological benefits to the rehabilitation process.

This chapter will answer the following questions:

1. *What elements make up a successful psychiatric rehabilitation intervention?*
2. *What is the role of the professional in the rehabilitation process?*
3. *What is the role of the consumer in the rehabilitation process?*
4. *Can consumers learn skills and can they apply the skills they have learned?*
5. *What role do environmental supports and modifications play in the rehabilitation process?*

Introduction

William Anthony and the staff of the Center for Psychiatric Rehabilitation at Boston University have been at a focal point of the psychiatric rehabilitation (PsyR) movement in this country for some time. Combining knowledge from areas such as psychology, occupational therapy, and rehabilitation counseling, as well as formulating and field-testing strategies based on scientific evidence, this group developed a PsyR "technology" or systematic strategy for rehabilitation. In addition, the Center for Psychiatric Rehabilitation has put a great deal of effort into training professionals in their PsyR technology both at Boston University and through consulting on a national and international basis. At times their efforts have met with resistance, due to misunderstandings about how their techniques worked as well as perceived threats to cherished beliefs and philosophies such as an adherence to psychodynamic principles. Today it is generally recognized, by any objective assessment, that the center's contribution to the successful rehabilitation of persons with severe mental illness has been incalculable.

Many others have also made important contributions in this area. For example, Robert Paul Liberman and his colleagues at UCLA have been strong proponents of a skills training approach for some time (Liberman et al., 1985; Liberman, DeRisi, & Mueser, 1989). Robert Drake and his colleagues at the New Hampshire–Dartmouth Psychiatric Research Center have taken a leading role in the movement toward evidence-based practices for psychiatric rehabilitation. In the relatively short time of several years, the efforts of this group to identify, define, and disseminate evidence-based practices have had a positive effect on the quality of service provided. Still, a major impetus for the development of the field of psychiatric rehabilitation must be directly credited to the work done at Boston University.

A successful rehabilitation process must be preceded by a thorough assessment of the consumer's readiness to participate in rehabilitation activities, his or her skill use, and the environments in which he or she operates or wishes to operate. Next, using the information from these assessments, a rehabilitation plan that outlines and prioritizes specific goals and objectives is formulated. Finally, the specific strategies to accomplish each goal or objective are identified. The Center for Psychiatric Rehabilitation characterizes these steps as the diagnostic phase, the planning phase and the intervention phase. We will cover each of these phases in more detail.

Consumer Choice

Consumer involvement in each and every aspect of the process is a basic ingredient of any successful rehabilitation. Consumer involvement is essential to ensure that the individual is ready to take action. Unlike the traditional approach to medical problems in which the doctor defines what is wrong and, therefore, what should be done, the rehabilitation process is designed to achieve the goals selected by the consumer. Goals that are set by the staff without real input from the consumer, even with the very best intentions, are not likely to be motivating. This may even be true in cases where a staff person selects the same goal the consumer would have if given the chance. Instead, the very act of its selection signifies ownership of a goal and helps to motivate a person to work toward its accomplishment.

A lack of involvement in the planning process might also cause problems later on due to incomplete information. For example, a person who likes animals and has some clerical and medical education might not be a good candidate for working in a veterinary hospital if he or she is highly allergic to cats.

The most important reason for maximum consumer involvement in the PsyR process may be to foster recovery. As Deegan (1988) describes this process, the task for the

---

BOX 5.1
William A. Anthony

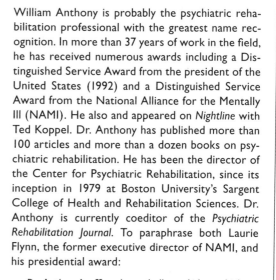

William Anthony is probably the psychiatric rehabilitation professional with the greatest name recognition. In more than 37 years of work in the field, he has received numerous awards including a Distinguished Service Award from the president of the United States (1992) and a Distinguished Service Award from the National Alliance for the Mentally Ill (NAMI). He also and appeared on *Nightline* with Ted Koppel. Dr. Anthony has published more than 100 articles and more than a dozen books on psychiatric rehabilitation. He has been the director of the Center for Psychiatric Rehabilitation, since its inception in 1979 at Boston University's Sargent College of Health and Rehabilitation Sciences. Dr. Anthony is currently coeditor of the *Psychiatric Rehabilitation Journal*. To paraphrase both Laurie Flynn, the former executive director of NAMI, and his presidential award:

> *Dr. Anthony's efforts have challenged ideas which have limited the potential of persons with mental illness. The innovative programs created through his leadership offer hope and opportunity by promoting the dignity, equality, independence and employment of people with disabilities.*

individual is the creation of a new self-image that incorporates the fact that one has a mental illness. This topic is covered in Chapters 4 and 12. The re-creation of a new self-image demands that the individual be included in every aspect of the PsyR process from the setting of goals and time frames to achieve those goals to the setting of the criteria for success. Recovery, after all, must be the ultimate goal of the PsyR process.

Environments of Choice

Unlike a medical evaluation, which assesses a person's overall health, PsyR interventions are targeted toward the consumers' environments of choice. In short, they are targeted toward what will enable the consumer to function in the specific environments where he or she chooses to live, work, and socialize. By targeting specific environments, the rehabilitation task is made both more relevant and more manageable. Only the skills and resources necessary for success in the environments of choice are developed. Symptoms or negative behaviors that are not problematic in the environments of choice may not be given high priority. This strategy represents a clear difference from the emphasis of some prevocational training efforts that have attempted to help consumers become vocationally ready in all areas without regard to the specific characteristics of a particular job.

An important goal of the PsyR process is to assist people to be successful and satisfied in the environments of their choosing. Rather than just focusing on the individual and his or her disability, PsyR includes an assessment of the requirements and characteristics of the environment and may attempt to modify these as part of the overall plan. Such modifications might consist of flex hours, more frequent breaks, or more obvious environmental cues. The importance of environmental assessment and modification was highlighted by the 1990 Americans with Disabilities Act, which calls for "reasonable accommodations" to assist individuals with disabilities on the job. These reasonable accommodations often take the form of environmental modifications or policy adjustments that aid the consumer in his or her job.

Psychiatric Rehabilitation Readiness

Psychiatric rehabilitation readiness refers to an individual's desire and motivation to pursue some aspect of psychiatric rehabilitation. Without such desire or motivation, an individual will not act to achieve a goal. Some degree of readiness is, therefore, a necessary element for rehabilitation success. This focus on readiness is in sharp contrast to much of medical and psychological practice. When a treatment is seen as superior for a particular condition, it is often prescribed without offering the patient any alternatives, since in many cases the doctor's view is that there are no realistic alternatives. In the case of psychiatric rehabilitation, the success of the process is dependent on the readiness of the individual to work toward the rehabilitation goals.

Rehabilitation is essentially carried out through a partnership between the individual and the psychiatric rehabilitation professional(s). As several theorists have pointed out, psychiatric rehabilitation is "a service that must be done *with* a person never *to* a person"

(Cohen & Mynks, 1993). This aspect of "working together" is one of the hallmarks of the profession.

Why would an individual be reluctant to choose and pursue a goal to improve his or her situation in life? Several possible factors may impede psychiatric rehabilitation readiness. As is often the case, when several of these negative factors are combined in one individual, the level of readiness for psychiatric rehabilitation is very low. Many candidates for psychiatric rehabilitation have experienced numerous and repeated failures in their attempts to improve their lives. These failures may come about because of relapses, lack of necessary skills, inadequate environmental supports, ineffective training, poor planning, and from setting goals inappropriate to the individual. Individuals often experience several of these problems at once, particularly if they are working with poorly trained or overworked PsyR staff. After several failures, an individual might be tempted to avoid getting his or her hopes up and just accept his or her lot in life. For these persons, positive change may not seem to be a real possibility. In short, they may lack the confidence necessary to participate in rehabilitation.

Some individuals become so habituated to the role of "psychiatric patient" that they do not want to change roles. Whether they are fearful of change or just stuck in their ways, these individuals would rather stay in their present situation than work toward change.

For example, important factors working against many persons pursuing an employment goal are a lack of knowledge about their own abilities, unfamiliarity with characteristics of various work environments, and a lack of awareness of the supports that are available. Consider the example of anyone looking for a career. Many people do not know enough about their own likes and dislikes, about the kinds of jobs that might be available and about the kinds of skills that are required for these jobs. For example, how many of your friends know about PsyR, the kinds of skills required, and what a PsyR professional would do all day? If the typical person lacks this vocational and self-knowledge, consider someone who has been coping with a major mental illness all of his or her adult life. A lack of knowledge of who we are and what is possible can narrow our choices and reduce our motivation.

Readiness Assessment

Several researchers (Cohen, Farkas, & Cohen, 1992; Cohen & Forbess, 1992; Cohen & Mynks, 1993) have stressed that one of the first steps in the psychiatric rehabilitation process should be a *readiness assessment*. The goal of this type of assessment is to evaluate the individual's readiness for entering a psychiatric rehabilitation process that has a good chance of success. If the individual is not ready for such a process, they recommend that services be targeted toward improving or developing the person's readiness for rehabilitation. These readiness activities, such as exploring goals, values clarification, and discussion of family expectations, would be targeted at the kinds of problems mentioned earlier.

A readiness assessment is much more than a practitioner concluding an individual consumer "is not ready." In fact, the judgments of professionals in this regard are often very inaccurate. Therefore, Cohen, Farkas, and Cohen (1992) recommended that a readiness assessment must look at five distinct factors:

- *Need for change.* This asks the question: Does the individual perceive a need for change? Or conversely, how dissatisfied is the individual with his or her current situation? This includes the influence of environmental issues such as how successful the individual is in his or her current environment and whether or not the environment is forcing a change (e.g., being evicted from an apartment).
- *Commitment to change.* This assesses the person's belief that change is (1) necessary, (2) positive, (3) possible, and (4) will be supported. Has the person taken concrete steps or actions to pursue change? Can the person see himself or herself making the change, or does the individual believe someone else or the circumstances have to change?
- *Environmental awareness.* This assesses the person's knowledge, including previous experiences, about the chosen environments in which they plan to operate.
- *Self-awareness.* This assesses the individual's knowledge about himself or herself. For example, his or her likes and dislikes, personal values, and strengths and weaknesses.
- *Closeness to practitioner.* This evaluates the relationship with the PsyR professional on dimensions such as trust. A close working relationship theoretically should contribute to a more effective rehabilitation process.

A person with high scores on each of these five dimensions is considered ready for rehabilitation and, more importantly, has a very good chance of success. If, on the other hand, a person has low scores on one or more of these dimensions, services need to be targeted toward improving those areas. Valid and reliable measures of rehabilitation readiness are now available (Roberts, 2006; Roberts & Pratt, 2006).

Increasing or developing individual readiness can take place in many ways. Beginning the rehabilitation process itself can encourage readiness by increasing a person's self-awareness and awareness of alternative environments. Educational and experiential efforts may be necessary to convince a person that recovery from a mental illness and achieving normalized role functioning such as being a worker, student, parent, or homeowner are realistic possibilities.

A lack of readiness does not imply that a person cannot benefit from psychiatric rehabilitation. Instead, low rehabilitation readiness should guide individualized services designed to increase readiness and prepare the individual for the choice and pursuit of goals. A lack of attention to the readiness issue may be at the root of some poor PsyR service outcomes.

Rehabilitation Diagnosis

The *rehabilitation diagnosis* is based on the consumer's choice of the environments in which he or she wishes to function. Identifying an *overall rehabilitation goal*, and conducting both a *functional assessment* and a *resource assessment* are all part of the rehabilitation diagnosis. The first step in the diagnosis process is setting the overall rehabilitation goal. One aspect of setting this goal is looking at the range of choices within the environment. For example, a person may consider several different housing arrangements (e.g., single apartment, shared apartment, group home) for a living environment. The requirements for each of these housing choices are then compared to the person's resources and characteristics. Once the possible options are determined, the individual's needs and preferences are considered in making the final choice of the goal. This goal-setting process is designed to increase the chances of success and ensure satisfaction once the goal is achieved. A person's desire to achieve a goal will influence his or her effort and perseverance. This process can be synthesized into three stages: (1) developing decision-making skills, (2) determining the requirements of the environment, and (3) determining what the individual needs to be successful in the chosen environment. Once these steps have been achieved, the match between the environment and the individual will be evident and an appropriate goal can be set. It is important to remember that the goal is based on the individual's preferences, not solely on the individual's skills.

Once a goal has been established, the PsyR practitioner and the consumer need to determine the skills and resources that the consumer will need to be successful and satisfied in his or her chosen environment. These skills need to be described in behavioral terms that allow for an objective evaluation of how well the consumer performs them and the necessary level of performance for success in the living, learning, working, or social environment. Once the skills and behaviors required for a certain environment are listed, an assessment of the consumer can take place.

The diagnostic process can be carried out in several ways. Most typically, it is carried out through individual meetings between the PsyR practitioner and the consumer. Some programs employ group meetings where several consumers will work together with a staff person or a team of PsyR professionals to arrive at rehabilitation goals and conduct assessments. When outside funding organizations such as a state vocational rehabilitation agency are involved, consumers may be referred for standardized skill and interest testing. These tests, which are usually expensive to administer and score, can provide detailed profiles of a consumer's basic areas of interest, skills, and skill deficits. In contrast, sometimes, they provide little useful information. Some of these tests employ task simulation strategies to evaluate skills such as dexterity, following directions, and problem solving. For example, a consumer who has expressed interest in studying to be an electrician might be given the tools, material, and instructions to build an electric circuit. His or her ability to follow directions, use the tools properly, and finish the task in a timely manner would be assessed. Although these tests are designed to achieve a clear assessment of a person's skills and abilities, they are hampered by the fact that they are not carried out in the actual job setting. Their principal advantage is that they can produce a fairly systematic and objective evaluation of specific skills.

By contrast, when a "place then train" approach is used, the on-the-job assessments that are carried out relate directly to that person's success on the actual job. Situational assessments in real environments are usually superior, but not always possible.

Functional Assessment

At this stage, the PsyR professional and the consumer can determine which skills and behaviors constitute either strengths or weaknesses for the environment of choice; in short, how well the consumer is functioning with respect to his or her environment of choice. Strengths are things that the consumer does well, meaning at or above the required level. Weaknesses are areas that need improvement or development. Because it is often more important to reinforce strengths than to emphasize weaknesses, the PsyR practitioner should focus first on consumer strengths.

Charles Rapp and his colleagues have made important contributions highlighting the importance of focusing on a person's strengths rather than weaknesses or disability (Rapp, 1997). Many people make positive changes in their lives when they feel strong enough to accomplish the change. Focusing on one's strengths helps provide a sense that change is possible and will be successful. A person's area of strength often identifies where that person will perform well and can be an important clue to the type of job that person will enjoy and be a success at. Finally, strengths are what a person has to offer on a job or in any environment. As Pat Nemec of Boston University points out, when a person has excellent "people skills" (a strength), but is also "disorganized" (a weakness), training and support can reduce the disorganization more easily than if the "people skills" were poor. And, "crabbiness," for example, can't be changed very easily.

Areas where the consumer's performance does not match the required level are identified for further assessment and future intervention. For example, Jane, who is the receptionist at her PsyR day program, wants to be a receptionist in a law office. Her strengths are a clear and pleasant telephone voice and a polite and professional manner when answering the phone. To be successful, she also needs to take clear messages listing who the call was for, the caller's name and number, the time of the call, and the message. A review of her work as the program receptionist indicates that of the 20 or so messages Jane takes on her 2-hour shift, one or two omit some of the needed information. For her new job Jane will have to be able to take messages without omitting the required information.

You may have noticed that before we can help Jane correct these messages we need to determine why she is omitting information. It could be, for example, that Jane has a slight hearing problem. Or, it may be that Jane doesn't know what information is most important to include in a message. Perhaps she is distracted by either having to field several calls at once or by other people speaking to her when she is trying to record a message. Whatever the case, Jane's message-taking ability won't be improved unless the problem can be clearly identified.

Resource Assessment

The availability of resources that can assist the consumer to achieve his or her goals must also be assessed. These resources, such as transportation, housing assistance, and special training, might relate either to a specific environment such as a job situation or to the needs of the individual. For example, because of scheduling constraints, it is not uncommon for a consumer to have to change her case manager, therapist, or psychiatrist when she gets a job. Such a resource adjustment should be planned for in advance to ensure that it does not cause unnecessary problems for the consumer. The goal of the resource assessment is to identify resource strengths, deficits, or problems so that they can be dealt with in the rehabilitation plan.

Rehabilitation Plan

The *rehabilitation plan* sets forth the skill and resource goals and objectives that consumers must achieve to operate in the environments of their choice. An important aspect of the rehabilitation plan is that these goals and objectives are prioritized by the consumer. Obviously, some skills need to be acquired before other skills. For example, someone who wants to do word processing should acquire some ability at keyboarding before he or she attempts to learn the intricacies of a word processing program. Another important aspect of this prioritization process is how it is experienced by the consumer. Everyone likes and needs to experience some success from their efforts. For persons who have gone through many previous failures, starting with the most difficult task first might not be the best strategy. Instead, it might be more motivating to start with a task that can provide some success in the short term and build up to the more difficult tasks. Unlike more traditional therapies, decisions about this kind of motivational issue are the responsibility of the PsyR professional and the consumer working as a team.

The rehabilitation plan is essentially an integration of (1) the decisions the consumer has made about what environments he or she wishes to operate in, (2) the functional and resource assessments, and (3) knowledge about the consumer and the best path to take to achieve his or her goals.

Rehabilitation Interventions

Rehabilitation interventions are the specific strategies for acquiring needed skills, behaviors, and resources. This is the information that is usually recorded in a consumer's rehabilitation plan (sometimes referred to as an *individualized service plan* or *treatment plan*). As such, these interventions need to be specific, objective, quantifiable, and time delineated. In short, they need to be very clear to everyone concerned, particularly the consumer. When behaviors and goals are described in quantifiable ways, they can be easily interpreted. For example, Jane may be maintaining a rate of 85% accuracy in her weekly message taking. A goal might be that Jane will improve her accuracy to a rate of 95% per week. By giving the goal a time frame, say, 2 months, Jane and her PsyR practitioner will be able to objectively evaluate her progress.

The Story of Paul (Continued from Chapter 1)

We first met Paul in Chapter 1. The following aspect of Paul's story covers his attendance at a program and his efforts, with the aid of his counselor Ruth, to achieve his goals. As you read the following story, look for the strategies that Ruth uses to help Paul move toward recovery.

Paul was nervous about what to expect on his first day at the program. After getting a short tour of the program from one of the members, he was directed to his counselor, Ruth. Ruth invited Paul to have a seat and then chose a seat for herself across from him rather than behind her desk. "You know, Paul, you and I have some important and exciting work to do. We have to figure out what you want your life to look like, what your goals are, and how to reach those goals. But before we get started on that, I wonder if you have some questions or concerns? I know the first day here can be confusing." Paul was reluctant at first to ask questions, but Ruth encouraged him to be honest with her, so he talked about the people who looked like they'd been at the program forever, about "schizophrenia," and about his terrible experience at college. Finally, Paul said "I can't believe my life is over. I don't want to come here for the rest of my life." "Good," said Ruth, "then let's talk about where you do want to be."

During the meetings that followed, Paul and Ruth talked about all areas of his life. Paul decided that he was happy living with his parents for now. They got along okay and he couldn't afford to pay rent anyway. They seemed happy to have him there even though they worried a lot about him and he wished they wouldn't. His social life was dismal. He'd pretty much alienated everyone he knew when he was "getting sick." Most important to Paul, though, was that he'd dropped out of school. His first love was still business. He couldn't imagine doing any other kind of work. Ruth and Paul agreed that going back to school was the area to start with.

Paul felt hopeful and scared at the same time. His goal of graduating with a degree in business had seemed out of reach a few months ago. Paul wondered if he was kidding himself. He imagined his professors seeing him back in class after he'd failed the first time and remembered the hurtful things he'd said to his friends. But Paul trusted Ruth. When he told her about these concerns she didn't dismiss them or accept them as evidence that he couldn't go to school. Instead she talked about making sure Paul had the supports and resources he would need to succeed in this goal.

Paul and Ruth listed the critical skills for him to reach this goal. Naturally, he'd have to meet all the requirements of the courses, so he would need to be able to focus on oral presentations and written materials, study for exams, and write coherent papers. Although Paul used to excel at these academic skills, he was concerned because both his concentration and stamina were diminished because of the illness and the medication. He'd also have to get some kind of transportation to school because he wouldn't be living on campus this time, and he'd have to learn to manage the symptoms he was still experiencing: hearing voices and feeling withdrawn.

With Ruth's encouragement, Paul contacted the registrar at the college he'd been attending. He found out that he'd withdrawn from some classes and failed others. In any case, he'd have to start over. He decided to take one course and he and Ruth agreed it should be Introduction to Marketing, since this was his area of interest and he'd be more likely to do well.

There was one month left until the start of the next semester. During this time, Ruth taught Paul how to use the public transportation system. To practice, Paul took the bus to the school a few times to help him feel less anxious about the trip. A few weeks before the course started, Paul contacted the professor and got permission to audiotape the class lectures. This way he could listen to the tapes to help organize his notes. He also got the reading assignments for the semester to help him plan his study schedule. He knew that his problems concentrating meant he'd have to start early because he'd need lots of breaks.

Ruth helped Paul set up a schedule that included study time, relaxation time, and meetings with her for support and problem solving. Paul's parents were skeptical about his plan to return to school. They were convinced that the stress of school is what had "pushed him over the edge." However, with Ruth's help, Paul was able to tell them how important school was for him and how important their support would be to his success. Paul's parents agreed to support his plan as long as they could figure out what to do if Paul got sick again. Paul, his parents, and Ruth made a list of things that would indicate that he was experiencing another episode of his illness and the things people could do to help.

Paul and Ruth had a meeting scheduled the day the midterm grades were posted. Paul arrived looking worried. "You look like your grade wasn't what you'd hoped for," Ruth offered. Paul looked surprised. "Oh, no," he chuckled, "I got a 'B'! It's just that, well, some of the guys in my class invited me out to sort of celebrate, you know. It means I'd have to cut our meeting short." "Go!" Ruth laughed. "Go and have fun! I'll see you next week. Call me if anything comes up before then. Oh, and by the way, Paul, good work!"

Skill Acquisition and Development

As you can see from the preceding example, a skill is the ability to successfully perform a behavior at a certain level, in a specific context. Acquiring and developing skills refers to teaching and refining specific behaviors so that they can be performed both correctly and frequently enough for success in the individual's environment of choice (Nemec, McNamara, & Walsh, 1992).

Effective skills teaching is much more involved than the kinds of didactic lectures usually experienced by high school and college students. This is particularly true when persons have been discouraged by repeated failures or when they have to simultaneously cope with other issues such as psychiatric symptoms.

Skills Training and Direct Skills Teaching

The two major proponents for a skills training approach to PsyR have been the Center for Psychiatric Rehabilitation at Boston University led by William Anthony and the Clinical Research Center for Schizophrenia and Psychiatric Rehabilitation at the University of California at Los Angeles (UCLA) led by Robert Paul Liberman. The UCLA group has simply titled their strategy *skills training*. Liberman's group has put a great deal of effort into the development of modules for teaching specific skills, for example, medication maintenance. Staff members at the Center for Psychiatric Rehabilitation call the technology they devised for teaching skills *direct skills teaching* (DST). The term *technology* conveys the importance this group places on the systematic application of the DST method.

Nemec, McNamara, and Walsh (1992) created an informative table in order to illustrate the subtle differences between skills training and direct skills teaching. The similarities should be apparent as you review the comparison between the two strategies presented in Table 5.1. Keep in mind that this table was formulated by researchers from the Boston University (DST) group.

TABLE 5.1
Skills Training versus Direct Skills Teaching

	Skills Training	**Direct Skills Teaching**
Purpose	Skills development	Skills development
Foundation	Learning theory, behavior therapy	Education "teaching as treatment"
Components	**Assessment**—determination of skill deficits in a targeted area (e.g., social skills).	**Assessment**—determination of skill performance requirements of consumer's performance in relation to environmental requirements.
	Acquisition—person can perform target behaviors.	**Acquisition**—person can perform the skill as needed.
	Generalization—person can perform target behaviors in the natural environment.	**Generalization**—person can perform the skill as needed in his or her preferred environment.
	Maintenance—person can continue to perform target behaviors over time.	**Maintenance**—person can continue to perform skills as needed over time.
	Impact—the new skill plays a meaningful role in improving the person's life.	**Impact**—the new skill increases the person's success and satisfaction in his or her preferred environment.
Techniques	**Instructions**—specific directions or requests to elicit behavior.	**Orient person to process**—comprehensive explanations and descriptions of skill performance.
	Modeling—demonstrated performance of skill and competent behaviors.	**Show**—demonstrations of performance of skill and competent behaviors.
	Role-Play—practice of skill.	**Do**—practice of competent behaviors and performance.
	Feedback—strengths, weaknesses of performance presented with encouragement and reinforcement.	**Critique**—interactive discussion about strengths/weaknesses of skill performance, with encouragement and reinforcement.
	Homework—assigned practice with feedback and reinforcement.	**Skill Programming**—identification of barriers to successful skill performance, of action steps and of self-rewards to use to eliminate barriers to skill performance.

Source: From Nemec, McNamara, & Walsh, 1992, p. 15–16.

Modeling

One of the most important and most common ways people learn is through modeling. Everyone has used modeling at one time or another to shape their behavior. Consider a time when you were entering a new environment, say, a new school, a new club, or some other place where you were not exactly sure how to behave, dress, or speak. Your probable response to this situation was to observe others to see how they were acting, how they dressed, who they spoke with, and so on. After observing for a time you probably began to feel more confident about how to behave in the new environment. You could model your behavior on the behavior you had observed. You can see how several of the steps in Bandura's learning theory (see Box 5.2) utilize modeling.

Modeling is also part of the reason that many PsyR professionals attempt to reduce obvious differences between themselves and the persons with whom they are working. It is easiest to follow a model if we perceive that the people we are modeling are like ourselves. It is unlikely that a consumer in a PsyR program would model his or her behavior on a staff person wearing a name tag and an expensive suit who keeps his professional distance. It is more likely that a staff person who eats lunch with the consumers, pitches in on some of the chores, and attends some of the social events will be seen as a good role model.

A Consumer-Centered Approach

Consumer-centered therapy, introduced by Carl Rogers in the 1940s, was a substantial departure from the traditional psychoanalytic therapies of that time. Sometimes called

---

BOX 5.2
Social Learning Theory

Albert Bandura (1977) formulated a social learning paradigm that defines five learning steps an individual goes through when effectively acquiring a new skill. These steps are very similar to the strategy adapted for skills training by both the Boston University (direct skills teaching) and UCLA (skills training) rehabilitation research centers. As you review the following steps notice how each one builds on the previous step so that the skill or behavior is approached gradually:

1. *Instruction.* This is the didactic part of the process. (For example, you get the bus on the corner of Main and 2nd Street. You need to have the exact change, etc.)

2. *Modeling.* Here the consumer watches the instructor perform the skill. (For example, the instructor takes the bus with the consumer, demonstrating how it is done and essentially taking care of everything.)
3. *Role Playing.* Here the consumer role plays the situation and skill in question outside the applicable setting. (For example, the consumer role-plays getting on the bus, paying the fare, etc.)
4. *Behavioral rehearsal.* Here the consumer actually carries out the skill. (For example, the consumer takes the bus, with the instructor present or not.)
5. *In vivo practice.* Here the consumer practices doing the skill in the real situation. (For example, the consumer uses the bus on a regular basis for practice.)

nondirective therapy, consumer-centered therapy proposed that the role of the therapist was not to direct or instruct the consumer based on the therapist's theoretical beliefs but to assist the consumer in understanding his or her own experience of the world and to promote positive change through a trustworthy relationship (Brammer, Shostrom, & Abrego, 1989; Krech, Crutchfield, & Livson, 1969). To accomplish this, the therapist has to hold the consumer in positive regard. In other words the therapist has to respect the consumer and empathize with him or her.

The basic tenets of consumer-centered therapy are highly compatible with psychiatric rehabilitation and have had an important influence on the field. Consumer-centered therapy is based on the belief that people will engage in activities leading to positive growth and development if given the opportunity (Krech et al., 1969). This belief is consistent with the PsyR value of optimism or hope. The practitioner believes that everyone has the potential for growth. Consumer-centered therapy asserts that the opportunity for growth exists within relationships that offer empathy, positive regard, and genuineness (Brammer et al., 1989). In PsyR, we know that the quality of the consumer–practitioner relationship is crucial to recovery and rehabilitation. Here, too, the relationship is an egalitarian one, based on empathy, positive regard, and acceptance.

Consumer-centered therapy focuses on the consumer's perception of his or her present circumstances and assists the consumer in identifying his or her own answers to problems or barriers (Brammer et al., 1989). A major strategy in consumer-centered therapy is reflecting back to the consumer the feelings, thoughts, and behaviors the consumer has communicated to the therapist but may not be fully aware of. Psychiatric rehabilitation also focuses on the here and now and uses active listening and reflection to assist consumers in understanding their experiences.

Finally, consumer-centered therapy places the major responsibility for successful change on the consumer (Krech et al., 1969). In PsyR, we recognize the value of self-determination in achieving personal life goals. The work of counseling psychologist Robert Carkuff, author of *The Art of Helping VIII* (2000), has been a great help to many PsyR professionals. Carkuff's writings help to simplify the helping process into comprehensible steps that are easily understood by the practitioner.

Behavioral Strategies

One of the basic ways we teach skills is through the application of behavioral strategies. Popularized by B. F. Skinner, *behaviorism* has often been accused of being an essentially inhuman or insensitive approach to education. In reality, some form of behaviorism underlies almost every teaching strategy or style.

A basic principle of behaviorism is that we encourage behaviors by reinforcing them and extinguish behaviors by not rewarding them or punishing them. We accomplish this by using either positive or negative rewards or positive or negative punishments. In this case, think of positive or negative as implying adding something or taking something away, respectively; for example, the same way you think of positive (something added) or negative (something lost or taken away) symptoms of schizophrenia. Behavior can be encouraged using positive rewards. For example, if you complete this project, you will receive a higher grade. A behavior can also be reinforced using negative rewards. For example, if you complete this project you will not have to take the final exam. A positive punishment means that something negative is added. For example, if you do not do well on this test you will have to write an additional paper. A negative punishment means that something positive is taken away. For example, if you do not do well on this test you will not be allowed to go on the class trip.

This theme of reward and punishment is a common element in education. One point that behaviorists have stressed is that reward is almost always preferable to punishment. Even though both strategies may be equally effective at either encouraging or extinguishing a particular behavior, the use of punishment often causes unwanted negative effects. People do not like to be punished and often feel resentment toward the person or source of their punishment. This resentment often expresses itself in other negative behaviors that can cause unexpected problems.

Rewards are more important when they are granted correctly. You may have noticed that you are less interested in playing a game when you know you will always win. When games are difficult to succeed at, we consider them a challenge and work harder for the reward of winning.

Rewards are very important in the context of rehabilitation. When staff members are uneducated about the importance of rewards, they often give rewards too freely in an effort to encourage a consumer, or to be liked. When a reward (e.g., praise) is given too freely, or at times when criticism is more appropriate, it loses its value. Rewards need to be given out after careful evaluation to ensure that they are timely and appropriate. People feel rewards are meaningful when they believe they represent real achievement. When handled carefully, providing rewards can be an important form of communication about a person's progress and can reinforce positive behavior.

Establishing a Rationale

An important cognitive strategy for effective skill acquisition and maintenance is establishing a rationale for the skill with the consumer (Bellack, Mueser, Gingerich, & Agresta, 2004). Similar to motivational interviewing, the issue of why it is worth the effort to learn a particular skill needs to be addressed so that the consumer is motivated to acquire that skill. Individuals may not grasp the relationship between a particular skill, for example, socially appropriate communication, and a vocational goal such as becoming a secretary/ receptionist. Clarification of the need for the skill is a necessary first step if the individual is going to make a concerted effort to acquire the skill.

Skill Generalization and Skill Maintenance

Skill generalization and skill maintenance are two important factors that need to be considered for any successful rehabilitation plan. Skill generalization refers to the fact that behavior (or skill performance) is situation specific. In simple terms, just because a person can perform a skill in one environment does not mean that he or she can or will perform the same skill in a different environment. This problem has been one of the main drawbacks to the prevocational training strategy practiced for so long by PsyR services trying to get people back into the workforce. Individuals who demonstrated successful acquisition of prevocational skills (e.g., proper grooming, punctuality, attention to detail) at a PsyR program often did not maintain these skills when they started regular employment. This failure to generalize skills to other environments or settings appears to be a common human failing rather than a characteristic of individuals with mental illness. More recent strategies for vocational rehabilitation that have taken this factor into account, most notably, supported employment, have demonstrated much higher rates of successful job placement. (Vocational rehabilitation will be discussed in Chapter 9.)

Assigning skill practice as homework is an effective strategy for increasing the generalizability of skills. Practicing skills in other settings helps to habituate the individual to using the skill in different settings. This also allows the individual and the practitioner to identify problems that may exist when the target skill needs to be applied in a new setting. At this stage it is important to reassess the skill performance to determine whether progress is being made.

Skill maintenance is another important consideration for successful rehabilitation. You have probably noticed that when you do not perform a complex or difficult task for some time your performance level goes down. You might have experienced this if you used to be a fast typist, a good chess player, a scratch golfer, or performed any task in which higher levels of practice are necessary to maintain peak performance. The common saying describing this effect is "use it or lose it." For the individual going through rehabilitation, it is just as important to maintain skills that the person already has as it is to acquire new ones. Persons attending PsyR programs that mainly focus on therapy, recreation, and prevocational skills—instead of work skills and practice—often had fewer skills when leaving the program than they had when they entered.

The PsyR principle of emphasizing strengths rather than deficits helps to identify and highlight the skills that consumers possess. Awareness that these skills must be reinforced through regular practice will help to ensure that they are not lost.

Lastly, most people take pride in the things they do well. Maintaining skills as a source of pride for individuals is an important element in the rehabilitation process. The fact that a person can do some things very well gives one confidence that, with some time and effort, she or he will be able to do other things as well.

Principles of Skill Development

Cohen, Ridley, and Cohen (1985, as cited in Anthony, Cohen, Farkas, & Gagne, 2002) formulated 11 principles that should be considered in the development of skill intervention strategies. Notice how these suggested principles incorporate the ideas put forth in Bandura's social learning theory as well as behavioral strategies. In addition, Anthony and his colleagues (2002) pointed out that the application of these principles may increase the individual's ability to generalize learned skills to new environments.

1. Use the natural reinforcers present in the relevant environment to reward appropriate responses in the training environment.

2. Provide support services to the consumer in the relevant environment.
3. Teach support persons to use the skill of awarding selective rewards in the relevant environment.
4. Teach the consumer to identify intrinsic motivation (enjoying the task) as a replacement for extrinsic reward (pay or benefits).
5. Increase the delay of reward gradually.
6. Teach skill performance in a variety of situations.
7. Teach variations of skill use in the same situation.
8. Teach self-evaluation and self-reward.
9. Teach the rules or principles that underlie the skill.
10. Use gradually more difficult homework assignments.
11. Involve the consumer in setting goals and selecting intervention strategies.

Resource Development

One important area of the rehabilitation process is resource development or acquisition. Resources might be thought of as any person or thing that can assist someone to achieve their goals or be successful in environments of choice. Basic examples of resources are public entitlements that provide someone with financial assistance to meet living expenses. A PsyR practitioner might assist someone in applying for Social Security benefits, rental assistance, a prescription plan to purchase medications at reduced rates, or any number of other entitlement programs. A resource might also be an item that improves someone's ability to function in a particular setting, such as a bus schedule, or a watch that can be set to beep when it is time to take medication. Sometimes resources are people. A job coach who provides work support, a peer counselor at a drop-in center, or a friend who provides transportation to the program might all be considered resources.

In the rehabilitation planning process, the consumer and the PsyR practitioner will identify any needed resources. In some cases a consumer may choose to access a resource instead of developing a skill if he or she is unable to develop that skill or doing so would take too long. For example, instead of learning the skills of job acquisition, someone might rely on a job coach to make contact with potential employers. After identifying needed resources, the consumer and practitioner will assess whether or not the resources are currently available and articulate a plan to acquire those which are not.

Environmental Modifications

Another important set of elements in rehabilitation is the modifications to the environments in which the consumer wants to operate. Environmental modifications share some similarities with resource development, since they can include supports such as the presence of a job coach. In the workplace, environmental modifications might include assistance from a job coach, changes in policy that make allowances for the medical needs of consumers, and communication with supervisors and coworkers so that they have a clear understanding about mental illness.

BOX 5.3
*Evidence-Based Practice and
Psychiatric Rehabilitation*

The adoption of evidence-based practices (EBPs) by psychiatric rehabilitation, a relatively new development, is already having profound effects on the field. These changes both offer the promise of improved services and raise issues about the future of PsyR. EBPs produce specific outcomes by maintaining high fidelity (similarity) to a specific service model. For example, research tells us that high-fidelity assertive community treatment (ACT) programs reduce hospital utilization rates. If a service planner wishes to reduce the number of state-funded hospital beds, which tend to be very expensive, an effective solution would be to develop ACT programs. Of course, to ensure that hospital utilization rates were reduced, those programs would need to have fairly high fidelity with the EBP ACT model.

A concern of many PsyR professionals is that future funding will be increasingly directed toward EBP-type services at the expense of other services, which, because they are too broad (e.g., clubhouse; see Chapter 6) or too new (e.g., supported education; see Chapter 10), have not yet received empiri-

cal support. This is of particular concern to those in the PsyR field wishing to promote recovery. Because recovery is a unique individual process that may take many forms, it is unlikely to be engendered by a specific EBP.

At the same time, the EBP movement is having a profoundly positive effect on PsyR by providing reliable standards for what can be achieved. The adoption of standards will either reduce the number of ineffective services provided or serve as an impetus for reforming those services. Consider the supported employment (SE) EBP. Numerous vocational strategies (see Chapter 9) have been shown to be less effective than SE. Focusing on the employment outcomes that can be achieved by SE will help reform or remove funding from those programs. Ultimately, the effect will be that better vocational services will be available and more consumers will obtain competitive employment.

Any emphasis on EBP must be balanced with opportunities to study other promising practices. Today's promising practices may be tomorrow's EBPs, once enough high-quality evidence is gathered. This will lead to greater understanding of those services that produce positive outcomes and those that should be abandoned. The EBPs and promising practices are discussed in greater detail in the remaining chapters.

Since passage of the Americans with Disabilities Act (ADA) in 1990, reasonable environmental modifications are the law. Some of the more visible results of this law are handicapped parking spaces, cutouts on curbs, and building ramps for wheelchairs. The ADA will be explained in more detail in the chapter on vocational rehabilitation (Chapter 9).

Evaluating Rehabilitation Progress

An important step in the process of rehabilitation service planning is the periodic evaluation of progress toward rehabilitation goals and objectives. PsyR service providers typically evaluate the progress of consumers every 3 months, although the length of the time period between evaluations often varies quite a bit depending on agency policy and the individual needs of a particular consumer.

The primary importance of establishing rehabilitation goals and objectives with a consumer is that these help clarify what she or he is specifically hoping to accomplish.

CONTROVERSIAL ISSUE
Independence, Dependence, or Interdependence

Independence versus dependence has been an issue in PsyR since deinstitutionalization. Because of their disabilities, many persons who have a severe mental illness require ongoing support to reside comfortably in the community. As demonstrated by the effectiveness of case management programs, described in Chapter 7, without effective supports many individuals would be hospitalized more often and for longer periods of time. At the same time, efforts to achieve community integration, self-determination, and empowerment all suggest that independence is an important goal for the individual. Recovery itself is based on the individual deciding what he or she wants in life, something that cannot happen without a degree of independence.

Anthony et al. (2002), dealt with the issue of independence versus dependence in their formulation of PsyR principles. One principle states:

The deliberate increase in consumer dependency can lead to an eventual increase in the consumer's independent functioning.

On the first reading this may seem like a contradiction. It is the same contradiction that has troubled the PsyR community for many years. On further consideration, we can see that in order for a consumer to gain the benefits of rehabilitation he or she must be willing to go through the process. Hence, the consumer must follow the lead of (read: be somewhat dependent on) the rehabilitation practitioner in order to achieve the eventual goal of acquiring independence.

In one way, this conception of the independence versus dependence issue may be too simplistic. Who among us is truly independent? In fact, although we all achieve degrees of independence, we all have some areas of dependence. We may be dependent on a spouse or loved one or an institution such as a school or a job or anything else in our life on which we rely. At the same time, these people and institutions may be dependent on us. In fact, the issue is more correctly defined as one of *interdependence*, that is, being simultaneously dependent on others while they are dependent on us. This balance, which is both normalizing and empowering is often absent in the lives of people with disabilities. To complicate matters further, our degree of interdependency with elements in our environment may go through constant changes. Consider the parents who want to protect their child and help her to grow up and be self-reliant, or the couple that supports each other in their different careers while being dependent on one another. The real goal seems to be much more complicated than simply achieving independence. Instead, we must learn to be simultaneously comfortable with a degree of dependence and comfortable with a degree of independence.

Long-range goals are reduced to specific tasks that must be undertaken in sequence, guiding the person through the rehabilitation process. When this is accomplished, the individual has a sense of his or her own progress.

Evaluating whether goals are achieved is a much simpler task when goals are objective, time framed, easily quantified, and measurable. For example, a consumer's goal may be to improve punctuality. As it stands, this goal is rather nebulous and it would be difficult to assess the consumer's progress. This goal can be made specific and measurable by stating it this way: The consumer will arrive at the PsyR program location at 9:30 A.M., five times a week. In a program where the arrival time of consumers is logged, it is easy to keep track of progress toward this goal. More important, the evaluation results would be unequivocal. When all the goals and objectives specified on an individual's rehabilitation plan are written in an easily measurable form, determining whether or not progress has been made is easily evaluated, providing clear feedback to the consumer.

If a consumer and practitioner have determined that progress has been made toward a goal, the progress should be acknowledged in a positive manner. Once a goal is achieved, a new goal may be set. However, if progress has not been made or is too slow, the crucial task is to determine why. Sometimes practitioners do not ask this question and instead assume that more time is needed to work toward the existing goal. Although this may be the case, one should not jump to such a conclusion until the practitioner and consumer have thoroughly explored possible reasons for lack of progress. It may be that the basis for a particular deficit was not clarified to begin with. For example, a practitioner could assume that the reason a consumer often arrives late to a program is because he is not used to taking responsibility for being someplace on time. The actual reason could be that the consumer does not own an alarm clock. When practitioners make inaccurate assumptions about the cause of a problem, it is very unlikely that the intervention they devise to solve the problem will be successful. In the preceding example, the practitioner's original intervention might have been to give the consumer positive reinforcement. This might consist of praising the consumer each time he arrived on time and rewarding him with a cup of coffee at the end of the week if his punctuality showed improvement. However, if the root of the problem is actually the lack of an alarm clock, positive reinforcement may have no discernible effect. The appropriate intervention is helping the consumer purchase an alarm clock, which happens to be a good example of resource acquisition.

A lack of progress is often very frustrating for both the consumer and the staff. Sometimes it is difficult to determine why progress is not being made. There are several reasons why a consumer might not be motivated to achieve a goal. The consumer may feel that the goal is not really what he or she wants. It may be that the consumer has lost interest in working toward a particular goal. Or, it could be that although the consumer wants to achieve the goal, he or she is not ready to work on it. This last issue relates to rehabilitation readiness, as discussed earlier in the chapter.

Staff members need to be very thoughtful and empathic when progress is eluding a consumer. Too many staff members automatically associate lack of progress with lack of motivation and then fail to productively address the motivation/readiness issue. Frustrated practitioners tend to place blame on the consumer and think, "If she only would try harder she could do it!" The reality is often that practitioners need to make a greater effort to gain a clearer understanding of a consumer's situation. In some cases, the answer may be to abandon an unrealized goal and return to the initial stage of the service planning process: helping the consumer to choose a rehabilitation goal that is consistent with his or her rehabilitation readiness, as well as the person's hopes and dreams.

Summary

Rehabilitation methodology begins with consumer choice. The first task of the PsyR practitioner is often to help a consumer understand what his or her potential choices are and how to make decisions that the consumer will find satisfying. Before rehabilitation takes place, a consumer's readiness to begin a rehabilitation process can be assessed. Increasing rehabilitation readiness can be an important first step for someone who lacks the confidence to work toward a goal. Once a goal has been established, the PsyR practitioner helps the consumer evaluate the skills that will be required, the environmental supports that will be required, and the resources that can be made available. This approach provides the greatest chance for success. This is in contrast to strategies that focus on a consumer's deficits without regard for the specific skills needed for success in a specific environment. Instead, only those skills required for success in the environments that the consumer chooses to operate in are addressed. Skill teaching and modification can be achieved through a number of strategies including role modeling, direct skills teaching, and behavioral techniques. The basic philosophy used by the PsyR professional is a consumer-centered approach that respects the consumer.

Class Exercise

This exercise is designed to give you some familiarity with the PsyR service planning process. You will begin by doing a mock functional assessment and then choose critical skills on which to focus. Finally, you will identify appropriate PsyR interventions aimed at the achievement of an overall rehabilitation goal.

Read the following case study, and then complete the assigned tasks:

Anne is a 27-year-old woman who has a severe mental illness. She has spent much of the last 8 years in and out of psychiatric hospitals. In between hospitalizations Anne had lived with her parents. However, the last time she was discharged she was placed in a boarding home, where she now resides. Although Anne is currently stable and doing well in her part-time job as a receptionist in a dentist's office, she is unhappy with her living situation. She would like to move to her own apartment.

Anne tells Bill, her PsyR practitioner, that she would like to live on her own in her own place. Bill assists her in the process of researching local housing opportunities that are affordable for Anne. They determine that even with her monthly Social Security check, and the salary from her part-time job, it will be difficult to afford a one-bedroom apartment. However, they are able to place her on a waiting list for a federally subsidized housing complex. A few months later Anne gets a call. An efficiency apartment will become available in 3 months! Anne is both excited and apprehensive, because she is not totally sure she is prepared to live successfully on her own. She is particularly concerned about money, because she has very limited experience with managing her own finances. At the same time she knows that she has some important strengths like being able to keep the place clean, do the shopping, and keep up with the chores. It does concern her that she is unfamiliar with the location of the apartment complex. She has grown comfortable with the neighborhood her boarding home is in, in part because she can catch a bus on the corner which takes her to her job and the mental health center.

Anne sits down with Bill to plan for the move. They begin by writing an overall rehabilitation goal: "Anne will move into an efficiency apartment at the Cedar Hill Apartments in May 2006." Their next steps are (1) complete a functional assessment of Anne's independent living skills; (2) choose critical skills to begin working on; and (3) determine strategies for helping Anne acquire the skills and resources she will need.

Task 1

Create a list of "independent living skills" that you think are critical to Anne's success in her new apartment. It may be helpful to think about what skills you actually use, if you live independently. However, keep in mind that some of these skills may be necessary for some people to be successful and satisfied in their own home, but are not necessarily critical to Anne's success. Be prepared to discuss the rationale for your choices with the class.

Task 2

Now, rank order your list of skills starting from the most important. Be able to explain why you think that one skill might be more important than another.

Task 3

Consider the two or three skills that you have ranked as most important. What specific strategies would you suggest to help Anne develop those skills?

References

Anthony, W. A., Cohen, M. R., Farkas, M. D, & Gagne, C. (2002). *Psychiatric rehabilitation* (2nd ed.). Boston, MA: Center for Psychiatric Rehabilitation.

Bandura, A. (1977). *Social learning theory.* Englewood Cliffs, NJ: Prentice Hall.

Bellack, A. S., Mueser, K. T., Gingerich, S., & Agresta, J. (2004). *Social skills training for schizophrenia: A step-by-step guide* (2nd ed.). New York: The Guilford Press.

Brammer, L. M., Shostrom, E. L., & Abrego, P. J. (1989). *Therapeutic psychology: Fundamentals of counseling and psychotherapy*, 5th ed. Englewood Cliffs, NJ: Prentice Hall.

Carkuff, R. R. (2000). *The art of helping VIII.* Amherst, MA: Human Resource Development Press.

Cohen, M. R., Farkas, M. D., & Cohen, B. (1992). *Training technology: Assessing readiness for rehabilitation.* Boston, MA; Center for Psychiatric Rehabilitation.

Cohen, M. R., & Forbess, R. (1992). *Training technology: Developing readiness for rehabilitation.* Boston, MA: Center for Psychiatric Rehabilitation.

Cohen, M. R., & Mynks, D. (1993). *Compendium of activities for assessing and developing readiness for rehabilitation services.* Boston, MA; Center for Psychiatric Rehabilitation.

Deegan, P. E. (1988). Recovery: The lived experience of rehabilitation. *Psychosocial Rehabilitation Journal, 11*(4), 11–19.

Krech, D., Crutchfield, R. S., & Livson, N. (1969). *Elements of psychology*, 2nd ed. New York: Alfred A. Knopf.

Liberman, R. P., DeRisi, W. J., & Mueser, K. T. (1989). *Social skills training for psychiatric patients.* Elmsford, NY: Pergamon Press.

Liberman, R. P., Massel, H. K., Mosk, M., et al. (1985). Social skills training for chronic mental patients. *Hospital and Community Psychiatry, 36*, 396–403.

Nemec, P. B., McNamara, S., & Walsh, D. (1992). Direct skills teaching. *Psychosocial Rehabilitation Journal, 16*(1), 13–25.

Rapp, C. A. (1997). *The strengths model: Case management with people suffering from severe and persistent mental illness.* New York: Oxford University Press.

Roberts, M. M. (2006). A construct validity study of the employment readiness of people with serious psychiatric illnesses. Unpublished doctoral dissertation, University of Medicine and Dentistry of New Jersey, 2006.

Roberts, M. M., & Pratt, C. W. (in press). Putative evidence of employment readiness. *Psychiatric Rehabilitation Journal.*

Part III

Applications of Psychiatric Rehabilitation Principles and Methodology

Chapter 6

Psychiatric Rehabilitation Day Programming

Introduction 166

The Origins of Day Programming in the United States 167

The Development of Clubhouse Programs 168

Clubhouse Standards 170

Some Selected Standards for Clubhouse Programs 170

The Story of Jill, Affinity House Member 171

Partial Hospitalization 173

The Development of Partial Hospitalization Programs 174

Milieu Therapy 175

Components of a Psychiatric Rehabilitation Day Program 176

Service Recipients 176

Staff 177

Space 178

Program Ingredients 178

Scheduling 178

Evaluating Psychiatric Rehabilitation Day Programs 180

A Day Program Taxonomy 180

The Effectiveness of Day Programs 180

State-of-the-Art Psychiatric Rehabilitation Day Programming 183

Day Programming and Evidence-Based Practice 186

Summary 186

Class Exercise 187

References 188

Much of the development of psychiatric rehabilitation has taken place in community-based settings where groups of consumers gather during the day for friendship, support, recreation, rehabilitation, and treatment. These settings are potentially most effective when their environments are designed to promote the recovery of persons with severe mental illnesses. This chapter will explore the historical roots of these programs. Starting from two distinctly different program types, each emphasizing different philosophies, characteristics, and program elements, we will trace their eventual synthesis into today's psychiatric rehabilitation day program. We will examine how these programs may be designed and operated to help facilitate specific rehabilitation outcomes. Finally, we will discuss the potential for improved services inherent in the advent of evidence-based practices and the recovery movement.

This chapter will answer the following questions:

1. *What is psychiatric rehabilitation day programming?*
2. *When did day programming begin and how did it develop?*
3. *What are the common elements that make up a day program?*
4. *What is milieu therapy and how does it work?*
5. *How can programs be designed to produce specific outcomes?*
6. *What impact will evidence-based practices have on these programs?*

Introduction

Psychiatric rehabilitation (PsyR) day programs are based on the premise that an environment can be created that can assist in the rehabilitation and recovery of persons with severe mental illness. This type of setting is intended to improve quality of life and promote community integration. These programs have their roots in at least three distinct philosophies or movements: (1) the clubhouse movement, (2) partial hospitalization, and (3) milieu therapy. Within the community mental health field, these three program types are seen as quite different. For example, traditional therapy is a common element in many partial hospital programs. Clubhouses, on the other hand, do not see themselves as treatment programs and do not perform therapy. Milieu therapy represents a treatment style or philosophy rather than a specific program model, and it uses the program environment as the intervention. In that sense, both the clubhouse and partial hospitalization movements are based on principles of milieu therapy. Despite these differences, each of these movements shares the belief that working together, people can help each other promote rehabilitation and recovery.

The clubhouse movement began in the 1940s and 1950s as a natural response to the needs and wants of ex-psychiatric patients living in communities around the country. Facing stigma, rejection, unemployment, and poverty, these individuals began to band together for mutual support and comradeship. As these groups became established, they became recognized community support networks for persons with mental illness. This chapter will describe the development of Fountain House in New York City, one of the first clubhouses in the country. From that modest beginning, a worldwide network of clubhouses was established. The ex-patients attending these programs are known as *members* rather than *patients* and have a real say in how the clubhouse is operated. In turn, clubhouses are very responsive to the needs of their members.

As the deinstitutionalization movement grew in the late 1960s and 1970s, the treatment of many persons with severe and persistent mental illness began shifting from hospitals to community mental health center (CMHC) programs called *partial hospitals*. The *partial hospital* label reflects these programs' initial similarity to inpatient psychiatric hospitals. At a typical partial hospitalization program, groups of patients received various

BOX 6.1

What's in a Name? The Ongoing Confusion about Program Terminology

Psychiatric rehabilitation programs designed to provide day programming have many different labels. These programs are called partial hospitals, psychosocial programs, day treatment centers, psychiatric day care centers, and clubhouses to list just some of the more common names. To complicate matters further, programs with the same label may actually be quite different from one another, depending on when programs were established, where they are located, who the director(s) is, funding source requirements, and other factors. Much of this confusion came about because no general definition of these programs existed before they became widely established to provide services. Hence, as they designed these services, program developers were free to attach the names they believed best exemplified the services they were providing.

Much of this confusion over program types and labels still exists today. Programs, particularly the better ones, change and evolve in response to

advances in our understanding of how to provide effective services and changes in the needs of the populations they serve. For example, over time many of the programs originally designated as partial hospitalization programs began to take on program characteristics more commonly attributed to clubhouse programs. Many partial hospitalization programs have abandoned formal group therapy in favor of prevocational and vocational services to respond to the needs of a population interested in returning to work. In turn, in some instances clubhouse programs have adopted so many partial hospitalization or sheltered employment strategies that they are no longer "true" clubhouse programs. For example, many clubhouses have added medication monitoring components and services for persons with substance abuse problems, elements that are not available in a traditional clubhouse. This chapter will describe in detail the differences between these and other program types. In an effort to steer a middle course, this textbook will use the term *psychiatric rehabilitation day programming* to make general reference to this type of PsyR service.

types of service such as group and recreational therapy, socialization, medication monitoring, and activities of daily living skills training.

At their inception, both of these community-based psychiatric rehabilitation program models represented important treatment innovations for persons with severe and persistent mental illness. Much of the early development of PsyR took place in these settings. This chapter covers the history and development of these day programs.

The Origins of Day Programming in the United States

Today's PsyR day programs often combine elements from two distinct and very different treatment elements and philosophies: the clubhouse movement and the partial hospitalization movement. The clubhouse movement started as a grassroots movement. With extensive support from private charities, ex-hospital patients in several major cities around the nation developed clubhouses as everyday places to congregate for social support, recreation, and to address community living needs and problems.

In contrast, partial hospitalization programs were part of a large, federally funded program. Initiated by the federal government, numerous partial hospitalization programs were developed as elements of community mental health centers. These essentially medical model programs typically provided deinstitutionalized consumers with therapeutic and medication monitoring services from Monday through Friday. As it turns out, both the clubhouse movement and the partial hospitalization movement had something to offer persons with severe mental illness.

The Development of Clubhouse Programs

During the late 1940s a group of ex-patients from Rockland Psychiatric Center in New York State formed a support group, which met on the steps of the New York City Public Library in Manhattan. The support group members called themselves "WANA" (We Are Not Alone). A private social welfare group, the National Council of Jewish Women, became aware of the WANA group and began supporting their cause. In 1948, with the help of Elizabeth Schermerhorn, a building on West 47th Street in New York City was purchased as a clubhouse for WANA (Dincin, 1975; Flannery & Glickman, 1996; Propst, 1992a). Because it had a small fountain in the backyard the group named it Fountain House. Fountain House, initially staffed and operated solely by its members and volunteers, was designed to provide social supports and serve as a meeting place for ex-patients. People who joined Fountain House were called *members* rather than *patients* and, like a club, they could remain members for as long as they wished.

As Fountain House grew, the members decided to hire professional, non-consumer staff to operate the program. The first professional, non-consumer mental health staff were recruited in 1955. Even with the addition of professionally trained staff, Fountain House retained its clubhouse atmosphere and philosophy. After trying out several directors with unsatisfactory results a social worker named John Beard was hired. Beard helped to change Fountain House (Beard, Propst, & Malamud, 1982) from what was essentially a social club into a truly comprehensive psychiatric rehabilitation facility, which became the model for the clubhouse movement (see Box 6.2).

The National Council of Jewish Women played a major role in the development of the clubhouse movement and psychiatric rehabilitation nationwide. During the 1950s this philanthropic group focused its attention on the plight of ex-mental patients. Capitalizing on the success of their efforts at Fountain House, they supported and encouraged the development of clubhouse model programs nationwide including Thresholds (Chicago, Illinois), Hill House (Cleveland, Ohio), Council House (Pittsburgh, Pennsylvania), and Bridge Haven (Louisville, Kentucky) (Dincin, 1975).

As awareness of the benefits of clubhouses grew, other centers were developed around the country, including Horizon House (Philadelphia, Pennsylvania), Fellowship House (Miami, Florida), Center Club (Boston, Massachusetts), and the Social Rehabilitation Center (Fairfax, Virginia), to name but a few. Most importantly, using a strategy similar to the mythical Johnny Appleseed, Fountain House and programs like it vigorously trained their staff and then sent them out to develop new clubhouses around the country and the world (Propst, 1992a; Vorspan, 1992). Today, literally hundreds of clubhouse programs worldwide can trace their roots back to either Fountain House or one of the other early clubhouse programs.

BOX 6.2
John H. Beard

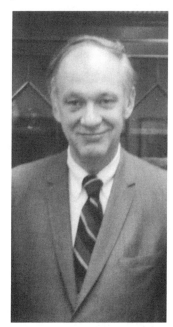

John Beard was the father of the worldwide clubhouse movement. Beard, who earned his master's degree in social work from Wayne State University in Detroit, Michigan, had worked at Wayne County General Hospital in Michigan as a social worker. In 1955, Elizabeth Schermerhorn and the board of directors of Fountain House hired Beard as their executive director. He led Fountain House until his death in 1982.

Beard focused on the members' strengths rather than on their illnesses. An excerpt from a video made in 1978 captures his attitude about working with members.

> I had no interest in why he was sick. That was not my job... I wasn't interested in trying to review his ... psychopathology. I had no interest in it at all. I was terribly interested in how normal we might get him to function. (Flannery & Glickman, 1996, p. 28)

Almost single-handedly at first, Beard's vision and efforts were the guiding force behind the creation of the clubhouse movement. Today there are over 300 clubhouses worldwide and the number is growing. Each of these programs is, in some small way, a symbol of Beard's caring and efforts. In 1982 he recieved the Extraordinary Service Award for Exceptional Commitment and Dedication in Serving the Mentally Ill of New York. The award reads as follows:

> His leadership has provided:

> Dignity where there was shame,
>   Belonging where there was alienation,
>   Empowerment where there was helpessness,
>   Self-respect where there was self-denigration,
>   Hope and opportunity where once there was only despair.

The clubhouse exists primarily to improve the quality of life of its members. Clubhouses began as places where members gathered to socialize and to give and receive support. As such, nothing designated as medical "treatment" took place there. Members were accepted without regard to their symptoms and did not have to "improve" in order to continue their member status. This focus on quality-of-life issues led to an emphasis on members' basic needs: housing, work, socialization, and recreation. *Length of stay*, the time an individual is in a program, is a good example of the difference in how a clubhouse operates in contrast to a partial hospitalization program. Clubhouse members can stay as long as they wish regardless of their clinical state; they are considered members for life. By contrast, many partial hospitalization programs have prescribed lengths of stay and clients are discharged if their clinical state improves.

Probably the most important difference between clubhouses and early partial hospitalization was the clubhouse's emphasis on work (Jackson, 1992; Vorspan, 1992). Clubhouse philosophy, embodied in the "work-ordered day," stresses the importance of work for providing a sense of meaning in life and a sense of belonging to a community. Performing meaningful work endows the worker with purpose. For clubhouse members, work begins with the day-to-day operation of the clubhouse itself, from custodial tasks and record keeping to paying bills and hiring new staff. The clubhouse emphasis on work leads to several other important outcomes such as member empowerment and the development of a sense of self-efficacy and self-esteem. Perhaps most importantly, it is intended to lead to competitive employment outside the clubhouse. Clubhouse members and staff emphasize many ways in which their programs differ from other types of psychiatric rehabilitation services. The following section about clubhouse standards highlights some of the most important ideas behind these programs and some of the ideas that make them different.

Clubhouse Standards

In 1988 the Robert Wood Johnson Foundation, Pew Charitable Trusts, and the Public Welfare Foundation funded the National Clubhouse Expansion Program (NCEP). One of the tasks of the NCEP was the development of standards for clubhouse programs. Starting in 1989, the staff of the NCEP and a group designated the Faculty for Clubhouse Development made up of 50 members and staff from clubhouse programs around the country set out to involve the entire clubhouse community in the development of standards (Propst, 1992a). This effort culminated in the establishment of the International Center for Clubhouse Development (ICCD; http://www.iccd.org).

The ICCD initially identified 35 standards that should be adhered to by programs that considered themselves clubhouses (Propst, 1992b). The ICCD reviews and amends these standards as needed every 2 years. The following section discusses a select group of standards that outline some of the aspects of clubhouses that set them apart from the more traditional psychiatric day programs. As of this publication, a list of the current standards can be reviewed at http://www.iccd.org/default.aspx.

Some Selected Standards for Clubhouse Programs

Program standards can tell us a great deal about the places they describe. As you read the standards for clubhouse programs listed next, try to imagine what such a place would feel like. You might also consider how these policies might be received in a highly formalized environment such as a hospital. More importantly, consider what attitudes about psychiatric treatment and rehabilitation are reflected by these standards. Finally, although clubhouses reject the notion of therapy, decide whether you think the clubhouse can be a therapeutic environment for its members.

Membership
- Membership is voluntary and without time limits.
- Members choose the way they utilize the clubhouse and the staff with whom they work. There are no agreements, behavioral contracts, schedules, or rules intended to enforce participation of members.

- Members, at their choice, are involved in the writing of all records reflecting their participation in the clubhouse. All such records are to be signed by both member and staff.

Relationships

- All clubhouse meetings are open to both members and staff. There are no formal member-only meetings or formal staff-only meetings where program decisions and member issues are discussed.
- Clubhouse staff have generalist roles. All program staff share employment, housing, evening, weekend, and unit responsibilities. Clubhouse staff members do not divide their time between the clubhouse and other responsibilities.

Space

- All clubhouse space is member and staff accessible. There are no staff-only or member-only spaces.

Work-Ordered Day

- The work-ordered day engages members and staff together, side by side, in the running of the clubhouse. The clubhouse focuses on members' strengths, talents, and abilities; therefore, the work ordered day is inconsistent with medication clinics, day treatment, or therapy programs within the clubhouse.
- All work in the clubhouse is designed to help members regain self-worth, purpose, and confidence; it is not intended to be job-specific training.

Employment

- The clubhouse enables its members to return to the normal work world through transitional employment and independent employment; therefore, the clubhouse does not provide employment to members through in-house businesses, segregated clubhouse enterprises, or sheltered workshops.

The Story of Jill, Affinity House Member

A great deal goes on each day in a typical day program. As you read about Jill's day, consider how she carries out her role as a program member and the role staff members' play. Is attending the program having a positive effect on Jill? Would she be better off returning to college? The answers to these questions are far from obvious. What is the right plan for someone like Jill? Is the day program the right place for her at this stage?

Jill, 27 years old, has been a member of Affinity House for 7 months. Diagnosed with schizophrenia at 17, Jill has been in and out of the hospital numerous times, all the while trying to earn a college degree in English and journalism. Two years ago, still a sophomore, she was hospitalized again for 6 months. While getting ready for discharge, a liaison worker visiting the hospital suggested that she might try Affinity House, because she would be discharged in the middle of the spring semester and could not return to school till the fall semester some 7 months away. While still in the hospital, Jill made a visit to Affinity House and it seemed like a warm place with friendly people, so she decided to give it a try.

Today, Jill is the assistant supervisor of the Clerical Unit, where she is mainly responsible for putting out the weekly Affinity House newsletter All Things Considered. The members and staff at Affinity House were really excited when Jill told them about her studies in journalism. Even though Jill hadn't always been able to complete her courses, she had learned a great deal about creating effective newsletters. Now she had the chance to put her knowledge to good use. Helping improve the newsletter was exciting and fun. She found that her ideas were well received and really made a difference in the quality of the publication, which over the weeks grew better and better.

The hardest part for Jill was that as more of her ideas were put into practice she became the one responsible for supervising other members working on the newsletter. This responsibility was something she had not experienced before or been trained for. The Clerical Unit supervisor, Emil (also a member of Affinity House), and the staff assigned to the unit were important sources of support for Jill in her new role as newsletter supervisor. Jill found it difficult to supervise people, mainly because her first impulse was not to say anything that would upset anyone. She wanted to be liked, but she also took great pride in the newsletter. She spent some time every week speaking to Emil or a staff member about how to motivate the Clerical Unit members or how, when someone had made a mistake, she could correct the person but be supportive and encouraging at the same time. After several months of supervising the newsletter Jill was gaining some confidence in her ability to supervise and be a leader.

The first scheduled event at Affinity House each morning is the unit meeting, which starts at 9:30 A.M. sharp. Unit members meet to plan the tasks of the day, see how other unit members and staff are doing, and evaluate how things are going. Unit meetings are also the time when new members who might be trying out the unit as part of their orientation are introduced. When a new member is introduced, Jill always remembers how nervous she was when she first came to the Clerical Unit for her orientation. Today a new member named Bob was introduced to everyone. Jill suggested that Bob might work with her on the initial layout of the next newsletter.

At 10:00 A.M. the unit work begins. Most unit members are clear about the tasks they have to perform, and Jill and Emil spend most of their time supervising the members and helping out when problems arise. Staff members are usually present and either working on clerical projects or working with members on their individual goals. With the members preparing the newsletter, writing outreach letters, and preparing mailings, the unit generally has a very busy, productive feeling in the morning.

Lunch, prepared by members in the Food Service Unit, is usually from 12:00 to 12:30 P.M. Jill often eats with other members from her unit or with a staff person who she had met several years ago in one of her classes in college. After lunch several of the members and staff go outside to smoke.

In the afternoon, in addition to the units there are meetings to attend both about program operations and about things of interest to members. Jill attends a 2 P.M. meeting.

This meeting is designed to orient members who are planning to get a transitional employment position. Members learn about transitional employment (TE), share some of their past experiences at work, talk about what kind of job they would like, and find out about jobs that may be available. Jill has only attended this meeting once in the last 2 weeks, so she is still getting to know the members and working up her courage to really talk about her concerns about work. Her work in the unit has built up her confidence in her ability to hold down a regular job. During the meeting a staff person invites anyone who is interested to attend that evening's TE Support Group. The TE Support Group is for members who are out working in the community. The staff person believes that attending this group will give everyone a better idea of the issues they will face when they get a transitional employment job. Jill isn't sure if she wants to attend the evening group. She is still debating whether she should return to college or try to work, and the idea of going to the group feels too much like ruling out college.

Back in the unit, Jill sees that Bob, the new member on orientation, has left early and not finished cutting out some of the illustrations for pasting up on the next newsletter. Jill enlists another unit member, Herb, and they finish the task together. Other members report that Bob said he was going out for a cigarette but didn't return.

At 3:30 P.M. the day is over and members head out to their rides or the van. Jill has made sure the computers are turned off and the supplies locked up for the night. Jill decides not to attend the TE Support Group this evening. It's her favorite TV night and she's tired. Maybe she will attend next month.

Partial Hospitalization

It is ironic that the first published reports on the principal treatment strategy employed for the massive deinstitutionalization of persons in the United States came from Stalinist Russia (Dzhagarov, 1937). During the early 1930s, after a revolution followed by a bitter civil war, there were too few psychiatric beds in Moscow to meet the demand. Out of necessity, Dzhagarov, the director of a psychiatric hospital, had some of the patients attend the hospital during the day but return to their own homes at night. Dzhagarov reported that his half hospital served more than 1,200 patients and achieved results equivalent to those produced by full-time hospitalization. Necessity, often the "mother of invention," led to an important innovation in psychiatric treatment and rehabilitation.

Shortly after World War II, similar programs emerged in Canada (Cameron, 1947, 1956) and the United Kingdom (Bierer, 1948). Cameron, who established a program at the Allen Memorial Institute of Psychiatry in Montreal in 1946, is generally credited with introducing the term *day hospital* to describe this emerging treatment modality (Luber, 1979). In the United States, programs were reported at the Yale University Clinic and the Menninger Clinic as early as 1948. Many of these early programs were organized from a psychoanalytic perspective, emphasizing individual and group therapy as well as expressive therapies such as art and dance. These pre-deinstitutionalization programs provided services to patients who were generally less symptomatic and less disabled than those relegated to continued institutionalization. Possibly, these "healthier" patients were deemed more appropriate for an insight-oriented therapeutic approach.

By 1963, according to a National Institute of Mental Health (NIMH) report, there were 168 operating day treatment programs in the United States (Taube, 1973). With the passage of the 1963 Community Mental Health Construction Act, the number of programs would grow by more than 700% in 10 years. By 1973 there were 1,280 programs in operation treating some 186,000 patients. This phenomenal growth helped make community treatment available to thousands of people who were deinstitutionalized. At the same time the meteoric development of this new treatment modality presented some very real challenges and problems. No one was completely sure how these programs should operate, who should staff them, or what kinds of services they should offer the patients. Because there was no clear definition of what a day hospital or day treatment program was, many programs began formulating their own strategies for the community treatment of persons with severe and persistent mental illness.

The Development of Partial Hospitalization Programs

The Community Mental Health Centers Construction Act (PL 88-164) passed in 1963, designated partial hospitalization as one of the five essential service modalities each CMHC must provide to be eligible for funding. The requirement that each CMHC must offer partial hospitalization was responsible for the tremendous increase in the number of these services around the country. The partial hospital programs were intended to be the main community-based treatment element for persons deinstitutionalized from state psychiatric hospitals.

This initiative represented a major change in policy regarding responsibility for persons with major mental illness. Up to that time the states had responsibility for providing treatment for this population through their institutions and asylums. With this act, the federal government was providing the states with some of the resources required to move the treatment of persons with severe mental illness from state hospitals into the community. This initiative was also supported on the federal level with the passage of the government-funded health insurance programs Medicaid and Medicare. These programs, especially Medicaid, helped to pay for services for a large proportion of this population.

To foster the continued development of CMHC's around the country, despite limited resources, the centers were placed on 8-year funding cycles. The plan was that with the help of Medicaid, Medicare, and other sources of funds these centers would learn to become financially self-sufficient. During the first 2 years of their existence, CMHCs were federally funded at 100% of their cost for providing services. From the third year to the eighth year, their funding was reduced, until the ninth year when they would receive nothing. The money that was saved as funding was reduced was earmarked for the funding of new CMHCs in identified areas of need around the country. This highly logical funding plan only worked for a time. The cost of the war in Vietnam combined with rising medical costs helped to scuttle the plan financially.

In the CMHCs themselves, many staff and administrators focused their efforts on the "higher functioning" clients with less serious disorders (Torrey, 2001). In some of these centers, people with severe mental illnesses were either ignored or assigned to poorly funded treatment programs operated by staff with little or no training. In short, in many centers the mission of treating people with severe mental illnesses was abandoned in favor of working with the "worried well."

These partial hospitalization programs were (and still are) essentially medical model programs. To bill Medicaid, Medicare, or other sources, program participants had to have a psychiatric diagnosis (ICD or DSM) conferred by a licensed psychiatrist. By government regulation, psychiatrists also had to supervise or prescribe many of the treatments provided. Medication, medication monitoring, and group, individual, and expressive therapies were emphasized, as well as recreation and socialization.

Milieu Therapy

Day programs and some psychiatric hospital wards were largely based on a treatment strategy for providing services called *milieu therapy*. *Milieu*, a French term that literally means "environment," refers in this case to the physical, social, and cultural setting of the program. Milieu therapy is a technique based on the idea that every aspect of a treatment setting or environment can be used to help achieve therapeutic or rehabilitation goals or results. Milieu therapy can be a very powerful tool for shaping behavior, encouraging self-awareness, and increasing self-confidence. In everyday terms, milieu therapy uses phenomena such as peer pressure, social support, public recognition, and social mores to help improve participants' social functioning, self-confidence, and ability to check their perceptions of reality. Some examples of the implementation of milieu therapy strategies are structuring a day around work tasks, community meetings, and skills training groups; ensuring that the physical environment is comfortable, inviting, and clean; and planning a recreational event that will encourage high levels of participation and interaction between people. Each of these tasks helps to shape the environment in order to make it conducive to achieving the goals of the individuals receiving services.

> *Milieu therapy—the use of the whole physical, social, and cultural environment in the therapeutic process. In milieu therapy the environment is the essential treatment component.*

Milieu therapy had its roots in inpatient treatment, where all aspects of the patient's life were under the control of treatment professionals. For persons with disorienting conditions (e.g., acute psychosis), various aspects of their surroundings and environmental cues can be very important. We have all experienced these environmental effects. Messy, hectic environments accompanied by loud noise tend to make people either anxious or withdrawn. Peaceful, calm environments accompanied by soft music tend to make people relaxed. For persons with severe mental illness, attention to all aspects of the milieu is critical because these effects can be greatly magnified.

Gunderson (1978), described five basic elements of successful treatment that were helped by milieu therapy: containment, support, structure, involvement, and validation. As you review these terms in the list that follows consider what it might feel like if each of these elements were absent. Then consider how important it is to an individual's sense of well being to help restore these elements.

1. *Containment:* A sense of being controlled by the environment
2. *Support:* A sense of being supported or affirmed by the environment
3. *Structure:* An ordered environment, where who, what, and where are predictable
4. *Involvement:* Participation and belonging to the social environment
5. *Validation:* Affirmation of the individual in the environment.

The benefits of these therapeutic effects for persons with severe mental illness were first observed in inpatient settings, but they are equally beneficial and important for persons in the community programs where milieu strategies are employed.

Washburn and Conrad (1979) suggest that a sixth important treatment element of milieu therapy is negotiation. Negotiation refers to the process a consumer goes through with treatment staff to determine treatment goals and plans. As PsyR has developed, so has the emphasis on consumer choice and involvement, making negotiation a very important skill. Numerous other benefits of milieu therapy have also been suggested by practitioners and researchers. Milieu therapy can be a powerful tool for reducing anxiety, improving self-awareness, and shaping and maintaining behavior.

Components of a Psychiatric Rehabilitation Day Program

The following are general components or characteristics of almost any PsyR day program: service recipients (e.g., clients, consumers, members), staff, space, program ingredients, and scheduling. By understanding these you will understand the core elements of these programs. As you read their descriptions, notice that there is room for a good deal of variability within each element. This variability and the lack of universally agreed-on principles of PsyR have helped create a situation where it seems that no two programs are truly alike. Many professionals regard the idiosyncratic nature of day programs as a major strength. These different program types are seen as the laboratories where new PsyR strategies are developed and refined. Others point out that program differences create nearly insurmountable problems for program evaluation and research. If no two programs are alike, how can we determine which are superior or even which program elements are effective?

Service Recipients

Service recipients of a program should be diagnosed with a condition that warrants participation in such a program. This relates to the principle of least restrictive setting. This principle states that all consumers of mental health services should be treated in the least restrictive setting that can provide effective services for them. For example, people should not be hospitalized if they are not a danger to themselves or others and they can receive comparable treatment in the community.

- Service recipients of a program should have a history of either long or repeated hospitalization or have repeatedly failed to function in the community without substantial structure and/or support. This also relates to the principle of least restrictive treatment setting. Service recipients who function well in the community should not be referred to such a program in most cases, despite symptoms or diagnosis.

- Service recipients of a program should not be a danger to themselves or others. Persons judged to be a danger to themselves or others are better served in a hospital setting where their behavior can be closely monitored.
- Service recipients of a program should be able to tolerate involvement in the milieu. The milieu of a day program, no matter how it is designed, can be a stressful place for some people. For such people the amount of stress generated by the milieu may offset any gains that the program has to offer.

Staff

Staff at a day program include the following:

- *Director:* The program director's role is critical, setting both the philosophical and administrative tone for the program. The specific tasks of the director may typically include setting the program design, supervising the daily operations of the program, supervising staff, and recruiting staff. Program directors usually have years of experience in PsyR and at least a master's degree in an appropriate field such as psychiatric rehabilitation, social work, psychology, or a related human service field.
- *Supervisory-level staff:* These staff members typically have responsibility for specific program staff, program elements (e.g., vocational units, intake), or consumer caseloads. These staff members often hold master's degrees in an appropriate field (psychiatric rehabilitation, social work, psychology, etc.). Supervisory-level staff may also be direct service workers such as case managers, team leaders, clinical supervisors, or unit leaders. These staff may also function as administrators responsible for subelements of the program such as intake or hospital liaison.
- *Counselors/case managers:* These workers, sometimes referred to as *line staff*, spend most of their time working directly with consumers. Their academic training may range from a high school education to a master's degree. These workers typically make up staff teams supervised by more experienced staff.
- *Mental health aides or paraprofessionals:* These workers typically have little relevant education or experience in the field. There are numerous tasks that aides can carry out effectively in the milieu. These staff members often work in prevocational units, help out with activities, drive vans, and conduct outreach to name just some of their roles.
- *Auxiliary and support staff:* A number of other staff are critical for the operation of a successful PsyR program. Auxiliary staff often includes medical staff such as psychiatrists and nurses, specialized therapists such as art and dance therapists, and other specialized professionals such as vocational counselors, job developers,

and residential counselors. Support staff includes secretaries, file clerks, accountants, and so forth.

Space

The program should have enough square footage to allow staff and members to function in groups and carry out different kinds of activities. It is usually necessary for there to be at least one space big enough for the entire program to meet. The program area should be safe and clean. It should be well lighted, have proper ventilation including heating and cooling, and have the necessary equipment and furnishings to carry out designated functions. There should also be appropriate auxiliary facilities such as toilets, washrooms, and kitchens. Last, but most important, the program should be located in a normalized environment and have reasonably easy access by public transportation. A program located on the locked ward of a hospital, for example, would not be in a normalized environment, even if the clients returned home every afternoon.

Program Ingredients

Program ingredients refers to the kinds of activities that take place during the program day. Some typical program ingredients are recreation; socialization; skills training including social skills, activities of daily living skills, and prevocational skills; education including basic remedial education and symptoms, illness management, and medication education; medication monitoring; case management; and vocational services such as transitional employment or supported employment. Sadly, despite years of progress, programs still exist where one might observe clients doing simple arts and crafts or playing Bingo when they are not in individual or group therapy. Better programs have a rational mix of skills training, vocational activities, support, and recreation depending on the individual needs of the program members. These programs also conduct periodic or ongoing needs assessments to ensure that their efforts are in line with the needs of the members.

Scheduling

Scheduling refers to issues such as what time the program opens, when activities take place, and whether members have to be on time. Programs frequently have evening hours for recreation, graduates, or consumers who work. What happens during the hours the program is operating is a matter of scheduling clients and staff. Scheduling may reflect a regular work environment or the looseness of a social club. A program's scheduling should be in line with its philosophy, goals, and ingredients. For example, a program that actively encourages its members to volunteer or take part-time jobs may be designed to provide members with very flexible schedules to accommodate time off on different days and at different times. Lastly, how schedules are set and who sets them can be an important empowerment issue. Figure 6.1 shows a sample weekly schedule.

COMPLETE IN PENCIL ONLY

Name: _____   Date: _____

TIME	MON	TUE	WED	THU	FRI	SAT
8:00 AM						
8:30 AM	← Breakfast (Optional) →					
9:00 AM	← Unit Meetings →					
9:30 AM	← Fresh Start (MICA Members Only) → ← Unit Activities →					
10:00 AM	Unit Activities (Cont'd.) ← →		Clubhouse Committee	Voice of Prospect House	Unit Activities (Cont'd.)	
10:30 AM	← Coffee Break →		↓	↓		SOCIAL
11:00 AM	MICA Education		Member Reps. Meeting		MICA Relapse Prevention	(OPTIONAL)
11:30 AM	← Unit Activities → ↓				↓	10:00 AM
12:00 PM	← Lunch →					TO
12:30 PM	← Community Meeting →					4:00 PM
1:00 PM	Continuing Education					
1:30 PM	↓	← Unit Activities (Cont'd.) →				
2:00 PM	Case Mgmt.	← Unit Activities →			Unit Activities	
2:30 PM	↓			Case Mgmt.		
3:00-7:00 PM			Social (Optional)		Social (Optional)	

Assigned Unit: _____   Days in Program: _____

SPECIAL GROUPS:

☐ MICA   ☐ Continuing Education   ☐ Member Reps   ☐ Voice of PH

☐ TE   ☐ Coping Groups   ☐ Fresh Start   ☐ Clubhouse Committee

☐ SE   ☐ Other   ☐ Clerical Research   ☐ Food Services

☐ House Services   ☐ Member Services   ☐ Seniors

FIGURE 6.1 Example of a weekly schedule.

═══ *Evaluating Psychiatric Rehabilitation Day Programs*

A Day Program Taxonomy

Several researchers have suggested that partial hospitalization programs and PsyR programs in general are most effective when they are specifically designed to produce a specific outcome for a particular type of consumer (Astrachan, Flynn, Geller, & Harvey, 1970; Neffinger, 1981; Solomon, 1992). For example, if a program had a primary purpose of helping consumers return to regular community life as quickly as possible, the emphasis might be on skills training and supportive therapy. Alternatively, a program with a primary purpose of helping individuals who are acutely symptomatic stay out of the hospital might emphasize support and medication maintenance. This idea might be summed up by the following question: What type of program is effective for what type of individual?

In 1981 Neffinger proposed a taxonomy of partial hospitalization (PH) programs (see Table 6.1). Neffinger's taxonomy identified three different primary purposes or functions for PH's: (1) an alternative to inpatient treatment, which he labeled *day hospital*; (2) a supplement to traditional outpatient treatment and vocational rehabilitation, which he labeled *day treatment*; and (3) functional maintenance in the community, which he labeled *day care*. Many programs today can still be classified using this taxonomy, although they would probably employ different terms to describe themselves. For example, today, programs designed to function as an alternative to inpatient treatment are typically called *acute partial hospitals.*

It is instructive to closely review the details of Neffinger's taxonomy in Table 6.1. Notice that the term *chronic*, which is no longer acceptable, is used. Also, review the variables or program characteristics Neffinger used to distinguish between program types. These variables are still an important consideration when evaluating programs, but their content has changed somewhat as the field has evolved. For example, intensive psychotherapy has been replaced by supportive psychotherapy. In addition, the characterization of day care patients as older is probably an artifact of the deinstitutionalization movement and is certainly less true today. The original exodus from the hospitals included many middle-aged and elderly patients who had spent the better part of their adult lives in institutions.

The Effectiveness of Day Programs

The first reports of effective day hospitals (Bierer, 1948; Cameron, 1947; Dzhagarov, 1937) stressed the innovative strategy of using these programs in place of inpatient treatment. This strategy had several obvious benefits in addition to the fact that it is much less expensive to provide day treatment than inpatient hospitalization. Day programs allowed patients to stay in the community, which reduced stigma and helped maintain normal contacts and supports. Day programs also eliminated the need for what was often a difficult transition back to the community after a long inpatient stay.

The first evaluations of day programs in the United States focused on the question of how this treatment strategy compared with inpatient hospitalization. This research was

TABLE 6.1

A Schematic Presentation of the Theoretical Spectrum of Partial Hospitalization Programs Subdivided into Three Parallel Continua Representing (A) General Taxonomy, (B) Primary Function, and (C) Differential Characteristics[a]

	Day Hospital	Day Treatment	Day Care
A. General Taxonomy	Day Hospital	Day Treatment	Day Care
B. Primary Function	Alternative to inpatient transitional setting	Supplement to traditional outpatient treatment, vocational rehabilitation	Functional maintenanace
C. Differential Characteristics			
Treatment Goal	Stabilize acute episode	Catalyze rapid improvement Minimize Subsequent treatment	Prevent further deterioration and rehospitalization
Treatment Modality	Psychopharmacology/ supportive therapy	Intensive psychotherapy and structure	Activity therapy, and advocacy
Symptom Intensity	Acute	Pre/post acute	Chronic
Age	Mixed	Younger	Older
Staffing Pattern	Medical mental health professionals	Nonmedical mental health professionals	Predominantly paraprofessionals
Patient/ Staff Ratio	4	6	15+
Maximum Census	12	20 to 40	50+
Treatment Duration	2 to 4 weeks	3 to 4 months	Indefinite
Organizational Relationships	Closely allied to emergency and/or inpatient unit	Separate from but available to inpatient or emergency unit	No necessary relationship to inpatient or emergency unit

[a]Reprinted with permission from Neffinger, G. G. (1981). Partial hospitalization: An overview. *Journal of Community Psychology, 9,* 263.

nearly unanimous in finding that day hospitalization was both clinically superior and more economical than inpatient hospitalization. In a 1971 study, Herz, Endicott, Spitzer, and Mesnikoff randomly assigned patients to either inpatient treatment or day hospitalization and found that day treatment was superior on each of their outcome measures.

A similar study by Washburn, Vannicelli, Longabaugh, and Scheff (1976) found that initially, day hospitalization was superior to inpatient hospitalization in reducing subjective distress, improving community functioning, and reducing family burden, total hospital cost, and length of stay in the program. At a 24-month reassessment, they found that there was no longer a difference between the day hospital and inpatient hospital groups. It is interesting to speculate why the differences between the day program and inpatient groups fade after 2 years. The most likely explanation is that for many of these individuals the disease process may have reasserted itself, blurring the advantages gained by attending day programming. An alternative explanation is that day programming improves outcomes faster than the usual natural course of the illness (as discussed in Chapter 3). Perhaps by 2 year's time, the functioning of those who were served in inpatient settings "naturally" reached the level of those served in day programming. As the advantages of day hospitalization became clear, the focus of research moved toward determining which elements of the day hospital were most effective. Neffinger's work cited earlier is one example of this effort. Probably the most important study in this area to date was done by researchers working for the Veterans Administration (VA). Taking advantage of the large number of day hospitals operated by the VA, Linn, Caffey, Klett, Hogarty, and Lamb (1979) randomly assigned patients from 10 different hospitals to receive either day treatment plus psychotropic drugs or psychotropic drugs alone. The positive results of day programming were not immediately apparent. At the initial 6-month follow-up, the researchers found no difference between the two groups. But, at the 18-month follow-up, they found that the combination of medication plus day treatment was superior to medication alone. Individuals who had received day treatment plus medication had fewer episodes of hospitalization, spent less time in the hospital, and had better social functioning. Day treatment plus medication was found to be clearly superior on almost every outcome measure. Interestingly, they also found that the overall treatment cost of day treatment plus medication was not higher than the treatment cost of medication alone. This might be considered a surprising result, since the recipients of day treatment with better outcomes were receiving more services than those receiving medication alone. The lower cost of their treatment was due to the fact that they used fewer inpatient services, spending fewer days hospitalized. These hospital services have a very high cost.

Analyzing the results further, the researchers found some sharp differences between programs on the outcome variables under study. They found that six of the day hospitals produced positive outcomes, while the other four day hospitals produced outcomes no better than medication alone. They proceeded to study which program factors were associated with both positive and negative outcomes. One important finding was that the six centers producing positive outcomes had costs that were not much greater than the cost of drugs alone, whereas the costs of the four centers with poor outcomes were significantly higher. After reviewing their findings the authors concluded that:

> High patient turnover and brief but more intensive treatment, particularly in terms of psychotherapeutic counseling by professionals, may lead to relapse for some schizophrenic patients. (Linn et al., 1979, p. 1061)

In short, group psychotherapy, which costs more because it requires more professionally trained and higher paid staff, also produced poorer outcomes. This evidence supports a more practical, supportive, skills training approach (in contrast to more traditional therapy), which is one of the hallmarks of PsyR.

Beigel and Feder (1970) had similar results, finding that persons with more persistent conditions do poorly in programs designed to provide treatment more appropriate for individuals experiencing acute symptoms. This indicates that certain types of programs are effective for persons in different phases of their illness and ineffective or even harmful for others. These findings also imply that depending on the stage of their illness, they have different treatment needs and goals, the attainment of which may best be achieved in specifically designed programs.

The more recent research has focused on achieving specific outcomes and has examined clubhouse programs. For example, a comparison of outcomes achieved by assertive community treatment programs (see Chapter 7) and clubhouse programs conducted by Stein, Barry, Van Dien, Hollingsworth, and Sweeney (1999) found strong similarities on measures of vocational activity, social relationships, social networks, and community integration. Similarly, Macias (2001) reported on a long-term experimental comparison of the employment results of a program of assertive community treatment (PACT) team (see Chapter 7) and an ICCD-certified clubhouse in Worcester, Massachusetts. Not surprisingly, the PACT team, considering its assertive outreach component, was clearly superior in retaining consumers in the program in contrast to the completely voluntary nature of the clubhouse. PACT was also superior with regard to the proportion of people who achieved employment, although this difference diminished with time. Clubhouse members actually worked more total days for higher hourly pay and earned more money over the length of the study. Interestingly, clubhouse member jobs were more likely to be "white collar and professional rather than manual labor" (Macias, 2001, p. 2). While the relatively lower employment rates among clubhouse members support criticisms of PsyR day programming as increasing dependency and lowering expectation regarding employment (e.g., Bond, Dietzen, McGrew, & Miller, 1995), the clubhouse results point to better, longer lasting, and more career-oriented employment (Macias, 2001).

State-of-the-Art Psychiatric Rehabilitation Day Programming

One of the most important contributions of organizations such as the United States Psychiatric Rehabilitation Association (USPRA) and publications such as the *Psychiatric Rehabilitation Journal* and the *American Journal of Psychiatric Rehabilitation* is that they bring together professionals, consumers, family members, and others from all philosophies of PsyR. This coming together, which has grown year by year, has helped to synthesize the best elements of these different program types into what we consider today's state-of-the-art program. PsyR services are still largely idiosyncratic, but the best programs contain many of the same elements, though in differing amounts.

From the clubhouse movement, we get a strong respect for each individual's quality of life and those things that support quality of life: employment, housing, social supports, and membership in the community. This translates into many support initiatives that go far beyond treating the mental illness itself. State-of-the-art programs are instrumental in securing housing for their members, have one or more vocational rehabilitation elements (see Chapter 9), support their members' efforts to further their education (see Chapter 10), and help provide opportunities for building social supports and networks. Clubhouses,

CONTROVERSIAL ISSUE
Psychiatric Rehabilitation Day Programming: An Effective Rehabilitation Setting or an Obsolete Service?

While psychiatric rehabilitation day programming is still a widely employed service modality, there are a number of researchers, service providers, and consumers who are strongly critical of its continued use. As you read about the pros and cons of day programming, consider what factors you think should be considered in settling this issue.

Psychiatric rehabilitation day programs were established all over the United States to address the needs of newly deinstitutionalized individuals. As such, they were some of the first widely employed community-based service modalities for persons with severe and persistent mental illnesses. In an effort to provide effective services for their recipients, many, but certainly not all, of these programs have evolved over the years. The clubhouse movement and advances in psychiatric rehabilitation knowledge have influenced much of this change. Today's PsyR day program should incorporate evidence-based practices, provide comprehensive and individualized services, have a recovery orientation, and be responsive to new knowledge and developments in psychiatric rehabilitation. Large numbers of persons with severe mental illnesses still receive services through this modality. Many rely on these programs for services, support, and recreation.

Strong criticisms have been raised concerning the continued use of PsyR day programs. Much of this criticism is based on the notion that the field has moved beyond the concept of providing treatment and rehabilitation in segregated facility-based settings and now has better ways to provide services. Newer models such as assertive community treatment, supported employment, and supported housing meet the individual needs of persons by design. These new services start by considering the preferences of the individual (e.g., what kind of job is desired, what kind of housing), are offered in the environments in which the individual wants to live, work, and socialize, and are less stigmatizing than attending a mental health clinic or program. In addition, services such as assertive community treatment and supported employment are evidence-based practices, which means they produce dependable results if they are carried out properly.

In studies of the conversion of day programs to supported employment programs, employment rates have increased without apparent negative outcomes in other areas such as hospitalization, homelessness, and incarceration rates (Bond et al., 2001; Drake et al., 1996). A study by Becker and her colleagues (2001) compared two Rhode Island psychiatric day programs that converted to supported employment programs with another Rhode Island program that did not and found the same results: Employment increased but negative effects did not. Those who were not served in employment received a comprehensive case management and outpatient service.

Proponents of day programming have argued that many consumers require a structured and supportive environment to prepare them to assume normalized roles in the community. The studies cited above suggest that day programming may not be a requisite component of a comprehensive mental health system.

for example, tend to be open in the evenings and on weekends because their members' social lives and recreation are important.

The development of a nationwide network of clubhouse programs helped give birth to the psychosocial rehabilitation movement. The clubhouse network was also instrumental in the creation of the International Association of Psychosocial Rehabilitation Services (IAPSRS), now USPRA. Today, some clubhouses belong to both USPRA as organizational members and to the national clubhouse movement, the ICCD.

From the partial hospitalization movement, our state-of-the-art program gets its emphasis on medication, medication management, and symptom and medication education for consumers and their families. This aspect is important because the major mental illnesses are biologically based diseases and their symptoms can be controlled with medication. It is also believed that the best long-term outcomes are achieved if psychotic episodes are dealt with effectively and in a timely fashion.

Although it would be wrong to give the impression of universal agreement about how things should be done, PsyR is no longer divided between groups with totally different philosophies and strategies. Rather, the field has matured to the point where we agree on most of the goals, values, and principles, but still debate the proper mix of these elements to address the needs of those receiving services. Take the idea of empowerment for example. Many people use this term and many professionals believe it is an important PsyR element. But, there is still little agreement as to just what the term *empowerment* means and whether it is a good idea in every situation. Consider the issues spelled out in Box 6.3.

BOX 6.3
Empowerment: Will We Know It If We See It?

Empowerment is something that comes from within a person, rather than something that is done to a person. Someone who is empowered may have a sense that what they think and feel counts, that their wishes are important, and that they have choices to make. The best a program can do is create an environment that encourages empowerment. In a PsyR day program member empowerment might manifest itself in many ways. There might be a strong consumer committee or governing body, members might hold supervisory positions, and they might help to collect data to evaluate the program. Staff members at some programs try to engender some of these activities but find that they are rejected by service recipients. Empowerment, like recovery, is a personal and complicated phenomenon.

Can you tell whether a program milieu empowers its members? In many programs the consumers and staff give a great deal of "lip service" to the importance of empowerment. In other programs, the issue of empowerment is not discussed unless it is raised by a visitor. Does speaking about empowerment indicate that a program is empowering? Apparently not. A study done by students of the first author of this text found an inverse relationship in programs between consumer empowerment and talking about empowerment. In short, programs that said they were empowering tended to be less empowering than programs that didn't mention the term at all.

Some measures have been devised to evaluate the program milieu (Wolfensberger, 1980; Moos, 1974). These scales do not claim to measure empowerment directly. Instead, they touch on many related issues such as normalization and control. While empowerment is considered an important ingredient of PsyR programming, there is still no agreement on an objective way to measure it. Using a participatory action research approach, which involves researchers working hand-in-hand with consumers, a group of researchers developed an empowerment scale that holds some promise of capturing the essence of this term for individuals diagnosed with severe mental illnesses (Rogers, Chamberlin, Ellison, & Crean, 1997).

Day Programming and Evidence-Based Practice

When carried out effectively, psychiatric rehabilitation day programs are complex entities providing a host of different services designed to meet the needs of individual consumers. For example, a program might provide its members with (1) case management services for advocacy and supports, (2) skills training, (3) medication evaluation and monitoring, (4) illness management training, (5) family education and support, (6) vocational services, (7) supported education, and (8) integrated services for persons with substance abuse problems. Each of these services, if carried out correctly, is either an evidence-based practice or being tested as a possible evidence-based practice. In fact, the ideal psychiatric rehabilitation day program would consist of a large set of high-fidelity, evidence-based practices that could be offered to consumers on an as-needed or as-requested basis.

Sadly, the current state of PsyR day programming is very far from such an ideal. Still, the advent of evidence-based practice in combination with the recovery movement may hasten change in this direction. System-wide and individual program change processes based on securing the positive and predictable outcomes obtainable with high-fidelity evidence-based practices have a high potential for success. Chances for positive change may also increase if consumers and consumer advocates demand that programs provide services with proven effectiveness (i.e., evidence-based practices) based on consumer choice.

Because an effective PsyR day program is necessarily composed of a constellation of evidence-based practices, as described above, PsyR day programming in and of itself will not be an evidence-based practice. The advantage of one program providing all of these services is very clear. Coordination of services is carried out more effectively and efficiently. The need for consumers to "negotiate" the system is greatly reduced, which minimizes the stress often experienced when trying to access needed services. Some may see a possible disadvantage since opportunities for community integration created by moving from service to service may be lost. In fact, good services work to connect people to natural community supports as much as possible.

Summary

Psychiatric rehabilitation day programming has roots in the clubhouse movement, the partial hospitalization movement, and milieu therapy. These programs were the principal treatment facilities for many of the people deinstitutionalized during the 1960s, 1970s, and 1980s. These programs are characterized by the belief that people coming together facing the same problems and issues can create an environment that is conducive to treatment, rehabilitation, and recovery. Research has demonstrated that some program designs (e.g., a focus on the here-and-now, less formal therapy) produce outcomes that are superior to medications alone (Linn et al., 1979). Research has also demonstrated that these programs are economically efficient. Today's programs are a combination of elements of the partial hospitalization movement (e.g., emphasis on medication, treatment) and the clubhouse movement (e.g., emphasis on quality of life, consumer empowerment). Some of these programs have grown into large multi-service agencies that attempt to provide for all if not most of the needs of individuals diagnosed with severe mental illnesses. While these programs are falling out of favor with many professionals and consumers, the advent of evidence-based practices and the recovery movement may supply the impetus and the standards necessary for effective reform.

Class Exercise

Psychiatric Rehabilitation Day Program Design Activity
The following nine variables or characteristics of day programs help to determine how the program functions:

Member/Staff Ratio

May range from low (2/1 to 6/1) to high (16/1 or more) depending on the type and philosophy of the program.

Program Size

May vary from small (20 to 40 members) to very large programs with hundreds of members.

Staffing

May vary from being predominantly paraprofessional to predominantly professional depending on the goals and type of program.

Staffing Pattern

May vary from being a generalist pattern where staff carry out multiple roles with little regard for academic or professional credentials, or a specialist staffing pattern in which staff carry out specified organizational or professional roles.

Attendance Requirements

May vary from laissez faire (consumers attend when they wish) to strict and mandatory similar to a regular work environment.

Scheduled Program Time

May be loose, varied, and flexible or may approximate a typical work environment.

Treatment Focus

May vary from no treatment other than concrete feedback about the task at hand to intensive and frequent group and individual therapy.

Program Ingredients

May offer differing amounts (from none to all day) of recreation, socialization, supportive individual and/or group therapy, expressive therapies (e.g., art, dance), pre-vocational

TABLE 6.2
Program Type by Program Variables Matrix

Program Variables	Program Type		
	Maintenance	Movement	Acute
Member/staff ratio			
Program size			
Staffing			
Staffing pattern			
Attendance requirements			
Scheduled program time			
Treatment focus			
Program ingredients			
Empowerment			

skills training, specific skills training, work units, and transitional or supported employment. These ingredients should be offered in an internally consistent pattern with respect to program type and philosophy. Some of these grouping variables might be:

- Vocational (work like) vs. non-vocational (supportive)
- High therapy vs. no therapy
- Skills training vs. social learning theory.

Empowerment

Programs range from being run by consumers to being totally controlled by the staff. Clues to the degree of empowerment in a particular program might be the degree of authority wielded by a member government, the presence of members in important meetings, and the ability of members to shape both their individual treatment plans and the program in ways important to them.

Instructions

Based on Neffinger's taxonomy of partial hospitalization programs, using the program type by program variables matrix shown in Table 6.2, fill in the value of each variable (e.g., member/staff ratio = low, staffing pattern = general, empowerment = high) under each program type. You should have a clear rationale for each decision.

References

Astrachan, B. M., Flynn, H. R., Geller, J. D., & Harvey, H. H. (1970). Systems approach to day hospitalization. *Archives of General Psychiatry, 22*, 550–559.

Beard, J. H., Propst, R. N., & Malamud, T. J. (1982). The Fountain House model of psychiatric rehabilitation. *Psychosocial Rehabilitation Journal*, V(1), 47–53.

Becker, D. R., Bond, G. R., McCarthy, D., Thompson, D. Xie, H., Gregory, G. J., & Drake, R. E. (2001). Converting day treatment centers to supported employment programs in Rhode Island. *Psychiatric Services*, 52(3), 351–357.

Beigel, A., & Feder, S. L. (1970). Patterns of utilization in partial hospitalization. *American Journal of Psychiatry, 126*, 1267–1274.

Bierer, J. (1948). *Therapeutic social clubs*. London: H. K. Lewis.

Bond, G. R., Dietzen, L. L., McGrew, J. H., & Miller, L. D. (1995). Accelerating entry into supported employment for persons with severe psychiatric disabilities. *Rehabilitation Psychology, 40*(2), 91–111.

Bond, G. R., Resnick, S. G., Drake, R. E., Xie, H., McHugo, G. J., & Bebout, R. R. (2001). Does competitive employment improve nonvocational outcomes for people with severe mental illness? *Journal of Consulting and Clinical Psychology, 69*(3), 489–501.

Cameron, D. E. (1947). The day hospital: Experimental forms of hospitalization for patients. *Modern Hospital, 69*(3), 60–62.

Cameron, D. E. (1956). The day hospital. In A. E. Bennett, E. A. Hargrove, & B. Engle (Eds.), *The practice of psychiatry in general hospitals*. Berkeley: University of California Press.

Dincin, J. (1975). Psychiatric rehabilitation. *Schizophrenia Bulletin, 13*, 131–147.

Drake, R. E., Becker, D. R., Biesanz, J. C., Torrey, W. C., McHugo, G. J., & Wyzik, P. F. (1994). Rehabilitative day treatment vs. supported employment. I. Vocational outcomes. *Community Mental Health Journal, 30*, 519–532.

Dzhagarov, M. (1937). Experience in organizing a half hospital for mental patients. *Neuropathologia Psikhatria*, 137–147.

Flannery, M., & Glickman, M. (1996). *Fountain House: Portraits of lives reclaimed from mental illness*. Center City, MN: Hazelden.

Gunderson, J. G. (1978). Defining the therapeutic process in psychiatric milieus. *Psychiatry: Journal for the Study of Interpersonal Process, 41*, 327–335.

Herz, M. I., Endicott, J., Spitzer, R. I., & Mesnikoff, A. (1971). Day versus inpatient hospitalization: A controlled study. *American Journal of Psychiatry, 127*, 1371–1382.

Jackson, R.(1992). How work works. *Psychosocial Rehabilitation Journal, 16*(2), 49–54.

Linn, M. W., Caffey, E. M., Klett, C. J., Hogarty G. E., & Lamb, H. R. (1979). Day treatment and psychotropic drugs in the aftercare of schizophrenic patients. *Archives of General Psychiatry, 36*, 1055–1066.

Luber, R. F. (1979). The growth and scope of partial hospitalization. In R. F. Luber (Ed.), *Partial hospitalization: A current perspective* (pp. 3–20). New York: Plenum Publishing.

Macias, C. (2001). An experimental comparison of PACT and clubhouse. Massachusetts Employment Intervention Demonstration Project, Cooperative Agreement No. SM51831.

Moos, R. (1974). *Evaluating treatment environments: A social ecological approach*, New York: John Wiley & Sons.

Neffinger, G. G. (1981). Partial hospitalization: An overview. *Journal of Community Psychology, 9*, 262–269.

Propst, R. N. (1992a). Introduction to special issue: The clubhouse model. *Psychosocial Rehabilitation Journal, 16*(2), 25–30.

Propst, R. N. (1992b). Standards for clubhouse programs: Why and how they were developed. *Psychosocial Rehabilitation Journal, 16*(2), 25–30.

Rogers, E. S., Chamberlin, J., Ellison, M. L., & Crean, T. (1997). A consumer-constructed scale to measure empowerment among users of mental health services. *Psychiatric Services, 48*(8), 1042–1047.

Solomon, P. (1992). The efficacy of case management services for severely mentally disabled clients. *Community Mental Health Journal, 28*(3), 163–180.

Stein, L. I., Barry, K. L., Van Dien, G., Hollingsworth, E. J., & Sweeney, J. K. (1999). Work and social support: A comparison of consumers who have achieved stability in ACT and clubhouse programs. *Community Mental Health Journal, 35*(2), 193–204.

Taube, C. A. (1973). *Day care services in federally funded community mental health centers* (Statistical Note No. 96). Rockville, MD: Survey and Reports Section, Biometry Branch, National Institute of Mental Health.

Torrey, E. F. (2001). *Surviving schizophrenia.* New York: Harper Collins.

Vorspan, R. (1992). Why work works. *Psychosocial Rehabilitation Journal, 16*(2), 49–54.

Washburn, S. L., & Conrad, M. (1979). Organization of the therapeutic milieu in the partial hospital. In R. F. Luber (Ed.), *Partial hospitalization: A current perspective* (pp. 47–70). New York: Plenum.

Washburn, S. L., Vannicelli, M., Longabaugh, R., & Scheff, B. J. (1976). A controlled comparison of psychiatric day treatment and inpatient hospitalization. *Journal of Consulting and Clinical Psychology, 44,* 665–675.

Wolfensberger, W. (1983). The definition of normalization: Update, problems, disagreements and misunderstandings. In R. J. Flynn and K. E. Nitsch (Eds.), *Normalization, social integration and community services.* Baltimore, MD: University Park Press.

Chapter 7

Assertive Community Treatment and Case Management

Introduction   192

The Need for Continuity of Care   193

Awareness of the Need for Care Coordination at the National Level   196

Case Management   196

   The Case Manager   198

Models of Case Management   199

   Expanded Broker Model   199

   Rehabilitation Model   200

   Strengths Model   200

   Full Support Model (Assertive Community Treatment) Model   200

The Story of Micky   201

Evaluating Case Management   203

The Development of Assertive Community Treatment   204

   Evaluating Training for Community Living   206

Evolution into ACT   206

When Is a Program Actually ACT?   207

Do Effective Case Management Programs Share Similar Characteristics?   208

Assertive Community Treatment: An Evidence-Based Practice   208

Critical Ingredients of ACT   211

Service Outcomes of ACT   211

Reviews of ACT Research   211

ACT as an Early Intervention Strategy   212

ACT and Persons in the Criminal Justice System   213

ACT Comes of Age as a Program and a Professional Specialty   214

The Future of ACT and Case Management Approaches   214

Summary   215

Class Exercise   215

References   216

Psychiatric rehabilitation (PsyR) responds to the variety of needs of persons with serious and persistent mental illness. Given the multifaceted nature of the disabilities caused by these illnesses and fragmented systems of care, it is necessary to coordinate both services and resources. This coordination is generally known as case management and it is an essential ingredient of all psychiatric rehabilitation. At the same time, some people with psychiatric illnesses who need a variety of services and resources may not receive them unless they are assertively approached. The most effective strategy for accomplishing this is known as assertive community treatment.

This chapter will answer the following questions:

1. *Why do psychiatric rehabilitation services require so much coordination?*
2. *What are case management, outreach, and assertive community treatment?*
3. *Why are these approaches essential to psychiatric rehabilitation?*
4. *How do assertive community treatment and case management differ?*
5. *What is the evidence that these approaches are effective?*

Introduction

Deinstitutionalization, the national policy of discharging people who were institutionalized back to the community, began in earnest during the early 1970s in the United States. Moving the site of treatment from large, long-term institutions to the community was an important milestone for persons with severe and persistent mental illness. In a 5-year period between 1970 and 1975, more than 100,000 individuals were discharged into the community for treatment. By 1985, the number of individuals in state and county psychiatric hospitals around the country had been reduced by 450,000.

As they deinstitutionalized their individual populations, psychiatric hospitals also began to reduce the length of stay of newly admitted individuals. Unlike the previous era, when long-term hospitalization was the rule, psychiatric hospitals began discharging individuals after very short stays. Sadly, many of those discharged returned to the hospital after equally short stays in the community. This created a new set of problems for these people and the psychiatric treatment system that was supposed to serve them.

The problem of individuals returning to the hospital, a phenomenon known as *recidivism,* was new. This cycle of frequent discharge and readmission to the hospital became known as the "revolving door" syndrome. While warehousing individuals in large psychiatric institutions was, in large part, a thing of the past, community treatment still had a long way to go to meet the needs of people with psychiatric disabilities. Compounding these problems was the fact that most of the money spent for hospital treatment stayed at the hospitals rather than following the individuals into the community to fund treatment there.

Mental health planners soon found that the concept of "cheaper by the dozen" applied to the hospital services they provided. As the number of people in the hospital decreased, most hospital costs tended to remain the same. In fact, it cost almost as much to run a hospital at 30% of its capacity as it had to operate that same institution at 110% of capacity.

As these problems became apparent, laypersons, professionals, and people with mental illness raised considerable criticism of the national policy of deinstitutionalization. One critical report questioned a policy that releases mentally ill individuals into community facilities that "don't exist" (Santiestevan, 1975). In 1986, *Newsweek* magazine wrote an exposé on the effects of deinstitutionalization. Labeled "Abandoned," the article pointed out that despite the good intentions of the deinstitutionalization reforms, thousands of people with mental illness were left to fend for themselves on the street:

> *Todd had his first psychotic episode at age 20, after a prep-school career marked by brilliance in science, baseball and the piano. His family spent his college tuition on private psychiatric care—and when their savings were exhausted, transferred him to a state mental institution. In and out of the hospital for years, Todd, now 37, recently was released to a boarding home in Worcester, Mass. Three weeks later he was mugged, an event that precipitated yet another psychotic breakdown. "He tried so hard to make it," his mother says. "They all try so hard, and they fail because they receive no care. It's torture for the families to watch that. These people are too sick to be let out into the community without any help. It's a national disgrace." (News-week, January 6, 1986, pp. 14–15).*

Many researchers at the time (e.g., Aviram & Segal, 1973; Kirk & Therrien, 1975; Klerman, 1977; Kohen & Paul, 1976) saw the deinstitutionalization movement as essentially an overambitious, unrealistic plan driven by rhetoric, myth, and good intentions, but lacking any real planning. Planners had underestimated the difficulties of recently released individuals. In fact, people with serious mental illnesses were often "ghettoized" or socially excluded (Aviram & Segal, 1973). One consumer wrote that the conditions she saw in the community were often worse than those in the hospital and that it was a myth that one treatment setting (i.e., community) was better than another (i.e., hospital) (Allen, 1974). In fact, for many of the people who were deinstitutionalized, the movement that was heralded as bringing important legal rights to individuals with psychoses was actually a major catastrophe in terms of the *quality of life* of many people with serious mental illness.

According to the President's New Freedom Commission report (2003), these problems persist today; the coordination of care in the community is often "fragmented" and is currently in need of significant repair.

The Need for Continuity of Care

As with any broadly disabling condition, the person coping with major mental illness often requires a wide scope of services. These include basic needs such as food, shelter, and clothing. Various types of treatment and rehabilitation are also required. Ideally, these services are delivered in an uninterrupted flow over time until the disability is corrected or compensated for. This concept of receiving all the services necessary for the length of time they are required is called *continuity of care*. The continuity of care issues for people experiencing severe and persistent mental illnesses are critically important and, because of the nature of the disability, often difficult to solve. Hospital environments had been designed to meet the basic needs of patients with serious mental illnesses. Major continuity of care problems first arose as individuals moved from the centralized, institutional environment of the psychiatric hospital to the decentralized, multiagency environment of the community. Some researchers believed that the continuity of care needs of individuals was an important hospital benefit that was inadvertently lost with the rush to deinstitutionalize (Kirk & Therrien, 1975). The hospitals usually included medical staff, housekeeping staff, and recreation workers, all integrated within one large institution. In contrast, community services are usually provided by different agencies and programs that often communicate poorly with one another. Today, more than 30 years later, a similar situation exists. In most areas, individuals' needs are addressed by several poorly coordinated services (President's New Freedom Commission, 2003).

On returning to the community, a typical consumer might find herself attending a partial care program or clubhouse during the day, receiving her medication from a private physician, and living in a private boarding home. Previously, within one organization, the hospital staff orchestrated even the smallest details of her life. In the community, she now has to deal with three or more separate organizations. In the hospital, her modest economic needs for food, clothing, and shelter were met. Outside the hospital, she has concerns about maintaining her income through disability or welfare payments. In addition, she now needs medical benefits, from Medicaid or a similar program, in order to pay for her physician, medication, and treatment services. Worse still, if she failed in any of these community settings she might find herself on the street, out of medication, or back in the hospital. In one sense, at the very moment she is trying to reestablish herself in the community, her opportunities for failure have been multiplied. Furthermore, the potential sources of stress in her life, which might aggravate her illness, have greatly increased. Paradoxically, improvements in her life might prove to be equally troublesome. A large reduction in symptoms or obtaining regular employment might make her ineligible for her disability benefits and perhaps medical coverage. A number of recent improvements in this area are reviewed in Chapter 9, but these concerns still persist.

In the early years of deinstitutionalization, the service delivery systems available in the community for released individuals were new and often uncoordinated. With several agencies or programs responsible for different aspects of an individual's treatment, a systemic kind of "diffusion of responsibility" problem arose. Diffusion of responsibility refers to a situation in which shared responsibility for an issue or problems allows each of the responsible parties to assume that another party will take care of it with the result that no one takes care of the situation (Daley & Latane, 1968). This social psychological phenomenon can be observed in large cities where bystanders have been known to literally step over someone lying on the sidewalk, or when drivers pass a broken down car by the side of the road, assuming that someone else has already called for help. In the context of community services for persons with severe and persistent mental illness, while every service or program had some degree of responsibility for some aspect of an individual's treatment and care, no one was responsible for the whole person. Staff at one agency would assume some other agency or person should be taking care of issues that his or her own agency was not designed or funded to deal with. This increased jeopardy created a situation by which consumers were said to "fall through the cracks" of the service delivery system. These consumers would often return to the hospital, end up living on the streets, or become homebound recluses.

In addition to the difficulty of connecting with needed community services, the newly discharged people often found that certain services simply did not exist (Test, 1979). Partly because of a lack of affordable housing, in many areas individuals were given bus tickets and literally discharged into the streets. Vocational programs were also in very short supply during the early stages of the deinstitutionalization process. In these situations continuity of care could not be achieved because of a lack of available services.

To appreciate the vast scope of this problem, we must multiply the plight of each individual consumer by the hundreds of thousands of deinstitutionalized individuals. The increased stress associated with dealing with a complex, often disorganized and unconnected treatment delivery system contributed to the high rates of recidivism experienced by the deinstitutionalized population.

In recent years substantial progress has been made in the development of community-based supports and services for people with psychiatric disabilities, yet many of the challenges faced by people discharged from institutions in the 1970s still exist for people being discharged today. There are still major gaps in the service systems, many of which remain poorly coordinated, and recidivism rates are still too high.

The risk of rehospitalization is highest during the first 6 months after a person is discharged from the hospital. People are hospitalized during the *acute phase* of their illness and this instability may extend past their discharge. The obvious stress related to psychiatric relapse or *decompensation,* and then the return to the community may also add to high rates of recidivism in the 6 months following discharge.

Probably the most important single cause of recidivism is failure to connect with needed services and supports in the community. Everyone is aware of the difficulties and

---

BOX 7.1
An Innovation in Psychiatric Rehabilitation

Just as with other fields, many of the innovations in psychiatric rehabilitation have emerged from seemingly casual observations and the initiatives of regular staff members "doing what comes naturally." The following description of the "discovery" of what would emerge as the assertive community treatment model, describes such an event.

About the fall of 1970, soon after Dr. Arnold Marx had assumed leadership of the Special Treatment Unit (a research unit of the Mendota Mental Health Institute), and after Mary Ann Test had been at the STU for two of what had become rather standard six-month-long studies, a critical event happened at the traditional staff party held to celebrate the end of each study and to generate ideas about what type of study to do next. Few staff came. Those present pulled their chairs into a circle and began to discuss why

others did not show up. Some staff did not come, it was observed, because their morale was low. They were discouraged because, despite their energetic efforts to create innovative inpatient treatments enabling discharge (Mendota is a Wisconsin state psychiatric hospital) recently discharged patients kept coming back to the hospital. Some aides suggested that they would not do another similar study.

In this discussion, one aide observed that when a social worker, Barb, followed patients into the community and provided aftercare, these patients tended not to come back to the hospital. As the evening wore on, they talked about how Barb did this. Someone suggested that the STU should do what Barb did and abandon the inpatient interventions. Eventually, it was agreed that this is what they would do, and the STU leadership, Drs. Marx and Test, stuck to this decision in the morning and thereafter. The next STU study was to be one about caring for persons with severe mental illness in the community. (Greenley, 1995, pp. 9–10) frustrations involved in dealing with large, impersonal bureaucratic systems. The newly discharged consumer often has to connect with new agencies, doctors, and staff persons. They have to make these connections at the very time when they may be least likely to cope with the frustrations and stress that we all experience when dealing with large organizations or new situations. It is little wonder that persons often become ill during the months directly after discharge.

Awareness of the Need for Care Coordination at the National Level

As the negative effects of massive deinstitutionalization became more widely known, the need for coordination of care in the community for persons with serious mental illness became a concern at the national level. The U.S. Congress passed PL 99–660 (1973), the Comprehensive Mental Health Services Act, which required each state to develop a plan for providing community-based services for persons suffering from severe and persistent mental illness. This act required each state to include case management services as an element of their plan. In an effort to respond to the obvious unmet needs of newly deinstitutionalized persons, in 1979 the National Institute of Mental Health (NIMH) created the Community Support Program (CSP). This program provided for nationwide demonstration projects to improve services to persons experiencing chronic (today we would say persistent) mental illness (Turner & TenHoor, 1978). CSP projects employed state-of-the-art solutions and strategies to meet client needs in the community. One strategy they employed to meet the comprehensive needs of people with a severe and persistent mental illness was case management.

Case Management

The term *case management* can mean widely different things to PsyR professionals from around the world. Despite the varied treatment procedures these differences usually represent, there is fairly good agreement about the goals of a case management system. Case management refers to any "process or method for insuring that the consumer is provided needed services in a coordinated, effective and efficient manner" (Baker & Intagliata, 1992, p. 215).

The use of the term *case management* has also become an issue for consumers, some of whom state that they are not a "case" and they do not need to be "managed." The International Association of Psychosocial Rehabilitation Services (IAPSRS) language guidelines (2003), for example, caution against the use of terms such as *case study*. Some people have even suggested that the term *care management* be used to replace case management. In this book, we have decided to continue use of the term case management for a couple of reasons. First, we believe it is a useful way to refer to all the issues surrounding individuals' treatment and rehabilitation. The term *case management* is widely understood and is used in the many informative articles that are referenced in this chapter. Clearly, *case* is not an appropriate term for the person served, but rather for the circumstances and conditions influencing the individual's life. Much of this chapter focuses on models of service provision described in the psychiatric rehabilitation literature and the research that has been done to examine their efficacy.

Baker and Intagliata (1992) have done extensive research on case management. They define four basic service objectives that are common to successful case management services. These programs ensure the following:

1. *Continuity of care:* The individual receives comprehensive services over an appropriate period of time.
2. *Accessibility:* The person can enter and use the services he or she needs.
3. *Accountability:* The system accepts responsibility for the services provided.
4. *Efficiency:* Services are provided in an economical fashion.

Providing consumers with needed services in a coordinated, effective, and efficient manner actually requires many distinct case management functions. Agranoff (1977) suggested that a good case management system should carry out five basic functions for its clients:

1. *Assessing:* identifying the client's needs
2. *Planning:* developing a comprehensive service plan for the client
3. *Linking:* connecting the client with services to be delivered
4. *Monitoring:* ensuring that the services are actually delivered to the client
5. *Evaluating:* assessing the client's response to services and providing follow-up.

Furthermore, Baker and Intagliata (1992) suggest that a good case management system may also (1) reach out to clients who are "service resistant," (2) advocate for clients so that they receive services at other agencies and programs, and (3) provide direct services to clients.

Of course, a case management program's ability to help consumers get their needs met depends in part on the resources available in a given community. An ideal *community support system* (CSS) offers a wide array of supports and services. The concept of a comprehensive CSS came out of NIMH's Community Support Program in the late 1970s and was used to help states plan their mental health systems. Consumers, family members, practitioners, and mental health administrators all helped to identify the components of an ideal CSS, which include the following:

- Client identification and outreach
- Mental health treatment
- Rehabilitation services
- Crises response services
- Housing
- Health and dental care
- Protection and advocacy

- Peer support
- Family and community support
- Income support and entitlements.

Case management is also an essential component. It has been described as the glue that holds a CSS together, ensuring that consumers get access to everything they need to live successfully in the community (Stroul, 1989).

The Case Manager

The case manager is both a psychiatric rehabilitation "Jack of all trades" and the "single point of responsibility" at the core of the case management service. This PsyR "generalist" carries out the functions listed earlier by performing many different roles, including but not limited to:

> case manager, integrator, expeditor, broker, ombudsman, advocate, primary thera-pist, individual representative, personal program coordinator, systems agent and continuity agent. (Baker & Intagliata, 1992, p. 217)

At its best, case management is the epitome of individualized service. Each consumer is met on his or her own ground and dealt with individually. The first task of the case manager is to comprehend the needs and aspirations of the individual. To accomplish this, the case manager must form a close working relationship with the consumer, based on trust. With this assessment also comes a clear understanding of the aspects of the psychiatric disability that must be addressed through the case management process to achieve the consumer's goals. Working together, the next step for the consumer and case manager is the development of a comprehensive plan. The plan should take into account strengths and weaknesses as well as environmental contingencies, which will help the individual reach his or her desired goals. Consumer input at this planning stage is critical for future success. The consumer will not achieve goals that are not "owned" by the consumer. This concept of service planning is explained in greater detail in Chapter 5.

The next step is for the case manager to help the consumer link up with the agencies, services, or organizations necessary for achieving the goals of the plan. This phase might be carried out by the case manager or by the consumer depending on the types of services needed and the ability of the consumer. Regardless of who makes the initial contact, it is important for the case manager to form and maintain an ongoing professional relationship with each of the services the consumer is utilizing. This will allow the case manager to perform other functions such as monitoring, advocating, and evaluating if they are needed. Some level of monitoring should take place even if no problems exist. If carried out unobtrusively, this process can have important benefits. The consumer may be reassured that someone is watching out for his or her interests. The agency or service will be reminded that the case manager is an available resource and can provide support if the need arises.

One of the most difficult tasks for the case manager is evaluating the consumer's progress toward his or her goal(s). Working with the consumer, the case manager needs to help assess progress and develop priorities for services and goals. Premature advancement to the next phase of a plan can be as much of a threat as failure to advance to the next step when the consumer is ready. Because of the difficulties inherent in assessing others and in being evaluated, the level of trust established in the working relationship between the consumer and the case manager is often tested at this stage of the process.

Finally, achieving goals may not signal the end of the process. Often, new needs and aspirations emerge as goals are achieved. An effective case management process is prepared to provide support for the consumer indefinitely.

Models of Case Management

There are a large number of case management programs around the country composed of service elements and philosophies borrowed from different program models. Despite this diversity, a number of identifiably unique models of case management exist and can be defined.

Solomon (1992) identified four general types of commonly practiced case management:

1. Expanded broker model
2. Rehabilitation model
3. Strengths model (Rapp, 1998)
4. Full support model (assertive community treatment).

A short explanation of each of these models is provided in the following subsections. These models have many common characteristics. When actually applied to the real world, program administrators and staff may combine one or more of these models. On the other hand, they may choose not to employ a particular element of a given model.

The full support model is given the most attention. Currently, it is most commonly referred to as *assertive community treatment* (ACT) or *program of assertive community treatment* (PACT). ACT is an evidence-based practice.

Expanded Broker Model

Staff members working in the *expanded broker model,* also called the *generalist model,* depend on making referrals to other agencies and services in the community for most of the basic services provided to their clients. This traditional case management model uses its staff primarily for assessment, planning, linking, and advocating. In general, the staff of the expanded broker model program acts as an agent for their client rather than a service provider. Staff members become resource persons steering their clients to different agencies or services to meet specific needs. Staff members also function as liaisons, advocates, and troubleshooters for their clients. For example, if a consumer is experiencing problems at his or her boarding home, the case manager might meet with the boarding home manager to discuss the problem and arrange for additional services, such as personal skills training (e.g., personal hygiene, clothes washing). It should be obvious from this example that for the staff member working in the expanded broker model, direct experience with existing community services (including knowing key staff persons, program rules and hours, etc.) is a must.

While its influence on the quality and emphasis of services provided is necessarily reduced, this model has the advantage of allowing for much larger caseloads than the other three models described here. Obviously, the effectiveness of the expanded broker model depends on the comprehensiveness and effectiveness of a community support system. In other words, this model has difficulty making up for the lack of available services because it can only link to what is currently available. The case management task in such an environment becomes one of ensuring that the consumer takes advantage of the services that are available.

Rehabilitation Model

The *rehabilitation model* follows a traditional rehabilitation approach. Emphasis is on helping clients achieve success in the environments of their choice rather than emphasizing a comprehensive program for improvement. Clients chose an overall rehabilitation goal and complete a *functional assessment* from which a rehabilitation plan is developed. Under this model the case manager focuses on skill development until the client establishes a support network (Goering, Wasylenki, Farkas, Lancee, & Ballantyne, 1988). In a sense, the rehabilitation model is case management within the context of the overall PsyR approach (Hodge & Drain, 1993). Chapter 5 provides a detailed overview of the PsyR assessment and service planning process.

Strengths Model

The *strengths model* is based on two assumptions (Modrcin, Rapp, & Chamberlin, 1985; Rapp, 1998). The first assumption is that to be a successful person, regardless of whether one has a serious mental illness or not, you must be able to use, develop, and access your own potential and have the resources to do this. The second assumption is that a person's behavior is dependent on the resources he or she has available. A focus on the individual's strengths, as opposed to his or her pathology, defects, and symptoms, is the defining element of this model, making it consistent with PsyR principles.

In this model, the case manager acts as a mentor who assists the client in problem solving and resource development (Hodge & Draine, 1993). Unlike many traditional approaches, the strengths and interests of the individual are the primary emphasis. Rather than emphasizing problems such as a lack of punctuality or poor personal appearance, interventions are focused on helping persons use their strengths to succeed in natural environments of their choice and their places within that environment known as *niches*. Through both assertive outreach to the individual as well as to gain support and resources, the case manager facilitates the person's pursuit of interests and opportunities of his or her choice in the community. Thus, the individual has both the reasons and the motivation to arrive on time and make a good personal appearance.

Full Support Model (Assertive Community Treatment) Model

In addition to providing the five basic case management functions, the full support model directly provides most or all of the necessary services for its clients. Thus there is little or no emphasis on referring clients to other existing community services. In other words, case managers utilizing the full support model are providing basic case management services plus a variety of rehabilitative and treatment services with a multidisciplinary team that typically includes a psychiatrist, nurse, rehabilitation counselor, substance abuse counselor, and perhaps a peer case manager. This team is composed of specialists from different service areas and is employed to ensure that clients have everything they need to make a good adjustment in the community.

The Story of Micky

The situation described in this story is a good example of the day-to-day challenges that face a PsyR professional working in case management. As you read, consider the strategies represented by the different models of case management.

1. What services did the members of the case management team employ to help Micky?
2. What do you think they could have done differently?
3. What could they have done that might have been more effective?
4. What model of case management does this team most resemble and how can you tell?

At 23 years old, Micky had been hospitalized six times since her 19th birthday. A bright student who got only average grades, Micky had spent most of high school writing poetry and smoking marijuana. She had her first full-blown psychotic episode a month after graduation and was hospitalized the next year with a diagnosis of schizophrenia, paranoid type.

Her psychotic episodes followed a predictable pattern. After being stabilized on medication in the hospital, Micky would be discharged to a residential program. Initially, Micky would exhibit an unusually high level of functioning and low level of symptomatology for a recently discharged person with her diagnosis. For several months she would make excellent progress toward the educational or vocational goals she had set with the help of her case manager at the mental health center. Then, as she neared her goal, Micky would typically stop taking her medication, because she was free from any symptoms and accomplishing a great deal. This was followed in several weeks by a psychotic episode, which usually included blaming her case manager for all her problems, dropping out of her job or school, and running away. When she was found, frightening hysterical outbursts would follow, which usually led to her being put out of her residence and hospitalized. Her doctors had tried long-acting, injectable medication but this did not break Micky's cycle of decompensation.

After discharge from the hospital, Micky was always very grounded in reality and rational. Because she was friendly and had a good vocabulary, many of her case managers scheduled individual therapy sessions with her. During these sessions Micky exhibited good insight about her cycle of decompensation. Many of her case managers believed that Micky's insight regarding the obvious pattern of her behavior would ensure that the same events would not happen again.

Now, being discharged for the sixth time in 4 years, Micky was being referred to a case management team. She first met two of the team members in the hospital. They had talked to her about where she wanted to live and what she wanted to do when she left the hospital. Before discharge one of the team members drove her to a garden apartment complex to meet a woman named Sylvia who she might share an apartment with there. Micky and Sylvia got along fine. Sylvia had been hospitalized once, 2 years ago. Since then she had completed her education and worked for a small company putting documents on microfilm for storage. Sylvia had been with the case management team since her discharge.

Micky had decided to go to work after discharge rather than go back to school. With the aid of one member of the case management team who seemed to know where to find jobs, Micky got a job as a billing clerk in a local heating oil company. The same team member visited Micky on the job for several weeks until she was sure that everything was going well. After discussing it with her case manager, Micky had decided to tell her fellow workers and the boss that she had been in the hospital. She was nervous about admitting her mental illness but pleased when she found that they were accepting rather than rejecting. Several days after telling the others about her mental illness, one of the other clerks called Micky aside. Swearing her to secrecy, she told Micky that she had been to a psychiatrist after her divorce and that he had given her pills to take. Micky felt accepted at work. She also got along well with Sylvia. Team members visited the apartment frequently when Micky first moved in. They helped arrange for special services like bank accounts and a telephone in her room. They also set up meetings so she and Sylvia could devise ways of sharing the household bills like the rent, telephone, gas, and electric. They divided the household chores such as cooking, cleaning, shopping, and clothes washing between them. At the end of each week, a team member would visit and ask how things were going, if there were any problems, and if there was anything special coming up during the following week. Micky and Sylvia became friends.

As the members of the case management team knew, rapid initial success after discharge was Micky's typical pattern. Their goal was to identify signs of decompensation and intervene as quickly as possible to prevent another decompensation and hospitalization. They informed Micky and Sylvia about this plan. They told Micky that if and when she began to decompensate they would arrange for her to see the team psychiatrist for evaluation and a possible increase or change in medication. They also told her that if necessary they would arrange for a leave of absence at her work and that they had a respite bed available if she needed more structure than she had at the apartment. Rather than try to elicit insight regarding her part in the pattern, the team members told Micky that her pattern of decompensations was caused by her illness. They stressed that she had a biological disease like diabetes or arthritis and that one of the symptoms of her illness was a periodic psychotic relapse. Her job was to recognize when she was becoming ill and to inform the team so that they could help her get more treatment.

Eight months after moving in with Sylvia, Micky decided to stop taking her medication. After a week, Sylvia noticed that Micky's medication had not been touched and asked her about it. Micky got very angry at first, but Sylvia reminded her of what the team had said about her decompensations. She said it wasn't her fault but that she needed to get more help. Micky called a team member and told them what had happened. An hour later the psychiatrist was at the apartment. After evaluating Micky he changed her medication, adding something to help her sleep better. He asked her to come and see him the next day at the office to see how the new medications were doing. When the team members left, Micky thanked Sylvia for helping her.

Micky continued to get worse for several days. She had several arguments with Sylvia and got into a dispute with a coworker. One evening she even felt so agitated that she asked to sleep at the respite bed where there was a 24-hour nurse for the night. During this crisis period, a team member visited the apartment every evening to see how things were going and monitor Micky's progress. A week and a half after she had seen the psychiatrist Micky began to feel better. She felt the same way she had each time she had been discharged from the hospital. But this time she hadn't been in the hospital; she still had her job and her apartment and Sylvia was still talking to her.

Evaluating Case Management

Numerous research studies have been carried out to evaluate the effectiveness and efficiency of case management. Partly because of the differences between case management programs, the results of these studies have been mixed and sometimes contradictory. Nevertheless, there is clear consensus that case management is effective for achieving certain results. This research literature answers specific questions about the effectiveness of specific types of case management programs (Bond, McGrew, & Fekete, 1995; Chamberlin & Rapp, 1991; Mueser, Bond, Drake, & Resnick, 1998; Solomon, 1992).

Mueser et al. (1998) identified 75 controlled studies of case management for review. Most of these 75 studies examined ACT programs or intensive case management (ICM) programs because other models of case management were less well represented in the research literature. The ACT and ICM program models are very similar with respect to design (see Table 7.1). The major difference between them is that ACT program staff share caseloads, whereas ICM program staff do not. This review provided clear evidence that these programs were effective at reducing time spent in the hospital and increasing clients' housing stability in the community. They also provided some modest evidence for improvements in quality of life and symptomatology.

Mueser et al. (1998) concluded that when case management services were reduced or withdrawn, for example when programs had a designated length of service, consumers showed reduced levels of functioning. This has very important implications for funding as well as the design of future case management services. Nevertheless, the gradual reduction of ACT services to a lower level of intensity is possible without the loss of the gains of the full model. This is known as a *step-down approach* and has been found to be successful (Salyers, Masterton, Fekete, Picone, & Bond, 1998).

TABLE 7.1
Features of Different Community Care Models

Program Feature	Community Care Model					
	Brokered Case Management	Clinical Case Management	Strengths Model	Rehabilitation Model	Assertive Community Treatment	Intensive Case Management
Staff:patient ratio	1:50?	1:30+	1:20–30	1:20–30	1:10	1:10
Outreach to patients	Low	Low	Moderate	Moderate	High	High
Shared caseload	No	No	No	No	Yes	No
24-hour coverage	No	No	No	No	Often	Often
Consumer input	No	Low	High	High	Low	Low
Emphasis on skills training	No	Low	Moderate	High	Moderate?	Moderate?
Frequency of patient contacts	Low	Moderate	Moderate	Moderate	High	High
Locus of contacts	Clinic	Clinic	Community	Clinic/ Community	Community	Community
Intergration of treatment	Low	Moderate	Low?	Low?	High	High?
Direct service provision	Low	Moderate	Moderate	Moderate	High	High
Target population	SMI	SMI	SMI	SMI	SMI high service utilizers	SMI high service utilizers

From Mueser, K. T., Bond, G. R., Drake, R. E., & Resnick, S. G. (1998). Models of community care for severe mental illness: A review of research on case management. *Schizophrenia Bulletin, 24*(1), 40.

The Development of Assertive Community Treatment

In the early 1970s Mary Ann Test, Ph.D., and Leonard Stein, M.D., working at the Mendota Mental Health Institute in Madison, Wisconsin, began developing strategies to solve the "revolving door" problem at their hospital and hospitals around the country. Test and Stein set out to reduce recidivism rates by supporting their patients in the community so effectively that they would not need to be continually readmitted for individual treatment. They started with the assumption that high readmission rates came about because the individual needs of people with serious mental illness were not being met in the community (Test & Stein, 1978). They believed that discharged hospital patients had the following needs that had to be met for them to be able to remain in the community:

- Material resources food, shelter, clothing, medical care, recreation, and so forth
- Coping skills to meet the demands of community life
- Motivation to persevere and remain involved with life
- Freedom from pathological dependent relationships
- A supportive system that assertively helps the individual with the preceding four requirements.

The original model they developed was called Training in Community Living (TCL). They implemented it in a program where they could conduct ongoing research, which eventually became known as Program for Assertive Community Treatment. TCL introduced an important innovation to psychiatric rehabilitation: a support system that takes an assertive stance in helping consumers to stay out of the hospital. TCL staff visited clients in the community, wherever and whenever they needed assistance, rather than asking them to come to a particular site. This approach has been referred to as "a hospital without walls" (Harron, 1993), because it was designed as an alternative to inpatient treatment.

Test (1992) reports that the Madison TCL program team consisted of 13 staff providing services for 115 persons diagnosed with schizophrenic disorders. The team's main goal was to meet the needs necessary to maintain people in the community. To accomplish this, the team developed individualized service plans for each individual. Whenever possible the team also carried out most aspects of the treatment plan. The interdisciplinary team, which was made up of specialists such as mental health technicians, nurses, and vocational rehabilitation counselors, worked together in a generalist staffing mode to meet each client's needs. A generalist staffing pattern implies that each staff person can and sometimes did do each task. A psychiatrist was also a part-time member of the team.

TCL services were provided in the community, at the individual's home, recreation, or job site. This is sometimes referred to as *in vivo*, or in the client's "real-life" environment. This approach has many advantages; for example, teaching a client a skill in the location where it will be used is a highly effective intervention (see Chapter 5 for more on this concept). Perhaps most importantly, staff used a very assertive outreach strategy to ensure that services were provided when and where they were needed. For example, if a client had difficulty remembering to take the correct dosage of medications, the team might visit him at home once or twice a day to deliver and monitor the medications. When appropriate, the TCL team also worked with families, community agencies, landlords, or whomever was involved in a client's support system.

Providing services to individual consumers in the community has the effect of ensuring that these services are individualized rather than watered down to meet the needs of a large group. The team provides individual consumers with symptom management in the form of medication, round-the-clock on-call assistance for crisis intervention, and brief hospitalization if necessary. The team also helps consumers obtain the basic needs of food and shelter and also social supports and assistance with family relations. Finally, the team helps consumers secure and maintain regular employment positions in the community. Initially, TCL was designed as a time-limited program. Follow-up research studies indicated that many consumers regressed when the program supports were removed. Rather than being time limited, the current program is designed to provide services indefinitely or on an as-needed basis.

The "revolving door" process of readmitting consumers for short-term hospitalizations and then returning them to the community for aftercare services was both ineffective and very costly. Test and Stein believed that it would be better for the individual—and less costly for the system—to provide intensive case management services and keep the individual in the community. Research study results (Stein & Test, 1985; Test, 1992) supported their beliefs, and TCL was soon replicated in other parts of Wisconsin, and eventually in other states and countries as well. When implemented in different locations, some agencies began to modify the TCL model in order to address the unique needs of their client population or in order to compensate for limited resources. For example, a program serving a high percentage of individuals with dual diagnoses (e.g., severe mental illness and substance abuse) might require several team members to be substance abuse specialists; or a program that lacks the financial resources to include psychiatrists and nurses on their teams might contract with another agency to provide medical and psychiatric services. While not strictly adhering to the full range of services provided by the original TCL program, these programs were strongly influenced by the work of Test and Stein.

Evaluating Training for Community Living

As the success of TCL became apparent, Test and Stein (1978) conducted research to test the effectiveness of their program compared with the traditional services offered in Madison. Their research design consisted of randomly assigning individuals newly admitted via hospital intakes to either the TCL program or traditional treatment. Traditional or "usual treatment" consisted of hospitalization and referral to a community agency. By the end of the first year, 130 individuals, evenly divided between TCL and traditional treatment, were included in their study. Of the 65 individuals assigned to TCL only 12 were hospitalized. This compared to 58 of the 65 individuals served in the traditional treatment who were hospitalized. In addition, TCL participants spent an average of 11 days in the hospital compared with the control group's average of 37 days in the hospital.

Evolution into ACT

Training in Community Living has evolved into assertive community treatment. Over the years, principles for the implementation of ACT have been established and its critical ingredients have been established. These have been outlined by Phillips et al. (2001) and Bond, Drake, Mueser, and Latimer (2001). ACT employs a multidisciplinary team approach with the capacity to provide services 24 hours per day, 7 days a week when needed. The team approach ensures that someone with knowledge of each individual receiving services is always available if needed. In addition, caseload sizes are kept small (approximate ratio of one ACT team member to 10 consumers). So a multidisciplinary team of six would serve a caseload of 60. All treatment and rehabilitation services are provided by the team including a part-time psychiatrist, nurse, case manager, substance abuse counselor, vocational specialist, and sometimes a peer/consumer provider. The team meets four or five times a week and is led by a team leader who is also a "front-line" practicing clinician. The entire team serves each individual. ACT teams provide the following services:

- Case management and coordination of services, primarily by direct provision of the services
- Psychiatric services, provided by an M.D. or nurse practitioner, including evaluation, prescribing medication, and monitoring symptoms and side effects

- All needed counseling and psychotherapy services
- Housing support services to help the individual maintain a stable residence
- Employment and rehabilitation services, similar to supported employment (see Chapter 9)

For consumers with addiction diagnoses, substance abuse counseling that is fully integrated with mental health services, using a stages of change or recovery model, is included (Bond et al., 2001). This treatment technique is covered in greater detail in Chapter 8.

As discussed earlier, all services are provided to consumers in the community, rather than at clinics. None of the services are arbitrarily time limited. All services are provided assertively; that is, individuals who do not respond or may initially refuse treatment are repeatedly contacted and offered the service. Service recipients are met or contacted wherever they can be found: at their homes, public places, and even in the streets. In ACT, there is no fixed length of stay and generally a "no close" policy—consumers can be served as long as they wish to be. Services are offered intensively, if needed, with contact between staff and clients averaging four times weekly, but at least 2 hours per week. As mentioned, supports are provided around the clock, including the availability of 24-hour crisis intervention. Generally, ACT teams control, in part or whole, the screening and evaluation for any needed psychiatric hospitalizations. They participate on hospital treatment teams, and facilitate discharge planning. In jurisdictions where permitted by law, ACT teams will collaborate with probation and parole officials. In addition, in some places, when someone is involuntarily committed to outpatient services, they are often enrolled in ACT.

An additional feature of many ACT programs is the inclusion of peer providers. Peer providers are persons who are themselves recovering from mental illness who serve as team members. Peer providers have been found to be as effective in some ways as non–peer providers. Added to teams, they bring unique strengths and sometimes produce better outcomes (Craig, Doherty, Jamieson-Craig, Boocock, & Godfried, 2004). The addition of a consumer or peer to an ACT or case management team successfully engages more consumers. Clients randomly assigned to teams with peer case managers were more engaged with treatment and had lower rates of nonattendance at appointments. They also had higher levels of participation in structured social activities and significantly fewer unmet needs in the domains of daytime activity, social activity, finances, transportation, and access to benefits. Employing peer providers also contributes to improved client engagement with services and improved outcomes in some areas.

The features and ingredients of ACT are summarized in ten principles stated by Phillips et al. (2001) and presented in Table 7.2.

When Is a Program Actually ACT?

How do you know an ACT program when you see it? A validated and widely used "fidelity scale" is the Dartmouth Assertive Community Treatment Scale (DACTS; Teague, Bond & Drake, 1998). Fidelity, as introduced in Chapter 1, is about "faithfulness" to a particular treatment or rehabilitation model. DACTS has been used to assess fidelity of programs to the ACT model (Bond et al., 2001).

TABLE 7.2
Ten Principles of Assertive Community Treatment

1. Services are targeted to a specified group of individuals with severe mental illness, usually those at high risk for hospitalization, rehospitalization, or relapse.
2. Rather than brokering services, all treatment and rehabilitation services are provided directly by the assertive community treatment team.
3. Team members share responsibility for the individuals served by the team.
4. The staff-to-consumer ratio is small (approximately 1 to 10).
5. The range of treatment and services is comprehensive and flexible.
6. Interventions are carried out at the locations where problems occur and support is needed, "in vivo" (in real life), rather than in hospital or clinic settings.
7. There is no arbitrary time limit on receiving services.
8. Treatment and support services are individualized.
9. Services are available on a 24-hour basis.
10. The team is assertive in engaging individuals in treatment and monitoring their progress.

Source: Based on Phillips et al., 2001.

Do Effective Case Management Programs Share Similar Characteristics?

Rapp and Goscha (2004) reviewed the relevant research literature on all forms of case management. They began by evaluating the quality of the research represented by each study. Applying very stringent criteria, they selected 22 research papers on case management and identified several important principles or active ingredients across effective case management approaches. These are described in detail in their article from *Psychiatric Rehabilitation Journal* in the spring of 2004 (pp. 345–359), and are summarized here:

- Case managers should deliver as much of the help as possible themselves rather than refer to other providers.
- Case managers should have primary responsibility for a person's services.
- Natural community supports (including people not paid to help the consumer) are the primary partners of the team.
- Case management work is done *primarily* in the community as opposed to an office or program site.
- Caseloads should be small enough to allow frequent contact.
- Services should be time unlimited, if needed.
- The availability of familiar people, 24 hours a day, 7 days a week, is helpful to consumers.
- Case managers should facilitate informed choice by the consumers they serve.

Assertive Community Treatment: An Evidence-Based Practice

Assertive community treatment is one of the most widely utilized evidence-based practices (EBP). As this chapter has pointed out, ACT has many positive characteristics for both the consumer and the service delivery system. Essentially, comprehensive services including medication, counseling, case management, rehabilitation, substance abuse services, and other specialized supports are provided to the consumer in the environments of his or her choice.

ACT is a highly normalized service. The stigma attached in attending a mental health center or a psychiatrist's office is eliminated, although some argue that having one or more professionals arriving at your home or job might be somewhat stigmatizing and intrusive. At the same time supports are provided on an as-needed basis to help the consumer achieve success in different settings such as school, work, and the community. Although ACT is a fairly high-cost community-based service, this increased cost is more than offset by the reduction in hospital utilization that is achieved. In fact, some states have employed ACT to help reduce the census of state psychiatric hospitals allowing for reductions in the number of needed hospital beds and the closing of some hospitals.

ACT employs a multidisciplinary team approach with the capacity to provide around-the-clock support. The team approach ensures around-the-clock availability of someone with knowledge of each individual receiving services. In addition, caseload sizes are kept small (approximate ratio of one ACT team member to 10 consumers) and support is provided to consumers as long as it is needed.

Randomized controlled clinical trials have consistently demonstrated that ACT is effective at reducing the number of hospital days (time spent in the hospital). ACT programs have also demonstrated an increase in housing stability for their clients. Results on improved quality of life and increased client satisfaction with services have been mixed. Some high-fidelity programs that are very faithful to the ACT model (see description of fidelity in Chapter 1 and earlier in this chapter) have achieved these outcomes, others have not.

CONTROVERSIAL ISSUE
Is Assertive Community Treatment Too Assertive?

An evidence-based practice, assertive community treatment (ACT), has consistently proven effective at reducing hospital utilization and increasing housing stability (Bond et al., 2001; Marshall & Lockwood, 2004). The fact that staff members actively seek out individuals in the community to ensure that they are receiving the services they need is considered an important ingredient in the success of this strategy.

This "assertive" approach on the part of staff has several important benefits. Frequent staff member visits may help remedy the lack of insight experienced by some individuals with severe mental illness. Xavier Amador, in his book *I Am Not Sick: I Don't Need Help* (Amador & Johanson, 2000), sees this lack of awareness as "anosognosia" a term referring to impaired awareness or ignorance of illness. This was discussed in Chapter 2 of this text. In short, the ill individual is unaware of the symptoms or presence of the illness. It is not uncommon for a floridly psychotic individual to state that he feels fine, has no problems and no illness. In these circumstances, left unchecked, the individual typically continues to deteriorate until hospitalization is necessary. Assertive outreach may also help to identify problems before they become full-blown crises. For example, a problem with the landlord may be dealt with in a timely fashion before it gets blown out of proportion and ends in eviction.

While the benefits of an assertive approach are obvious, an increasing number of consumers and professionals have raised concerns about the coercive effects this can have on individuals (e.g., Ahern & Fisher, 2001; Diamond, 1995). Because of the strong emphasis on medication compliance in some ACT services, some have questioned whether ACT is a "medical model" program rather than psychiatric rehabilitation. In addition, some individuals have complained that ACT is intrusive and occasionally coercive (Ahern & Fisher, 2001). The implication is that the principles of consumer choice and empowerment so strongly held by psychiatric rehabilitation are less emphasized in medical model programs. Ahern and Fisher consider ACT so coercive that they devised an alternate form of case management they call PACE (Personal Assistance in Community Existence). Diamond points out that assertive outreach falls along the same continuum as court-ordered treatment, which he sees as highly coercive and paternalistic. The point is very simple. An individual who, without requesting it, is frequently visited by a team of professionals who ask prying questions may reasonably feel coerced.

Diamond (1995) is correct; this issue is similar to court-ordered treatment and outpatient commitment. When, if ever, should the principles of choice and respect for the individual be violated in an effort to help? Should society be paternalistic and intrusive when an individual is not aware that he or she is putting himself or herself or others at risk?

What is the evidence that ACT is too assertive or even intrusive? Bond et al. (2001) in their study reported that only 11% of the consumers enrolled in ACT found it to be intrusive, confining, or fostering dependency. Rosenheck and Neale in two reports (Neale & Rosenheck, 2000; Rosenheck & Neale, 2001(a,b)) studied 40 ACT teams serving more than 1,500 consumers within the Veterans Administration system to determine the extent to which "limit-setting" coercive interventions were offered. Coercive interventions included assigning a representative payee (someone other than the consumer to manage his or her money), contingent withholding of services or supports until a desired behavior was established, invocation of external authorities such as parole or probation officers, and enforced "voluntary" or involuntary hospitalization. These coercive interventions were used with 10% of the ACT consumers. The coercive interventions tended to be used with individuals who had a more difficult course of their illness and recovery and were actually associated with poorer outcomes. Thus, there is some evidence showing that for a small minority of consumers ACT is viewed as a coercive approach.

BOX 7.2
Gary Bond, Ph.D.

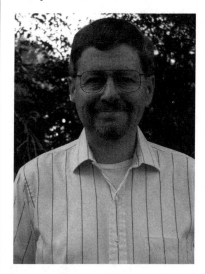

The research and writing of Gary Bond, Ph.D., Chancellor's Professor of Psychology at Indiana University–Purdue University Indianapolis, has contributed to the field of psychiatric rehabilitation since 1979. Since entering the field as director of research at Thresholds, a large PsyR agency in Chicago, he has worked to understand how services can be more effective and to train professionals to work in the field.

When he went to Thresholds for the first time, Dr. Bond found that the practical and egalitarian orientation appealed to him, as did the real-world relevance of the research questions. Does psychiatric rehabilitation help people get jobs? Does it help them to live independently? His interest in the answers to such questions has a personal side as well. Inspired by his sister's determination in coping with symptoms of schizophrenia, Dr. Bond is convinced that people with psychiatric disabilities can and should achieve full community integration.

Dr. Bond's research has focused on evidence-based practices, including studies of supported employment, assertive community treatment, and assessment of fidelity of implementation of evidence-based practices. Gary Bond's work is some of the most frequently cited research in the psychiatric rehabilitation literature.

Critical Ingredients of ACT

Here are some of the critical ingredients of the ACT model:

1. Services are provided to consumers in the community rather than at clinics.
2. Services are provided by a multidisciplinary team, including a psychiatrist, nurse, social worker or other case manager, and vocational specialists. This team meets four or five times weekly.
3. Services are not time limited, with no fixed length of stay and a "no close" policy.
4. The staff-to-client ratio is low.
5. Services are offered fairly intensely with contact between staff and clients averaging four times weekly, at least 2 hours per week.
6. Supports are provided around the clock, including the availability of 24-hour crisis intervention.
7. Services emphasize medication management and practical everyday issues.
8. ACT controls, in part, the screening and evaluation for any needed psychiatric hospitalizations, participates on hospital treatment teams, and facilitates discharge planning.

Service Outcomes of ACT

ACT service outcomes include the following:

1. Reduced hospital utilization (fewer instances and shorter stays)
2. Increased housing stability
3. Possible increased quality of life
4. Possible increased consumer satisfaction with services.

Reviews of ACT Research

The most comprehensive, rigorous, and up-to-date assessment of assertive community research was carried out by the Cochrane reviews, which looked separately at experimental, random assignment studies of assertive community treatment and case management (Marshall & Lockwood, 2004). According to Marshall and Lockwood, ACT has been demonstrated to be an effective way of caring for and providing rehabilitation to persons with severe and persistent mental illness living in the community. People in ACT are twice as likely as those in other types of services to maintain contact with their treatment providers. ACT also drastically reduces the use of inpatient hospital care, sometimes by as much as 20% of the hospitalization days compared with other approaches. Many consumers of ACT are satisfied with the care.

Because ACT is a relatively expensive approach, sometimes it is only offered to high users of psychiatric inpatient care. In these cases, there is pretty good evidence that the program's success in reducing costs is sufficient to justify the increased cost of the ACT teams. In other areas, ACT teams are being funded with resources formerly used on less effective forms of community care.

The findings from the Cochrane review (Marshall & Lockwood, 2004) are summarized next. Compared to other approaches, ACT produces superior outcomes in some clinical and social areas (e.g., living accommodations, employment, and satisfaction). Those receiving ACT were more than twice as likely to remain in contact with services as were those receiving standard community care. With respect to likelihood of hospital admissions, those receiving ACT were significantly less likely to be admitted to hospital than those in the standard community care groups. That is, their occasion for hospitalization was 60% of that of comparison approaches. With respect to living arrangements, ACT clients were twice as likely to be living independently and were four times less likely to become homeless. Those receiving ACT spent more days in independent living accommodations (Test, 1979), fewer days homeless, and more days in stable living arrangements (Bond et al., 2001; Lehman, Dixon, Kernan, & Deforge, 1995). With respect to employment, ACT recipients were three times more likely to be employed. There was no evidence of a clinically significant effect on mental state, symptoms, and overall social functioning (Marshall & Lockwood, 2004).

Compared to case management, people served by ACT teams consistently spend fewer days in hospitals than those provided by standard case management approaches (Marshall & Lockwood, 2004). The cost of hospital care was consistently less for those in ACT, so the extra expense of the ACT service itself proved cost effective.

ACT as an Early Intervention Strategy

Increased attention has been directed at the amount of time it takes before someone with psychotic symptoms receives appropriate treatment. The period between when a person becomes psychotic and when they first receive treatment for the psychosis has been labeled *duration of untreated psychosis* (DUP). Not surprisingly, the DUP for some individuals can be quite long. Studies have found average rates of DUP of about 1 year (McGlashan, 2000). This situation may be partly due to the fact that many of the individuals in question are in their late adolescent or early adult years, which are periods of significant change in one's development (Holloway & Aitchison, 2003) or because many persons with psychosis are unaware of their condition (Amador & Johanson, 2000).

Some researchers have theorized that untreated psychosis may have neurotoxic effects (e.g., McGlashan, 1996). In other words, when someone is actively psychotic, he or she may be losing healthy brain neurons (see Chapter 2). Thus, the longer one is acutely ill, the more damage is being done to the number, structure, and function of one's neurons. The evidence in this area is mixed and inconclusive. It is clear, however, that for many individuals being actively psychotic can be very unpleasant, frightening, and stressful and that longer periods without treatment simply compound the situation (Melle et al., 2004). Being in a psychotic state also has a detrimental effect on an individual's social relationships, job performance, and family life (Drake, Haley, Akhar, & Lewis, 2000; Melle et al., 2004). Longer DUP has also been related to an increase in the negative symptoms of schizophrenia such as anhedonia (Malla & Norman, 2002).

Many researchers have speculated that reducing an individual's DUP will result in improved short-term and long-term outcomes (e.g., McGlashan, 1999; Meller et al., 2004). Intervening to halt the psychotic process should reduce neurotoxicity, reduce the individual's suffering due to fear, anxiety, and stress, and improve performance socially, on the job, and in the family. There is fairly good evidence that, at least in the short term, shorter DUP is related to better outcomes (Malla & Norman, 2002). Several studies report that shorter DUP is related to longer remissions and lower symptom rates in the future, whereas longer DUP is related to increased negative symptoms and poorer quality of life. These relationships become weaker as the length of the research follow-up periods increase.

What is the best way to provide services to someone experiencing his or her first psychotic episode? The first problem is to identify people who are candidates for early intervention. The most common strategy yet employed has been to develop systems for community case detection and then employ mobile outreach teams (Malla & Norman, 2002). In England, where the government is beginning to mandate such service (Holloway & Aitchison, 2003), and in Canada, this issue has been addressed by using teams of professionals that are similar to ACT teams.

To be effective, as a first step these teams need to establish working relationships with persons who have recently become ill and their families, who are often still in a state of denial about the illness. Once a relationship is formed, the teams provide education about the illness, medication, and side effects. They also ensure that the treatment is begun and complied with, reducing the DUP. Denial is a typical response to these illnesses, which makes ACT with its assertive and in-the-community components an excellent helping strategy.

ACT and Persons in the Criminal Justice System

In the past several years, the principles of ACT have been applied to serve persons with severe and persistent mental illness involved in the criminal justice system. Examples of two nationally recognized models are the Thresholds Jail Program in Chicago, Illinois, and Project Link in Rochester, New York (Lambert et al., 2001; Lamberti & Weisman, 2004). Both of these programs use ACT to engage clients through assertive outreach in clinical, residential, and social services. The Thresholds Jail Program is a collaboration between Chicago's largest PsyR provider and one of the nation's largest jail systems, Cook County, Illinois. These programs coordinate with the many components of the criminal justice system, and provide services 24 hours per day. Use of ACT to engage offenders who are severely mentally ill is a strategy that is becoming increasingly more common. Both Thresholds Jail Project and Project Link have (1) demonstrated decreased arrest and incarceration rates, (2) lengthened the time individuals spend in the community, and (3) decreased overall costs. This new approach can be understood as an emerging forensic assertive community treatment or a "FACT" model (Lamberti & Weisman, 2004), although this acronym has also been used for a family assisted assertive community treatment program.

ACT Comes of Age as a Program and a Professional Specialty

In addition to being an EBP, the field of assertive community treatment is a specialty program that has come of age with its own professional association, Assertive Community Treatment Association (ACTA). On its website (http://www.ACTassociation.org), one can learn about ACTA annual conferences, training, and program standards. In the United States, special training and technical assistance centers are sponsored by state mental health agencies (e.g., ACT Center of Indiana and the Bridgeway Training & Technical Assistance Center, Elizabeth, New Jersey). Some version of ACT services are funded in dozens of U.S. states, Europe, Australia, and New Zealand.

The Future of ACT and Case Management Approaches

What is the future of ACT and related approaches? Gary Bond and his colleagues (2005) have made a number of predictions (see box for a profile of Gary Bond). They believe the "basic" ACT model will continue to improve in two ways. First, ACT will systematically incorporate EBPs such as illness management (Chapter 3), motivational interviewing for dual disorders (Chapter 8), supported employment (Chapter 9), and family psychoeducation (Chapter 13) into its service package. Second, ACT will be enhanced by the development of new strategies. For example, another service that may be integrated within ACT teams is supported socialization. Supported socialization employs volunteers or staff members who go on social and recreational outings with clients. The social isolation and loneliness of many persons with severe and persistent mental illness is well known. Bond et al. (2005) pointed out that ACT has had very little impact on social functioning. Yet most ACT clients deeply desire friendships and social contact. Peer support services, such as drop-in centers or support groups, may provide easily accessible social outlets (see Chapter 12).

In addition, Bond et al. (2005) predict that the scope of ACT may change in two separate directions. First, they believe, given its cost effectiveness, ACT services for the general population of people with severe and persistent mental illness will become more widespread. The second development that is very likely is the wider implementation of specialty ACT teams for specific target populations, particularly for persons with mental illness involved in the criminal justice system.

It is not surprising that the use of case management strategies for the community treatment of severe mental illness has steadily increased. Case management has obvious economic and quality-of-life advantages. *Although case management, particularly ACT, can be more expensive than traditional community-based services, it is considerably cheaper than psychiatric hospitalization.* Planners on the state and national level see increasing evidence that employing case management strategies reduces hospital usage. Numerous states have adopted case management strategies in an effort to reduce hospitalizations and close some of their state hospitals (see Chapter 14). These new strategies have also proven to be effective for reaching those consumers who have "fallen through the cracks" in the system. Whether because of their illness, underlying personality issues, past experiences that have alienated them from the system, or any number of other reasons, a large number of consumers are unconnected with the mental health system. Today, we know that treatment and psychosocial interventions have a positive effect on the long-term outcomes of these conditions. Assertive community treatment and other intensive case management approaches have proven to be the most effective strategies for reaching out to this group with the treatment and services they need.

Finally, and most importantly, case management models that provide services to consumers in the community are a more normalized form of treatment delivery than the traditional day programs or supervised residences. Such case management strategies allow the consumer to reside and work in the environment of their choice and receive services there. Consumers are not stigmatized by frequently attending a mental health center or vocational workshop. The services provided have a direct relationship to the here and now issues involved with coping with their illnesses and succeeding in the community. This consistency with the PsyR principle of normalization makes case management attractive to many consumers and PsyR professionals.

Summary

Assertive community treatment and case management programs were developed in response to the high rate of hospital recidivism often caused by substandard, underfunded, uncoordinated, and incomplete community-based services. These programs are characterized by the fact that services are provided to the consumer in the community where they live, rather than in a mental health center, clinic, or so forth. The role of the case manager may vary according to the model of program where they work. Some case managers act as brokers or agents arranging services for their clients. Others may be direct service providers working one to one with their clients in the community to help meet their needs. By either arranging for or directly providing services, case management systems strive to ensure that client needs are met in an appropriate and timely manner. Evaluation of these programs has demonstrated that they are effective at reducing the length of time of hospital stays. They have also been used effectively to reach out to those segments of the population with severe mental illness that are most resistant to treatment.

Class Exercise

1. Consider the four major models discussed in this chapter: case manager as broker, rehabilitation case management, strengths model case management, and assertive community treatment (ACT). How is each model consistent with the principles of psychiatric rehabilitation described in Chapter 4? Are they ever inconsistent with these principles?
2. Is it possible that the ACT model, its all-inclusive comprehensive nature, its aggressive outreach, the sometimes heavy emphasis on medication compliance and its no-close policy might be interpreted by some as unduly coercive or intrusive? Why might that be?
3. In many locales, ACT is reserved for the most high-risk persons who already have histories of many relapses and often have just been released from the hospital.
   a. Speculate why this might be the chosen target group for ACT in many states.
   b. Is this the best use of ACT? Why or why not?
   c. If ACT were used as standard treatment (as it is in a few places), what might be its effects?
   d. If ACT were used as an early intervention, as opposed to a relatively later intervention implied above in this question, what might be its effects?
4. Should ACT be used for the community treatment and rehabilitation of persons with mental illness in the criminal justice system beginning with their arrest, through their experience in jails and prisons, and after discharge? What might be the effects of such a program?
5. In a few states, ACT is used to serve for persons who live in the community, but have been committed to involuntary treatment in the community. What do you think of this application of ACT?

References

Agranoff, R. (1977). Services integration. In W. F. Anderson, B. J. Frieded, & M. J. Murphy (Eds.), *Managing human services*. Washington, DC: International City Management Association.

Ahern, L., & Fisher, D. (2001). PACE: Personal assistance in community existence. Lawrence, MA; The National Empowerment Center.

Allen, P. A. (1974). A consumer's view of California's mental health care system. *Psychiatric Quarterly, 48*, 1–13.

Amador, X., & Johanson, A. (2000). *I am not sick: I don't need help*. Peconic, NY: Vida Press.

Aviram, U., & Segal, S. P. (1973). Exclusion of the mentally ill: Reflection on an old problem in a new context. *Archives of General Psychiatry, 29*, 126–131.

Baker, F., & Intagliata, J. (1992). Case management. In R. P. Liberman (Ed.), *Handbook of psychiatric rehabilitation* (Vol. 166, General Psychology Series). Boston: Allyn & Bacon.

Bond, G. R., Drake, R. E., Mueser, K. T., & Latimer, E. (2001). Assertive community treatment for people with severe mental illness: Critical ingredients and impact on patients. *Disease Management & Health Outcomes, 9*(3), 141–159.

Bond, G. R., McGrew, J. H., & Fekete, D. M. (1995). Assertive outreach for frequent users of psychiatric hospitals: A meta-analysis. *The Journal of Mental Health Administration, 22*(1), 4–16.

Bond, G. R., Salyers, M. P., Rollins, A. L., & Moser, L. L. (2005). The future of ACT. In C. L. Mulder & H. Kroon (Eds.), *Assertive community treatment: Evidence-based bemoeizorg voor patiënten met ernstige psychiatrische aandoeningen*. Arnhem, The Netherlands: Cure & Care Publishers.

Chamberlin, R., & Rapp, C. A. (1991). A decade of case management: A methodological review of outcome research. *Community Mental Health Journal, 27*(3), 171–188.

Craig, T., Doherty, I., Jamieson-Craig, R., Boocock, A., & Godfried, A. (2004). The consumer-employee as a member of a mental health assertive outreach team. I. Clinical and social outcome. *Journal of Mental Health, 13*(1), 59–69.

Daley, J. M., & Latane, B. (1968). Bystander interventions in emergencies: Diffusion of responsibility. *Journal of Personality and Social Psychology, 8*, 377–383.

Diamond, R. J. (1995). *Coercion in the community: Issues for mature treatment systems* (New Directions for Mental Health Services No. 65). San Francisco: Jossey-Bass.

Drake, R. J., Haley, C. J., Akhar, S., & Lewis, S. (2000). Causes and consequences of duration of untreated psychosis in schizophrenia. *Psychiatry, 177*, 511–515.

Goering, P., Wasylenki, D., Farkas, M., Lancee, W., & Ballantyne, R. (1988). What difference does case management make? *Hospital and Community Psychiatry, 39*, 272–276.

Greenley, J. R. (1995). *Implementation of an innovative service in Madison, Wisconsin: The program of assertive community treatment (PACT)* (Research Paper Series 49). Madison, WI: Mental Health Research Center.

Harron, B. (Producer/Director). (1993). *Hospital without walls* [videotape]. Available from Duke University Medical Center, Durham, NC.

Hodge, M., & Draine, J. (1993). Development of support through case management services. In R. W. Flexer & P. L. Solomon (Eds.), *Psychiatric rehabilitation in practice*. Boston: Andover Medical Publishers.

Holloway, F., & Aitchison, K. (2003). Early intervention in psychosis: From government prescription to clinical practice. *Psychiatric Bulletin, 27*, 243–244.

International Association of Psychosocial Rehabilitation Service. (2003). *Language Guidelines*. Columbia, MD.

Kirk, S. A., & Therrien, M. G. (1975). Community mental health myths and the fate of former hospitalized individuals. *Psychiatry, 38*, 209–217.

Klerman, G. (1977). Better but not well: Social and ethical issues in the deinstitutionalization of the mentally ill. *Schizophrenia Bulletin, 3*(4), 617–631.

Kohen, W., & Paul, G. L. (1976). Current trends and recommended changes in extended-care placement of mental individuals: The Illinois system as a case in point. *Schizophrenia Bulletin, 2*, 575–594.

Lamberti, J., Weisman, R. L., Schwarzkopf, S. B., Price, N., Ashton, R. M., & Trompeter, J. (2001). The mentally ill in jails and prisons: Towards an integrated model of prevention. *Psychiatric Quarterly, 72*(1), 63–77.

Lamberti, J., & Weisman, R. L. (2004). Persons with severe mental disorders in the criminal justice system: Challenges and opportunities. *Psychiatric Quarterly, 75*(2), 151–164.

Lehman, A. F., Dixon, L. B., Kernan, E., & Deforge, B. (1995). Assertive treatment for the homeless mentally ill. Paper presented at the 148th Annual Meeting of the American Psychiatric Association, Miami, FL.

Malla, A. K., & Norman, R. M. G. (2002). Early intervention in schizophrenia and related disorders: Advantages and pitfalls. *Current Opinion in Psychiatry, 15,* 17–23.

Marshall, M., & Lockwood, Al. (2004). Assertive community treatment for people with severe mental disorders. In *The Cochrane Database of Systematic Reviews Issue 2* (The Cochrane Library). New York: Wiley Interscience.

McGlashan, T. H. (1996). Early detection and intervention in schizophrenia: Research. *Schizophrenia Bulletin, 22,* 327–345.

McGlashan, T. H. (2000; 1999). Duration of untreated psychosis in first-episode schizophrenia: Marker or determinant of course. *Biological Psychiatry, 46,* 899–907; Correction. *Biological Psychiatry, 47,* 473.

Melle, I., Larsen, T. K., Haahr, U., et al. (2004). Reducing the duration of untreated first-episode psychosis. *Archives of General Psychiatry, 61,* 143–150.

Modrcin, M., Rapp, C., & Chamberlin, R. (1985). *Case management with psychiatrically disabled individuals: Curriculum & training program.* Lawrence: University of Kansas School of Social Welfare.

Mueser, K. T., Bond, G. R., Drake, R. E., & Resnick, S. G. (1998). Models of community care for severe mental illness: A review of research on case management. *Schizophrenia Bulletin, 24,* 37–74.

Neale, M. S., & Rosenheck, R. A. (1995). Therapeutic alliance and outcome in a VA intensive case management program. *Psychiatric Services, 46*(7), 719–723.

Neale, M. S., & Rosenheck, R. A. (2000). Therapeutic limit setting in an assertive community treatment program. *Psychiatric Services, 51*(4), 499–505.

Phillips, S. D., Burnes, B. J., Edgar, E. R., Mueser, K. T., Linkins, K. W., Rosenheck, R. A., et al. (2001). Moving assertive community treatment into standard practice. *Psychiatric Services, 52,* 771–779.

President's New Freedom Commission. (2003). *Achieving the promise: Transforming mental health care in America.* Available from http://www.mentalhealthcommission.gov.

Rapp, C. A. (1998). *The strengths model.* New York: Oxford University Press.

Rapp, C. A., & Goscha, R. J. (2004). The principles of effective case management of mental health services. *Psychiatric Rehabilitation Journal, 27,* 345–359.

Rosenheck, R. A., & Neale, M. S. (2001a). Intensive psychiatric community care in the Department of Veterans Affairs [references]. In B. Dickey & L. I. Sederer (Eds.), *Improving mental health care: Commitment to quality* (pp. 183–192). Washington, DC: American Psychiatric Publishing.

Rosenheck, R., & Neale, M. S. (2001b). "A critique of the effectiveness of assertive community treatment": In reply. *Psychiatric Services, 52*(10), 1395–1396.

Salyers, M. P., Masterton, T. W., Fekete, D. M., Picone, J. J., & Bond, G. R. (1998). Transferring clients from intensive case management: Impact on client functioning. *American Journal of Orthopsychiatry, 68*(2), 233–245.

Santiestevan, H. (1975). *Deinstitutionalization: Out of their beds and into the streets.* Washington, DC: American Federation of State, County and Municipal Employees.

Solomon, P. (1992). The efficacy of case management services for severely mentally disabled clients. *Community Mental Health Journal, 28*(3), 163–180.

Stein, L. I., & Test, M. A. (1985). The evolution of the training in community living model. *New Directions for Mental Health Services, 26,* 7–16.

Stroul, B. (1989). Community support systems for persons with long-term mental illness: A conceptual framework. *Psychosocial Rehabilitation Journal, 12*(3), 9–26.

Test, M. A. (1979). Continuity of care in community treatment. *New Directions for Mental Health Services, 2,* 15–23.

Test, M. A. (1992). Training in community living. In R. P. Liberman (Ed.), *Handbook of psychiatric rehabilitation* (Vol. 166, General Psychology Series). Boston: Allyn & Bacon.

Test, M. A., & Stein, L. I. (1978). Training in community living: Research design and results. In L. I. Stein and M. A. Test (Eds.), *Alternatives to mental hospital treatment.* New York; Plenum.

Teague, G. B., Bond, G. R., & Drake, R. E. (1998). Program fidelity in assertive community treatment: Development and use of a measure. *Am J Orthopsychiatry, 68,* 216–232.

Turner, J. C., & TenHoor, W. J. (1978). The NIMH community support program: Pilot approach to a needed social reform. *Schizophrenia Bulletin, 4*(3), 319–344.

Chapter 8

Dual Diagnosis: Substance Abuse and Mental Illness

Introduction 220

History of Dual Diagnosis Treatment 221

Sequential Services 222

Parallel Services 223

Integrated Services 224

Fundamental Treatment Strategies in Providing Integrated Dual Disorders: Stages of Treatment 225

Precontemplation 225

Contemplation 225

Preparation 226

Action 226

Maintenance 226

Stages of Change: A Case Study Applying Motivational Interviewing 227

Principles of Treatment for People with Dual Diagnoses 228

Dual Diagnosis Treatment in Groups 229

Integrated Services: An Evidence-Based Practice 230

Elements of the Evidence-Based Practice: Integrated Dual Disorder Treatment 230

Outcomes of the Evidence-Based Practice 232

Limitations on the Research Evidence 232

Roger's Story 234

Discussion of Roger's Story 238

Summary 238

Class Exercise 238

References 240

This chapter deals with the treatment and rehabilitation of persons who have a severe and persistent mental illness and a substance abuse disorder. The person with a severe mental illness has a much greater risk of developing a substance abuse disorder than someone without a mental illness. The difficulties inherent in having two potentially disabling conditions (which we refer to as having a dual diagnosis) are confounded by the fact that the mental illness and substance abuse disorder may interact, each exacerbating or aggravating the other. In addition, coming from different philosophical and educational backgrounds, the service providers for these different conditions often have conflicting and sometimes contradictory approaches. Services have been developed to address these problems and other issues involved in helping this dually diagnosed population.

This chapter will answer the following questions:

1. *What unique problems are faced when providing services to someone dually diagnosed with a mental illness and a substance abuse disorder?*
2. *Why are such a large proportion of persons with mental illness at risk for substance abuse?*
3. *What barriers prevent the effective treatment and rehabilitation of individuals who are dually diagnosed?*
4. *What is the best way to provide services to persons with this dual diagnosis?*

Introduction

During the 1980s mental health providers witnessed the emergence of a seemingly new population of service recipients, the "young adult chronic patient." These individuals had not experienced the prolonged hospitalizations that were common prior to the deinstitutionalization movement (Caton, 1981; Drake & Wallach, 2000; Pepper, Ryglewicz, & Kirshner, 1981). Instead, remaining in the community, they experienced greater exposure and access to alcohol and street drugs. Over time, it became apparent to mental health providers and funding agencies that a large proportion of individuals with severe mental illness were also engaged in substance abuse (Drake & Wallach, 2000). Studies have indicated a wide incidence of substance abuse among people with psychiatric illness ranging from 14% to 70%, depending on psychiatric diagnosis and the specific populations being studied (Evans & Sullivan, 1990; Regier et al., 1990). Regier and colleagues found that for persons diagnosed with schizophrenia, 47% meet the criteria for a substance use disorder at some time in their life and that at any given point in time the incidence (individuals who meet the criteria for both diagnoses at a given moment) ranges between 25% and 35% (Cuffel, 1996; Mueser, Bennett, & Kushner, 1995). This is compared to a 7% incidence rate of an active substance disorder diagnosis in the general population (Evans and Sullivan, 1990). The population of people with this dual diagnosis is fairly heterogeneous with a variety of combinations of different psychiatric diagnoses and substances of choice (Drake and Wallach, 2000). Frequently, an individual with a dual diagnosis is a polysubstance abuser (using more than one substance). Although substance abuse is not unique to young persons, increased incidence of use has been found to relate to factors such as age (younger), gender (male), and education level (lower) (Drake & Wallach, 1989).

This phenomenon has been variously labeled *co-occurring disorder, coexisting disorder, dual diagnosis disorder, mentally ill chemical abuser (MICA),* and *mentally ill substance abuser (MISA),* among others. Regardless of the label, these conditions present serious problems for both the individual and the service system. To begin with, the disorders interact and worsen each other, complicating the clinical, rehabilitative, medical, and social needs of the dually diagnosed person (Drake, Mueser, Brunette, & McHugo, 2004; Drake and Wallach, 1989, 2000; Evans and Sullivan, 1990; Mueser, Noordsy, Drake, & Fox, 2003a; Regier et al., 1990). These individuals have been found to be at greater risk for medication noncompliance, hospitalization, homelessness, suicide, and illness including HIV infection. They tend to have more family problems and to exhibit more hostility, more disruptive behavior, and more violence than individuals with a single disorder. Furthermore, systems designed to provide services for specifically either a substance abuse or psychiatric disorder are often not particularly skillful at assessing or treating the other disorder.

Another important characteristic of persons with both a mental illness and a substance abuse disorder is that they often have greater *sensitivity* to substances than persons without a mental illness. This factor may reduce the ability to detect a substance abuse problem because workers who are unaware of this increased sensitivity may judge reported usage levels as well within the normal range (i.e., similar or less than their own levels of use). For example, the consumer who tells his counselor that he has two beers a night, an amount the counselor thinks is normal and within reasonable limits since he drinks that much as well, may have a substance abuse problem. In fact, the consumer may be several times more sensitive to alcohol than his counselor. This phenomenon, labeled the *supersensitivity hypothesis* by Mueser, Drake, and Wallach (1998b), makes it difficult for individuals in normal social gatherings to avoid negative consequences related to their substance use. It is also the likely reason for the high proportion of persons with severe mental illness reporting substance abuse problems.

History of Dual Diagnosis Treatment

People with a psychiatric disorder who abused substances have not always been thought of as having two psychiatric disorders. Psychiatric symptoms were seen as signs of an illness, but substance abuse was often considered bad behavior (Evans & Sullivan, 1990). Many mental health clinicians believed that their clients would cease abusing substances if they received adequate treatment for the psychiatric disorder. Substance abuse counselors often mistook psychiatric symptoms for evidence of substance abuse because abuse of drugs and alcohol may cause symptoms that mimic those of mental illness (Evans & Sullivan, 1990; Miller, 1997).

The mental health and substance abuse treatment systems were both unsuccessful in treating individuals with dual disorders. The mental health service provider found that the person with dual disorders was difficult to engage and did not respond to typical mental health treatment. Many in the substance abuse treatment system endorsed *abstinence* and considered even psychotropic medications to be mood-altering drugs. Service providers in both systems often refused treatment to people until the other disorder was under control. It was not uncommon, for example, for community mental health clinics to refuse services to an individual who exhibited signs of alcohol or drug intoxication. Such individuals might be admonished to "return when you are sober." Many people with a dual disorder found themselves inadequately treated by one system or the other or, in a "Catch-22"–like situation, simply not eligible or accepted for services at all because they needed both mental health and addiction services simultaneously.

Primarily because separate systems already existed for serving either persons with mental illness or persons with substance abuse problems, the first strategies for treating persons with a dual diagnosis consisted of either a *sequential* approach or a *parallel* service approach.

Sequential Services

In *sequential services* a person with a dual diagnosis first receives treatment for one of the disorders. When the first disorder is successfully dealt with or "under control," the individual is referred for treatment for the subsequent disorder. This method has been found to be largely ineffective since the disorder that is *not* being treated often undermines the treatment for the disorder being addressed (Drake, Bartels, Teague, Noordsy, & Clark, 1993).

Traditionally, mental health treatment consists of psychotropic medication (Chapter 3), individual and or group counseling, perhaps day program services (Chapter 6), and case management services (Chapter 7), which are typically used for persons with severe and persistent mental illness. Traditional substance abuse treatment often requires *abstinence* (refraining from the use of all drugs), sometimes including abstinence from psychotropic medication, attendance at Alcoholics Anonymous (AA) or Narcotics Anonymous (NA) meetings, and working a 12-step process based on the AA *12-step model* (Evans & Sullivan, 1990).

A popular misconception on the part of mental health providers has contributed to this method of treatment. Many providers believe that people with mental illness engage in substance use solely as an attempt to self-medicate. In other words, drugs or alcohol are used to provide relief from their psychiatric symptoms. If this is the case, it follows that adequate treatment of the psychiatric disorder would eliminate the need for the use of substances. This theory has not proven to be helpful for many people with dual disorders. Studies of motivation for using substances indicate that people with psychiatric disorders use substances for a variety of reasons other than relief from symptoms such as to feel relaxed, to improve social interactions, to be accepted by their peer group, and to alleviate boredom (Bellack & DiClemente, 1999; Nishith, Mueser, Srsic, & Beck, 1997; Spencer, Castle, & Michie, 2002). Not surprisingly, it appears that people with mental illness use substances for some of the same reasons as other substance abusers and users.

Treatment for the psychiatric disorder in the absence of treatment for the substance abuse is ineffective for both disorders. People engaged in substance abuse experience resulting impairments that interfere with their ability to engage in rehabilitative activities, manage a medication regimen, or even keep appointments with doctors and other treatment practitioners (Mueser et al., 2003a). It is not difficult to imagine the difficulty in monitoring the effect of a medication regimen, the most important agent for symptom control, at the same time someone is engaged in substance abuse. In addition, there is some evidence that substance abusers are more likely to lower or increase their prescribed psychotropic medications at their own discretion, compared to other individuals (Heyscue, Levin, & Merrick, 1998; Krystal, D'Souza, Madonick, & Petrakis, 1999).

Likewise, substance abuse treatment in the absence of mental health treatment is equally ineffective. Besides the obvious problem of untreated psychiatric symptoms, unaddressed functional impairments related to the psychiatric illness will interfere with the ability to address the substance abuse issues.

Parallel Services

With the *parallel services* approach, both disorders are treated simultaneously by different staff members who may be working in different programs or agencies. While this approach addresses some of the problems inherent in the sequential approach, it introduces several additional issues and often results in "fragmented, contradictory and inadequate care" (Drake et al., 1993, p. 607).

In the absence of specialized knowledge and training, the mental health provider lacks an understanding of the addictive behavior, while the addictions specialist lacks an understanding of mental illness. Furthermore, the traditional treatments used in each of these approaches tend to contradict each other. Mental health treatment often emphasizes empathy toward the individual and the development of a trusting working relationship. This empathic counseling is used to assist the person to gain insight and to set and achieve goals. Substance abuse treatment tends to take a more confrontational, no-nonsense stance toward the client.

An individual's failure to do follow through on substance abuse treatment is typically seen as a lack of commitment and confronted by the counselor or group members. This approach is in stark contrast to mental health services, which employ active outreach to engage clients in services when they might drop out of treatment. The person with a dual disorder finds himself or herself dealing with systems that may be quite different from each other in terms of philosophies, goals, strategies, and approaches. This dual diagnosis service strategy forces the individual to attempt to integrate these contradicting treatment approaches (Mueser et al., 2003a).

In some cases, these contradictions cause problems for the treatment systems as well. Confusion may arise concerning who is responsible for advocating for the individual, assisting with housing or social services, and other outside supports. For example, a traditional addiction treatment model might wait to let a person reach "rock bottom," that is, lose everything as a consequence of the addiction, so he or she might be motivated to get treatment. Mental health staff may be intervening in an opposite manner to prevent just such a scenario. A substance abuse professional might label this "enabling" a person to continue to use substances without negative consequences, while mental health staff will call it case management or crisis intervention.

Treatment plan goals and interventions may conflict with each other. The same issues that stem from the different approaches to these conditions manifest themselves in how the individual's relationship to the community is understood. Contradictions due to differences between these two service systems may emerge at many levels. Although these are not insurmountable, the lack of coordination of services and mutual awareness of these problems make them difficult to overcome for the individual with a dual diagnosis.

Table 8.1 summarizes the disadvantages just discussed of the traditional sequential and parallel treatment approaches.

Integrated Services

The integrated approach favored today was developed to overcome the shortcomings of the sequential and parallel approaches. Research literature surveys (e.g., Ridgely, Goldman, & Willenbring, 1990) supported the notion that parallel or sequential services are less effective than an integrated approach. With integrated services, the person with both a substance abuse disorder and a psychiatric illness receives treatment for both disorders in the same place, at the same time, by the same practitioners. These practitioners are knowledgeable about both disorders as well as about the complications resulting from co-occurring disorders.

Early efforts at integrating mental health and substance abuse services added substance abuse groups into mental health day treatment. These groups often followed the 12-step model adhering to features such as confrontation and the focus on abstinence. Still, practitioners found that some group members, who were often at different stages with regard to their readiness to recover or change, were not ready to make a commitment to changing their behavior (Drake et al., 2004; Drake, Mercer-McFadden, Mueser, McHugo, & Bond, 1998).

Today's integrated service model for dual disorders is an evidence-based practice and will be described in detail later in this chapter.

TABLE 8.1

Disadvantages of Traditional Sequential and Parallel Treatment Approaches to Dual Disorders

---

Sequential Treatment
- The untreated disorder worsens the treated disorder, making it impossible to stabilize one disorder without attending to the other.
- There is a lack of agreement as to which disorder should be treated first.
- It is unclear or impossible to know when one disorder has been "successfully" treated because both disorders may need long-term, perhaps lifelong, attention and/or treatment. Therefore, the second treatment may never commence. The client is never referred for further treatment.

Parallel Treatment
- Mental health and substance abuse treatments are not integrated into a cohesive treatment package.
- Treatment providers fail to communicate with each other.
- The burden of integration falls on the client.
- Funding and eligibility barriers to participating in both treatments simultaneously exist.
- Different treatment providers have incompatible treatment philosophies.
- A client "slips between the cracks" and receives no services, due to failure of either treatment provider to accept final responsibility for the client.
- Providers lack a common language and treatment philosophy.

Source: Based on Mueser, Noordsy, Drake, and Fox (2003a).

Fundamental Treatment Strategies in Providing Integrated Dual Disorders: Stages of Treatment

Early efforts at substance abuse treatment for persons with a dual disorder often consisted of demanding abstinence and teaching consumers about the many dangers of drug and alcohol abuse. While some people responded to this approach, for many it was a failure. This service approach was ineffective for those who did not want to stop using substances or lacked the awareness of the consequences of their substance use. Clearly, another approach was needed.

Working in the area of addictions treatment, Prochaska, Norcross, and DiClemente (1994) developed the transtheoretical model of behavior change. They identified five stages through which one progresses in making life changes:

1. Precontemplation
2. Contemplation
3. Preparation
4. Action
5. Maintenance.

Prochaska and his colleagues found that although the amount of time spent in each stage may vary for different people, the process, sequence, and the tasks of each stage do not.

According to Prochaska et al. (1994), in each of the five stages the individual is concerned with different tasks. To be effective, services designed to assist people to make changes (e.g., to reduce or eliminate substance use) must be relevant to the stage the person is in. We now take a look at descriptions of these five stages.

Precontemplation

In the *precontemplation* stage, people do not believe they have a problem and they are therefore resistant to change. They may not be aware of the negative consequences of their behavior (e.g., substance use) or they may be demoralized by their circumstances and unable to envision alternatives. People with dual disorders in the precontemplation stage are likely to deny that their substance use causes problems. Conflict within their personal relationships, inability to meet obligations, poor health, and other consequences are blamed on others or circumstances beyond their control.

The treatment task with a person at this stage is to help them become aware of the problems associated with their use of substances; in other words, to raise doubts within the individual. This may best be accomplished by using a technique called *motivational interviewing,* which will be addressed later in this chapter.

Contemplation

In the *contemplation* stage, people are experiencing ambivalence about their problem. They are aware that there are costs associated with continuing with their problem behavior, but these costs are still outweighed by perceived benefits. They are not ready to take action to change. Individuals with dual disorders in this stage may, for example, begin to recognize that their substance use is interfering with their sleep, which in turn is exacerbating their psychiatric symptoms. However, they are also convinced that substance use is an important part of their social interaction with friends.

In this stage individuals are weighing the benefits and costs of their behavior against the benefits and costs of change. They will move toward change when they perceive that the benefits of changing outweigh the costs of change, or the costs associated with their behavior outweigh its benefits. Thus, the treatment task at this stage is to help the individual understand that the benefits of change outweigh the benefits of continued substance abuse. This may also be accomplished by reinforcing or increasing the benefits of change, for example, by getting a job or acquiring new friends.

Preparation

In the *preparation* stage people recognize the need to change. They have decided to make changes in the near future and are ready to take small steps toward that change. They still experience a certain amount of ambivalence, but most of the time they can see that the benefits of change outweigh the costs of change. A program or practitioner who mandates abstinence will be unsuccessful with these persons. The more successful approach consists of helping to identify the steps to take and supportive counseling to sort through the continued feelings of ambivalence and the difficulties of taking even small steps.

Action

In the *action* stage people are taking definite steps to change problem behavior and are acquiring new behaviors. Although their commitment to change is strong, some level of ambivalence continues and supportive strategies that help individuals remember their reasons for change are useful. The person with dual disorders in this stage might be learning new avenues for social interaction, taking on new responsibilities, or accessing educational or employment opportunities.

Maintenance

In the *maintenance* stage, people have sustained change for a while and are working toward preventing relapse. Besides supports, effective maintenance depends on realistic expectations of the possibility of relapse and continual reinforcement of the motivational factors that encouraged the change.

Prochaska and his colleagues (1994) have found that at any given time, fewer than 20% of people expressing a desire to change are ready to take action toward making the change. Furthermore, their research indicates that interventions designed for a stage different from the one the client is currently at will be unsuccessful. For example, as you read about the stages of change in the following section, you will see that services that mandate abstinence as a condition of receiving treatment will not work for individuals in the precontemplation or contemplation stages. These individuals are not ready to take action. Prochaska and his colleagues found that although the amount of time spent in each stage may vary for different people, the process, sequence, and the tasks of each stage do not.

Stages of Change: A Case Study Applying Motivational Interviewing

If an individual's treatment process consists of passing through stages, the psychiatric rehabilitation professional's task becomes helping the individual move from one treatment stage to the next. In short, the professional helps the individual accomplish the tasks of the stage he or she is currently in and encourages movement to the next stage. A specific strategy to accomplish this, *motivational interviewing,* has been developed by Miller and Rollnick (2002).

Defined as "a client-centered, directive method for enhancing intrinsic motivation to change by exploring and resolving ambivalence" (Miller & Rollnick, 2002, p. 25), motivational interviewing is an empathic communication method. According to this strategy, rather than imposing change, the practitioner using motivational interviewing is nurturing the individual's intrinsic motivation to change by assisting the person to see discrepancies between her behavior and her personal goals.

Effective motivational interviewing is based on four principles: (1) express empathy, (2) develop discrepancy, (3) roll with resistance, and (4) support self-efficacy (Miller & Rollnick, 2002, p. 36). In expressing empathy the practitioner is communicating acceptance and an understanding of the person's behavior from the person's perspective. First, the practitioner assists the person in identifying his own goals and values. Then the practitioner helps the individual examine whether there is any discrepancy between his goals and his behavior. The practitioner does not argue for change when met with resistance, but rather accepts ambivalence as natural and assists the person in recognizing the discrepancy between his stated goals and behavior. The practitioner expresses belief in the person's ability to change.

Motivational interviewing is an especially good fit with the values and principles of psychiatric rehabilitation (PsyR). It can be an effective strategy for helping individuals in nearly every aspect of PsyR from complying with their medication regimen to getting a job. Many of the evidence-based practices described in this text call for practitioners to employ motivational interviewing with their clients.

Consider, John, who has been working with his counselor and has identified obtaining employment as his most important goal. In reviewing John's work history, his counselor learns that John has attempted several jobs in the past and has lost each of them because he missed too many days of work. His missed days always followed nights out drinking with his friends. John's counselor asks if John thinks his drinking is an obstacle to reaching his goal of employment. John does not think so but admits it sometimes gets him into trouble.

Rather than confronting John's perspective (e.g., "It seems to me that your drinking is a problem. You've lost several jobs because of it and you've been arrested twice for public

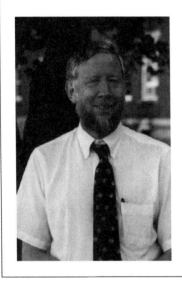
intoxication. I don't see how you can hold a job until you get control of your drinking problem."), using motivational interviewing the counselor engages John in a review of past work experiences and in an exploration of what would need to be different in order to make this next employment attempt successful. The counselor might ask John to list the benefits and costs of using alcohol. In this way the counselor could help John find alternative ways of getting the benefits (e.g., socializing with friends, feeling relaxed) while also examining the costs (e.g., missing work and other appointments, feeling ill, losing money) and helping John to see the discrepancy between his goals and his behavior.

Principles of Treatment for People with Dual Diagnoses

As integrated treatment programs have evolved, much has been learned about effective program components. In 2004, based on clinical research findings, Drake and his colleagues articulated nine principles that they believe to be critical to effective treatment for people with dual disorders (Drake et al., 2004):

1. *Integrated treatment*: Mental health and substance abuse services are provided concurrently by the same clinician or clinical team. The clinician(s) is knowledgeable

about both disorders and the interaction of these. The services are modified to address the specific needs of the individual and characteristics of their dual disorders.

2. *Stage-wise treatments*: Services are relevant to the person's stage of change similar to the work of Prochaska and colleagues (1994) described earlier. Drake and colleagues (2004, p. 368) describe the stages as engagement, persuasion or motivation, active treatment, and relapse prevention.

3. *Engagement interventions*: Services use strategies that increase the likelihood of engagement in treatment for this group of people who typically have difficulty engaging and sustaining participation. Examples of these strategies include active outreach, motivational interviewing (also known as motivational counseling), flexibility, practical assistance, and culturally competent services (Drake et al., 2004, p. 368).

4. *Motivational counseling interventions*: Services use counseling techniques that develop readiness for movement toward individual goals. These interventions are primarily based on the work of Miller and Rollnick (2002).

5. *Active treatment interventions*: Services include interventions such as motivational counseling, cognitive-behavioral counseling, or family interventions that are meant to assist individuals to manage their own illnesses by helping them to develop the needed skills and supports (Drake et al., 2004, p. 369).

6. *Relapse prevention interventions*: It is well known that there is an increased danger of substance abuse relapse for people with dual disorders. Some experts assert that relapse is almost inevitable. Services that assist the individual in planning strategies to address relapse are recommended.

7. *Long-term perspective:* Services are designed to promote retention (provide active outreach, are flexible enough to tolerate periods of relapse, etc.) recognizing that recovery is a long-term process.

8. *Comprehensive services*: Services address the individual's needs in all life areas. As stated earlier in this chapter, people with dual diagnoses are at greater risk for hospitalization, homelessness, illness, and incarceration.

9. *Interventions for treatment of nonresponders*: Services include specialized or modified options based on the unique needs of the individual. Some of these may include residential treatment, family interventions, trauma interventions, and money management.

Dual Diagnosis Treatment in Groups

Several models of group treatment for people with dual disorders have emerged either within day services for people with psychiatric illness or as stand-alone programs. These models may incorporate a combination of elements including (1) a 12-step recovery approach based on Alcoholics Anonymous, (2) stages of treatment as developed by Prochaska and colleagues (1994), (3) motivational interviewing strategies developed by Miller and Rollnick (2002), (4) social skills training, (5) cognitive-behavioral interventions, and (6) relapse prevention strategies (Mueser & Noordsy, 1996).

The *12-step models* are modifications of the 12-step AA model, incorporating the principles and philosophy of AA with mental health care. The groups are generally run by professionals, some of whom have personal experience with addictions. Although it is not required, group members are also encouraged to attend self-help groups in the community. *Professionally assisted pre-AA groups* prepare group members for attendance at community AA groups. These groups address education and motivation while adhering to the concepts of AA (working the 12 steps, facing denial, overcoming rationalization, surrendering to a higher power, etc.) (Mueser & Noordsy, 1996, p. 34).

Broad-based educational support groups are based on the belief that people with dual disorders lack the information needed about the effects of substance use and lack the social support needed for sobriety. These groups provide information in a supportive environment and are time unlimited.

Social skills training groups for people with dual disorders teach group members the skills needed to maintain a substance-free lifestyle (e.g., skills to refuse substances, manage conflict).

Stage-wise treatment groups provide interventions relevant to the different stages of recovery from substance abuse: engagement, persuasion, active treatment, and relapse prevention. Typically, clients in the engagement stage do not attend these groups although they may attend the persuasion groups. The persuasion groups use education and motivational interviewing to increase awareness of the consequences of substance use and to examine the discrepancy between behaviors and personal goals. People in the active treatment and relapse prevention stages attend active treatment groups. These groups include mutual support, skill building including social skills, relapse prevention strategies, and encouragement to use community self-help programs (Mueser & Noordsy, 1996).

Integrated Services: An Evidence-Based Practice

An evidence-based practice (EBP) is a treatment practice that has been shown to have positive consumer outcomes through controlled research studies across a variety of treatment sites. When someone has two simultaneous disorders such as substance abuse and mental illness, the integration of treatments for both disorders has consistently been shown to have better treatment outcomes than traditional treatment. Specifically, this integration refers to the concurrent treatment of both conditions by the same clinicians trained in both disorders. While developed primarily for co-occurring mental illness and substance abuse problems, service integration is generally considered the preferred strategy when faced with other co-occurring disorders (e.g., mental illness and development disability). In general, evidence leans toward the integration of all services regardless of the presence of an additional disorder (e.g., simultaneously providing psychiatric treatment and supported employment).

Elements of the Evidence-Based Practice: Integrated Dual Disorder Treatment

Since integrated treatment is associated with positive outcomes, programs that are carried out according to the integrated dual disorder treatment (IDDT) model are predicted to produce better outcomes for the consumers they serve. To determine how faithful or how well a program resembles the IDDT model, the IDDT Fidelity Scale was developed. (This scale can be downloaded from the Substance Abuse and Mental Health Services Administration website at http://mentalhealth.samhsa.gov/cmhs/communitysupport/toolkits.) Some of the items on the IDDT Fidelity Scale include the following:

1. *Concurrent treatment of both conditions by the same clinicians:* As described earlier, having the same clinicians simultaneously address both conditions is the core element of this EBP. This requires clinicians to have extensive training in both conditions as well as how the conditions may interact with one another. As you might imagine, the clinical picture presented by the individual with co-occurring conditions is more complicated than the clinical picture presented by someone with either condition alone.

2. *Assertive outreach:* Actively seeking out clients in their own environments, assertive outreach is an element of many of the EBPs. Given the propensity of individuals with either mental illness or substance abuse disorders to drop out of treatment, assertive outreach is often necessary to maintain contact.

3. *Motivation-based interventions:* Strategies for engaging the dually diagnosed client will be more effective if they are based on the motivational interviewing strategies described by Miller and Rollnick (2002). This approach takes into account how the client feels about her condition and her readiness to address it. This also incorporates the concept of stages of change put forth by Prochaska and colleagues (1994). Agencies that do not apply this approach tend to find that only a segment of their client population is responsive to their services.

4. *Reduction in negative consequences (harm reduction):* In general, the idea is that the focus should be on reducing the harm or negative consequences of substance use rather than insisting on abstinence. In short, if a client can be helped, for example, to drink less or less frequently the harm caused may be reduced. This is a controversial issue in the substance abuse community where abstinence has been considered the "gold standard" for some time. Still, based on Prochaska and colleagues' work (1994) it seems likely that many individuals in early treatment stages with respect to readiness for change are more likely to respond to a *harm reduction* approach than a request for abstinence.

The substance abuse concept that some people need to "hit bottom" before they get serious about dealing with their addiction is tacit recognition that readiness for change is an important factor in dealing with these conditions. In addition, "hitting bottom" in the sense of using substances in a destructive fashion can be very dangerous (e.g., contracting an HIV infection). Finally, someone who begins treatment based on an initial approach emphasizing harm reduction may, in time, arrive at the understanding that total abstinence is preferable to any substance use for achieving recovery.

5. *Comprehensiveness:* This is the idea that all of the related issues in a client's life need to be dealt with simultaneously. Clients often need to make fundamental changes in many aspects of their lives as they move through the recovery process. For example, it has long been recognized that a recovering substance abuser may need to change his habits including the places he frequents, the friends he hangs around with, and how he spends his time. Successfully addressing the addiction may require changes in all of these areas. To assist consumers in making such global changes, a wide array of services must be

available such as residential programs, supported employment, and social skills training.

6. *Cultural sensitivity and competence:* This element of the EBP should be present in all services. Whenever persons of different cultures work together, there is the possibility of miscommunication of meaning. When co-occurring conditions are present this danger is greatly increased and needs to receive special attention.

Outcomes of the Evidence-Based Practice

Integrated approaches for co-occurring mental illness and substance abuse problems have been found to be superior to nonintegrated approaches. Studies have demonstrated positive outcomes such as reduced substance abuse, reduction of psychiatric symptoms, increased housing stability, reduced hospitalizations, fewer arrests, improved functional status, and improved quality of life (Drake et al., 2002). While the integrated approach is not a panacea with respect to the conditions it is designed to address, it has been shown to be superior to either the sequential or parallel service models described earlier in this Chapter (Mueser et al., 2003b).

Limitations on the Research Evidence

Though the evidence cited in the literature has tended to support the effectiveness of IDDT, questions have been raised about the validity of the research studies. One important source that has questioned the validity of IDDT comes from the Cochrane Review. First becoming widespread in the 1990s, Cochrane reviews focus on specific medical specialties or subspecialties, systematically gathering all relevant data generated from controlled clinical trials. Named for one of the earliest proponents of this idea, Professor Archibald L. Cochrane, the reviews are commissioned by the Cochrane Collaboration (http://www.cochrane.org). Formed in 1993, the collaboration which is based in Oxford, England, currently has 10,000 collaborators from more than 80 countries around the world. A number of Cochrane reviews have focused on treatment and rehabilitation services for severe mental illness, including the issue of integrated treatment for persons with severe mental illness who are substance abusers.

A Cochrane review conducted by Jeffery, Ley, McLaren, and Siegfried (2000, 2003), reviewed six studies they deemed relevant to the issue. While they reported that the design quality of the studies was not high and several clinically important outcomes such as mental illness relapse, satisfaction, and social functioning were not assessed, they found no clear evidence supporting one strategy of providing care over another. In short, they concluded that the current trend toward integrated programming is not based on good evidence. This challenges the basis of an integrated treatment strategy for persons with dual disorders.

Why did the Implementing Evidence-Based Practices group described in Chapter 1 determine that integrated treatment strategies were superior while the Cochrane review team found no evidence for this advantage?

The most obvious answer to this question is that each group looked at somewhat different evidence. The Cochrane group accepted data for review from only six of the most rigorously designed studies (e.g., controlled trials with random assignment), whereas the EBP group looked at results from 26 studies with all types of study designs. In both cases reviewers commented on the quality of the studies under review. Clearly, the EBP reviewers applied more liberal criteria for inclusion. One might speculate whether a large amount of data from all different types of studies may or may not outweigh a much smaller amount of data generated by stricter criteria. Given the emphasis EBP places on outcome assessment, it is likely that this question and those like it will be answered shortly.

CONTROVERSIAL ISSUE
Total Abstinence versus Harm Reduction

The notion that substance abuse is a disease and that state and federal governments should provide funding for its treatment and rehabilitation is a relatively new idea. Today it seems clear that different people have different levels of tolerance for substance use, some are more prone to addiction than others, and substance abuse has a number of related physiological manifestations. Recognition of the physiological, social, and spiritual damage caused by substance abuse is worldwide. Still, a good deal of controversy surrounds whether the goal of services for substance abusers should be total abstinence or harm reduction.

One of the most successful models for dealing with substance abuse, Alcoholics Anonymous was begun in 1935 in Akron, Ohio, by a New York City stockbroker, Bill W., and an Ohio surgeon, Dr. Bob (http://www.alcoholics-anonymous.org). Based on self-help in the form of mutual support and a 12-step process, the goal of AA is total abstinence from alcohol. In fact, the first step of the process is to admit that one is powerless over alcohol. The AA website reports having more than 2,000,000 members attending 100,000 AA groups worldwide. AA has helped virtually millions of people with alcohol addiction.

Today, many substances besides alcohol, both legal and illegal, are abused. In the 1950s a similar organization based on the principles of AA, Narcot-

ics Anonymous, emerged (http://www.na.org). NA simply substituted the word "addiction" for "alcohol" in the first step of the 12-step process: One is powerless over the addiction. The NA website reports that by 2002 there were some 20,000 groups worldwide conducting more than 31,000 meetings per week. Recognition that one is powerless over either alcohol or drugs implies that abstinence is the best solution for achieving and maintaining sobriety. Not everyone is in agreement with this position.

Reducing, the negative consequences, or harm reduction, is the idea that the goal of treatment or rehabilitation should be to reduce the harm caused by the substance abuse rather than require total abstinence (Marlatt, Blume, & Parks, 2001). The harm reduction strategy, which fits well with motivational interviewing and Prochaska and colleagues' (1994) stages of change, has the advantage of meeting people where they are with respect to their substance abuse problem. It is no secret that many substance abusers have no intention of quitting (Marlatt, 1998). In fact, the drug rehab adage that someone has to "hit bottom" before they can start to recover from their addiction is based on just this recognition. The idea seems to be that not until someone hits bottom will he or she decide that the costs of using substances outweigh the benefits.

Interestingly, harm reduction is not as uncommon as one might first suspect. Methadone maintenance, the provision of free methadone to heroin addicts, is a successful harm reduction program.

Needle exchange programs to reduce the spread of HIV are another harm reduction strategy. Even ensuring that an intoxicated person does not drive is a harm reduction strategy. In the area of alcohol addiction, one self-help group, Moderation Management, uses a nine-step program to help people modify and manage their drinking (http://www.moderation.org). Starting in the 1980s in Rotterdam, the Netherlands, harm reduction was a natural outgrowth of liberalized drug laws that allowed drug users to organize publicly. This organization, "Junkiebond," began advocating for harm reduction strategies for drug users and was able to establish the first needle exchange program in 1984 (Saladin & Santa Ana, 2004).

The research on harm reduction appears to show that while some people benefit (e.g., suffer fewer negative consequences), others do not and would be better served by adopting the goal of total abstinence. The question may be how to best engage individuals in rehabilitation and then help them to decide whether they should have a goal of harm reduction or total abstinence. As Rusty Foster (personal communication, October, 2005) an experienced professional in this area puts it:

> The problem for the severely mentally ill population is their sensitivity to even small amounts of a substance. Though it is important to recognize that most consumers begin reducing substance use gradually rather than moving right to abstinence, and it is important to recognize and reward these changes, in the long range the treatment goal usually is abstinence. But here the movement to abstinence is seen as a process not an event.

Roger's Story

Roger's story has some similarities with many of the homeless persons you might encounter on the streets of big cities. With a mental illness and co-occurring substance abuse problems, Roger has had a lifetime of difficulty understanding his conditions and trying to fit into society. While some people seem to "get all the breaks," others, like Roger, seem born under a dark cloud. As you read about Roger you might consider whether his life to date would have turned out the same had he been born at a later date. You should also be considering the following questions:

1. What might the outcome have been if Roger had received more attention for his problems when he was in school?
2. What were the system problems that made Roger's first attempts at treatment difficult and how might they have been corrected?
3. What were the important worker and system characteristics of the last program that successfully engaged Roger in treatment and why were they effective?
4. Finally, based on what you know about Roger and the treatment he is receiving, what would you guess his future holds?

Roger is a 45-year-old man with a dual diagnosis of bipolar disorder and substance abuse disorder. He jokes that he's recovering from substance abuse and "the system," meaning the school system, the foster care system, and the legal system. As a child he moved from one foster home to another. Roger's school performance was generally mediocre. He occasionally did well on tests or assignments but more often barely passed. Most of the time in school he seemed gloomy and withdrawn. When he did emerge from this withdrawn state, he was animated and loud, arguing with his foster parents, teachers, and fellow students. During these arguments he frequently became physically aggressive, slamming doors, plates, textbooks, even punching or kicking holes in walls. He hardly slept at all during these periods. His classmates thought he was weird and dangerous. His teachers routinely kicked him out of the classroom for his behavior until finally he ended up in a special school for kids who are emotionally disturbed. Here, he found other kids he thought were as weird as he was. He learned how to cope with his mood swings: cocaine when he needed to perk up, pot when he needed to calm down, and alcohol when he couldn't get anything else.

Roger's first arrest was for shoplifting a six pack of beer. He had no trouble convincing the judge that it was a teenage prank. The third time he was arrested the judge decided to keep him in jail overnight. The school refused to be involved since Roger had "dropped out" a few months earlier when he turned 16. In the jail cell Roger went wild; screaming, cursing, punching his fists, and finally slamming his body into the cell wall over and over again. Roger only vaguely remembers what happened next—the restraints with belts, the ambulance, the injection. He woke up in the psychiatric ward of the local hospital. He was discharged a week later with a diagnosis of conduct disorder and a bottle of pills that he had no intention of taking. It wasn't until his second hospitalization following a suicide attempt that he was diagnosed with bipolar disorder.

Roger was mandated to mental health treatment and sent to the local day treatment center. He'd almost forgotten about his appointment with the "intake worker" the night before while he got high with his friends. He awoke feeling tired and groggy, not wanting to go to the mental health center, but not wanting to go back to the hospital or to jail either. He arrived only 10 minutes late. While he waited in the front hallway, he could see the people who went to this place. A few looked happy, talking, joking with each other. Many more looked like zombies, sitting and staring. Almost no one looked like they were even near his age.

The intake worker took Roger to an office. She was quiet and calm and seemed nice enough. She did not seem upset that his clothes were a mess and he looked like he had just rolled out of bed. She asked him a lot questions. He was surprised that she asked so much about drugs and alcohol and even more surprised when she said he had a "substance abuse problem." He was not disappointed when she told him he could not get services from them until he "stopped using." She would give him the name of a drug and alcohol treatment program. Roger felt great. The social worker from the hospital assured him he was not off the hook and that he would have to go to the drug and alcohol treatment program in order to leave the hospital. Roger was discharged from the hospital and went to live in a boarding home. She set up an intake for him. The one thing Roger was most sure of was that he did not have a "substance abuse" problem. He used stuff when he wanted to have fun or relax but it was social. As if to prove it, he went to bed early the night before the second intake having had only one marijuana joint. The man at the substance abuse treatment program who did the intake was mostly friendly, a little bit gruff. He asked Roger why his clothes were dirty and when he had last had a shower. He also asked a lot of the same questions about his use of drugs and alcohol and a lot more questions too. This time, Roger was more careful with his answers. He said he occasionally smoked pot but only for fun. In spite of this the intake worker said Roger should plan to start the program next Monday when he would do a drug screening, which would take place every so often afterward. He was warned that if he used any drugs he would be kicked out of the program, and if he were kicked out he would be going back to the hospital. Over the weekend Roger could feel himself getting anxious. He couldn't sleep. He could barely sit still. He knew he could calm down if he could score some pot. He wondered if it would show up in the drug screening he was led to believe he'd have to go through on Monday. He did not want to go back to the hospital. Feeling somewhat desperate, Roger decided to try one of the pills they'd given him when he left the hospital. He popped one. An hour later when he didn't feel any different, he angrily tossed the pills in the garbage. Monday morning he arrived at the program. They were expecting him. He met with a counselor who asked if he was on anything. Roger said no. The counselor sent him to the men's room for a urine sample and then to the group room to attend what he called a 12-step group. Later, the counselor called Roger into his office. "I thought you said you weren't using." "What do you mean?" Roger asked. "You know what I mean. What did you take?" "Oh," Roger remembered. "I took a pill they gave me at the hospital." "Listen," the counselor told him, "Substance free. This is a substance-free environment. You want to come here, you can't use." Roger thought, "Who said I want to come here!" Instead he said, "Who cares, I threw the pills away yesterday." The counselor wanted him to attend 30 groups in 30 days. He could barely sit through the one group today. He was up all night, pacing around his room at the boarding home, walking the streets. He showed up at the program the next morning. "You look like hell," the group leader said. "I didn't sleep last night." "Your eyes are bloodshot," said one of the group members. "I told you!" Roger shouted, "I didn't sleep!" "Yeah?" responded the group member. "Well, it looks like you've been using." Roger jumped up knocking over his chair. Heading right for the loudmouthed "know it all" guy, he thought better of it and smashed his fist into the wall. Back in the counselor's office Roger was told he was out of control. His erratic behavior was a sign to him that he'd been using. He was suspended for 3 days. He should return next Monday.

The final note in Roger's chart read "Lost to contact." Roger slipped away. Over the subsequent few years he lived on the street, in shelters, and occasionally spent brief periods in jail. He picked up odd jobs when he could and worked long enough to get money for drugs. He moved back and forth between sullen isolation and angry, aggressive outbursts. One cold winter night during a period of isolation while trying to warm himself in a doorway Roger was approached by a guy named Henry. Henry was carrying two cups of coffee and offered one to Roger. "Hey man, you must be cold. Here have some coffee." Roger was startled. Most people passed him on the street as if he were invisible. Henry declined Roger's request for money. Roger declined Henry's offer of food.

Roger was happy to be left alone, but Henry came back night after night, always with a cup of coffee and, after that first night, also with a sandwich. Roger kept pretty much to himself but Henry talked plenty, mostly about himself. He told outlandish stories about things he did during his "drinking days" and some stories about months in the "loony bin" after he tried to kill himself. Depression he called it. After a while, Roger started to let his guard down and told some of his own tales. Talking this way with Henry reminded Roger of his two best friends from junior high school. They did not get along any better with their fathers than Roger had with his, but they all thought things would be different when they grew up. They talked about it—about what their lives would be like. Roger joked with Henry about how different it had all worked out.

Eventually, they got around to the whole point of Henry's nightly visits. "So, Roger, is this really the way you want to spend your life?" "Oh God, what are you? Some kind of social worker?" "No, not exactly. Well in a way. Where I work they call me a MICA counselor. And if you want your life back, I think I can help." Roger shook his head no. "You don't have to make any promises." Henry told him. Here's my address, I'm there every day. Just come to my office and meet some other guys a lot like you and see what goes on there." A few days went by. Henry didn't come back. Roger kept thinking about his question, "Is this the way you want to spend your life?" "Maybe," he thought. "At least nobody's telling me what I can and can't do."

"Oh what the hell." Roger decided to stop in at Henry's place. Henry invited Roger to sit in on a meeting he was about to start. One guy in the meeting said he was beginning to feel really down, had no energy, and was afraid he was going to start using again. Henry said, "So, that's pretty scary when you feel yourself slipping and you're afraid you'll lose control." They went on to talk about depression, the guy's meds, seeing his psychiatrist, and the people he could call if he was thinking about using and needed support. In a private meeting Henry and Roger talked about bipolar disorder, what it is, what the meds he was given were supposed to do. They talked about addiction, about what Roger liked about using, about the downside of using. They talked about Roger's future.

Roger's been coming to this program for a year now. He's been taking lithium and that's helped, although he was hospitalized once for a week because of depression. Stopping using has been tough. He's tried repeatedly and has succeeded for brief periods. Right now he's been clean for 90 days. That's the longest he has gone and he feels pretty hopeful. Henry hooked him up with a GED prep course and a supported employment program. Henry says it's all Roger's doing, but Roger remembers what Henry told him that cold night when he was still living on the street. "If you want your life back I think I can help."

He did not have to lie about his drug use. In fact, other people seemed to understand the reasons he used drugs and drank. Gradually, his counselors and peers made him doubt he was doing the right thing with his life. The program found him a safe place to live. They introduced him to a psychiatrist who said if he controlled his drug use, he could take medication that would control his mood swings, and he began to try to do this. When he did take this medication, he did feel better, less down and moody. Before Roger realized it, over a number of months, he was actually on the road to recovery.

Discussion of Roger's Story

Roger apparently went though much of his adult life with little or no insight into his many problems. Sadly, this is quite common for dually diagnosed persons like Roger. One might effectively argue that in some ways Roger exhibited personal strength, some might still call it ego strength. Not believing he was sick, when the system was going to hospitalize him he left and began a life on the streets. Yet, while he was resourceful enough to survive on the street, that "strength" relegated him to the life of a reclusive outsider living alone and in poverty. The problems Roger had with his first encounters with the treatment system have been experienced by many people. Initially, a mental health system of credentialed professionals generally funded based on medical diagnoses and an emerging substance abuse system mostly staffed by ex-alcoholics and addicts and funded by grants and private donations represented two very different worlds. Recognition of the increasing number of dually diagnosed individuals has spurred the integration of these two services to provide effective treatment for people like Roger. The services he needed probably did not exist when he was in school and may not have existed the first time he was hospitalized. They do exist today and it is hoped that they will soon be available to everyone, like Roger, who needs them.

Summary

Recognition that persons with severe mental illness are also highly vulnerable to substance abuse did not come about until after the deinstitutionalization movement. For a period of time, there were few if any services for persons with a dual diagnosis of substance abuse and severe mental illness. The programs initially developed to address this issue were either sequential, requiring treatment of one condition before the other was addressed, or parallel, treating both conditions using different staff or different agencies. For a host of reasons, neither of these initial strategies was particularly effective.

Integrated treatment for persons with a dual diagnosis, providing simultaneous treatment for both conditions using the same professionals working in the same program, is the preferred service and is an evidence-based practice. Employing treatment stages and motivational interviewing techniques, the EBP deals with the individual's attitudes regarding these conditions and assists his or her progress toward recovery. Our current understanding of the treatment and rehabilitation of these difficult conditions suggests that much more research is needed in this area.

Class Exercise

For this exercise assign one or more individuals to play the role of substance abuse workers and others to play the role of mental health workers. Everyone should read the following vignette, select what they believe is the best response and be prepared to explain their reasoning behind the selection.

William, a 38-year-old white male, has been a resident of a residence for persons with dual diagnosis (mental illness and substance abuse) for 2 months. He has a history of extensive opiate and alcohol abuse as well as a diagnosis of schizophrenia, undifferentiated type, persistent. He is currently maintained on Prolixin decanoate (injectable) 1.5 mL, twice a month, and has not required other medication.

William, who has some college education, has been working in the clerical unit of a psychiatric day treatment program and is reported to be doing well there. He attends the Double Trouble group (a 12-step group for people with mental illness) and other substance abuse–related groups at the day program. William has fit in very well at his residence, forming friendships with other residents and staff members. In general, his adjustment seems to be very good. Usually he presents no problems at the residence or the day program and has been drug and alcohol free as well as free from psychiatric symptoms.

During the last week the staff noticed alcohol on William's breath. When confronted about this, he denied drinking. A staff person from the day program called the residence to report that William had been making vague excuses and leaving the program early. They also reported that he has become more withdrawn and may be responding to voices. When confronted by staff members of the day program, he denied hearing voices. Several other residents reported that they had seen William leaving a local liquor store with a brown bag. When asked about this, William responded that he knows that they want him to go back to the hospital and refuses to discuss it further.

Which is the best response to this problem? Read all of the options below and discuss their benefits and weaknesses.

- *Response A:* William is obviously using alcohol again. If he refuses to admit he is using he should have a blood test to settle the issue. If he tests positive he should be denied privileges. If he refuses to comply he should be sent back to the hospital.
- *Response B:* Even though he is on injectable medication, William is probably getting sick again. He should be evaluated by a psychiatrist to see if he needs an increase or change of medication. Confrontation about his drinking should be postponed until after the evaluation.
- *Response C:* William should be confronted about his drinking at a house meeting with the other residents and the staff present. Peer and staff support will probably help him to open up. Once he admits that he is drinking again, the problem can be dealt with openly.

After considering these three responses, can you craft a better plan, consistent with the principles of treatment presented in this chapter?

References

Bellack, A. S., & DiClemente, C. C. (1999). Treating substance abuse among patients with schizophrenia. *Psychiatric Services, 50*(1), 75–80.

Caton, C. L. M. (1981). The new chronic patient and the system of community care. *Hospital and Community Psychiatry, 32,* 475–478.

Cuffel, B. J. (1996). Comorbid substance abuse disorder: Prevalence, patterns of use and course. In R. E. Drake & K. T. Mueser (Eds.), *Dual diagnosis of major mental illness and substance abuse, Volume 2: Recent research and clinical implications* (pp. 93–105; Vol. 70, New Directions for Mental Health Services). San Francisco: Jossey-Bass.

Drake, R. E., Bartels, S. J., Teague, G. B., Noordsy, D. L., & Clark, R. E. (1993). Treatment of substance abuse in severely mentally ill patients. *Journal of Nervous and Mental Disease, 181*(10), 606–611.

Drake, R. E., Essock, S. M., Shaner, A., Carey, K. B., Minkoff, K., Kola, L., et al. (2002). Implementing dual diagnosis services for clients with severe mental illness. *Psychiatric Services, 52*(4), 469–476.

Drake, R. E., Mercer-McFadden, C., Mueser, K. T., McHugo, G. J., & Bond, G. R. (1998). Review of integrated mental health and substance abuse treatment for patients with dual disorders. *Schizophrenia Bulletin, 24*(4), 589–608.

Drake, R. E., Mueser, K. T., Brunette, M. F., & McHugo, G. J. (2004). A review of treatments for people with severe mental illnesses and co-occurring substance use disorders. *Psychiatric Rehabilitation Journal, 27*(4), 360–374.

Drake, R. E., & Wallach, M. A. (1989). Substance abuse among the chronic mentally ill. *Hospital and Community Psychiatry, 40*(10), 1041–1045.

Drake, R. E., & Wallach, M. A. (2000). Dual diagnosis: 15 years of progress. *Psychiatric Services, 51*(9), 1126–1129.

Evans, K., & Sullivan, J. M. (1990). *Dual diagnosis; Counseling the mentally ill substance abuser.* New York: The Guilford Press.

Heyscue, B. E., Levin, G. M., & Merrick, J. P. (1998). Compliance with depot antipsychotic medication by patients attending outpatient clinics. *Psychiatric Services, 49,* 1232–1234.

Jeffery, D. P., Ley, A., McLaren, S., & Siegfried, N. (2000, 2003). Psychosocial treatment programs for people with both severe mental illness and substance misuse [review]. *The Cochrane Database of Systematic Reviews.* Available online at http://www.cochrane.org

Krystal, J. H., D'Souza, D. C., Madonick, S., & Petrakis, I. (1999). Toward a rational pharmacotherapy of comorbid substance abuse in schizophrenic patients. *Schizophrenia Research, 35*(Suppl), 35–49.

Marlatt, G. A. (1998). Basic principles and strategies of harm reduction. In G. A. Marlatt (Ed.), *Harm reduction: Pragmatic approaches to managing high risk behaviors.* New York: The Guilford Press.

Marlatt, G. A., Blume, A. W., & Parks, G. A. (2001). Integrating harm reduction therapy and traditional substance abuse treatment. *Journal of Psychoactive Drugs, 33,* 13–21.

Miller, N. S. (1997). Clinical approach to diagnosis of comorbid addictive and psychiatric disorders. *Psychiatric Rehabilitation Skills, 2*(1), 77–90.

Miller, W. R., & Rollnick, S. (2002). *Motivational interviewing: Preparing people to change addictive behavior* (2nd ed.). New York: The Guilford Press.

Mueser, K. T., Bennett, M., & Kushner, M. G. (1995). Epidemiology of substance abuse among persons with chronic mental disorders. In A. F. Lehman & L. Dixon (Eds.), *Double jeopardy: Chronic mental illness and substance abuse* (pp. 9–25). New York; Harwood Academic.

Mueser, K. T., Drake, R. E., & Noordsy, D. L. (1998a). Integrated mental health and substance abuse treatment for severe psychiatric disorders. *Journal of Practical Psychiatry and Behavioral Health, 4,* 129–139.

Mueser, K. T., Drake, R. E., & Wallach, M. A. (1998b). Dual diagnosis: A review of etiological theories. *Addictive Behaviors, 23,* 717–734.

Mueser, K. T., & Noordsy, D. L. (1996). Group treatment for dually diagnosed clients. *New Directions for Mental Health, 70,* 33–51.

Mueser, K. T., Noordsy, D. L., Drake, R. E., & Fox. L. (2003a). *Integrated treatment for dual disorders: A guide to effective practice*. New York: The Guilford Press.

Mueser, K. T., Torrey, W. C., Lynde, D., Singer, P., & Drake, R. E. (2003b). Implementing evidence-based practices for people with severe mental illness. *Behavior Modification, 27*(3), 387–411.

Nishith, P., Mueser, K. T., Srsic, C. S., & Beck, A. T. (1997). Expectations and motives for alcohol use in a psychiatric outpatient population. *The Journal of Nervous and Mental Disease, 185*(10), 622–626.

Pepper, B., Ryglewicz, H., & Kirshner, M. C., (1981). The young adult chronic patient: Overview of a population. *Hospital and Community Psychiatry, 32,* 463–469.

Prochaska, J. O., Norcross, J. C., & DiClemente, C. C. (1994). *Changing for the good*. New York: Harper Collins.

Regier, D. A., Farmer, M. E., Rae, D. S., Locke, B. Z., Keith, S. J., Judd, L. L., et al. (1990). Comorbidity of mental disorders with alcohol and other drug abuse: Results from the epidemiologic catchment area (ECA) study. *Journal of the American Medical Association, 264*(19), 2511–2518.

Ridgely, M. S., Goldman, H. H., & Willenbring, M. (1990). Barriers to the care of persons with dual diagnoses: Organizational and financing issues. S*chizophrenia Bulletin, 16,* 123–132.

Saladin, M. E., & Santa Ana, E. J. (2004). Controlled drinking: More than just a controversy. *Current Opinions in Psychiatry, 17,* 175–187.

Spencer, C., Castle, D., & Michie, D. T. (2002). Motivations that maintain substance use among individuals with psychotic disorders. *Schizophrenia Bulletin, 28*(2), 233–247.

Chapter 9

Vocational Rehabilitation

Introduction 244

Barriers to Employment 245

    Stigma and Discrimination 245

    Misguided Services 246

    Lack of Vocational Experience 247

    Lack of Education 247

    Psychiatric Disability 247

    Possible Loss of Benefits 248

Developing Vocational Services 250

    Features of Effective Vocational
      Services 250

Vocational Service Modalities 255

    Transitional Employment 256

    Fairweather Lodges 256

    Hospital-Based Work Programs 257

    Job Clubs 257

    Sheltered Workshops 257

    Affirmative Industries 258

Supported Employment 258

Carl's Story 260

    The Role of the Job Coach 262

Models of Supported Employment 264

    Individual Placement Models 264

    The Enclave or Work Crew Model 266

    Supported Employment in Assertive
      Community Treatment 266

Other Vocational Preparation
Services 267

    Vocational Exploration Services 267

Supported Employment: An Evidence-
Based Practice 268

    Critical Ingredients of Supported
      Employment 268

    Service Outcomes of Supported
      Employment 268

Summary 269

Class Exercise 270

References 271

Many people respond to questions about what they do or "who they are" by talking about their job, position, or profession. Whatever a person does that is productive or meaningful contributes greatly to his or her sense of identity. Such information often conveys the individual's interests, values, aspirations, and socioeconomic status. A person who has a severe mental illness but does not have a job or profession is often relegated to the role of mental patient. This chapter outlines some of the problems associated with helping to achieve vocational goals and some of the strategies that have proven to be effective.

Persons with severe mental illness can complete school, be effective workers, and have a profession. When they accomplish these goals, their condition becomes something that they have overcome rather than defining who they are.

This chapter will answer the following questions:

1. *What are the barriers to employment for people with a psychiatric disability?*
2. *What skills, resources, or experiences are related to vocational success?*
3. *What constitutes quality vocational services?*
4. *What kinds of vocational services have been developed?*

Introduction

Employment is an essential adult activity. If we are fortunate, the work we choose to do reflects our interests, skills, and talents. Working, especially working and earning a paycheck, promotes self-confidence, self-esteem, status in the community, and economic well-being. Because of all these obvious advantages, our culture understandably puts great value on the role of wage earner. In addition, the role of wage earner provides access to other valued social roles including that of friend, spouse, parent, homeowner, neighbor, customer, and taxpayer (Carling, 1995). For most adults, having a job or profession is an essential element in defining who they are and for achieving a positive quality of life.

Does work have some additional benefits for people with mental illness? It certainly seems logical that successful employment would have a positive impact on other areas such as symptom reduction, community integration, and improved functioning. The results of a number of studies suggest this may be true (Arns & Linney, 1993; Bell, Milstein, & Lysaker, 1993; Bond et al., 2001; Drake, McHugo, Becker, Anthony, & Clark, 1996; Krupa, 2004; Lysaker & Bell, 1995). One study that specifically looked at this issue was conducted by Mueser and his colleagues in 1997. In this study, the researchers examined the relationship between competitive employment and nonvocational domains. Data were taken at the beginning of the study, and at 6, 12, and 18 months. The results indicate that

> ... formerly unemployed psychiatric patients who obtained competitive employment while participating in a vocational program tended to have lower symptoms, better overall functioning, higher self-esteem, and higher satisfaction with vocational services and finances. ... (p. 423)

In contrast, a more recent study by some of these same researchers (Torrey, Mueser, McHugo, & Drake, 2000) failed to find a relationship between employment status and self-esteem. Responding to this finding, Casper and Fishbein (2002) examined the contribution of job satisfaction and success as moderators of self-esteem. Their findings suggest that employment status is related to self-esteem when job satisfaction and success are taken into account. That is, self-esteem was not improved by simply having a job, but it was improved in individuals who reported feeling satisfied and successful in their jobs. More studies on this topic are needed to confirm and further illuminate these findings.

Persons with severe mental illness, however, rarely get to experience the positive results of having a regular job. Employment rates for people with a psychiatric disability are very low, ranging from 0% to 30% (Anthony & Blanch, 1987; Anthony, Cohen, & Danley, 1988; Anthony, Cohen, & Farkas, 2002). More problems than the mental illnesses themselves contribute to the high unemployment rate among people with severe mental illness.

Barriers to Employment

Stigma and Discrimination

One of the greatest barriers to employment for people with a psychiatric disability is stigma, which was discussed in detail in Chapter 1. This stigma has several sources. The most obvious source of stigma, which we have all experienced, is the frequently negative characterization of people with mental illness by the mass media. This is reflected in many of the attitudes about mental illness held by laypersons. Media reports often leave the false impression that a person with mental illness is frequently emotionally unstable, irrational, and dangerous.

An informal review of articles about mental health issues appearing in a large newspaper over a period of a year may be instructive on the issue of stigma in the media (Roberts & Rotteveel, 1995). The review found that more than 60% of the articles portrayed people with mental illness as criminals or in other undesirable roles, whereas only 4% of the articles presented a positive image of any kind. This kind of portrayal, as well as many seen in movies and advertisements, has a profound effect on the attitudes of both members of the community at large and of the business community. A Harris poll regarding attitudes of the general public toward people with disabilities found an overall improved acceptance of people with disabilities in the community, but also a continued feeling of "uneasiness" about people with mental illness (Chapman, 1992). A more recent Harris poll found that people with disabilities were significantly less likely than people without disabilities to be involved in their communities. Fifty-four percent of respondents with disabilities and 64% of those with more severe disabilities reported the primary reason for this isolation to be that they do not feel encouraged or invited to participate by community organizations (Harris Interactive, 2000).

Another, more subtle source of stigma is reflected in the beliefs (both conscious and unconscious) of professionals regarding the ability of people with psychiatric disability to work or to work in any but the most menial jobs. These beliefs are reflected in some of the vocational services and choices made available for persons with major mental illnesses.

Finally, the most insidious form of stigma may exist within persons with mental illness themselves. When society reduces access to good jobs, and staff people give subtle or overt messages of doubt about a person's ability to perform on the job, these negative beliefs can be internalized (Rehab Brief, 1993). This "self stigma" may be the hardest form of stigma to detect and is often the most difficult form of stigma to overcome (Ritsher, Otilingam, & Grajales, 2003; Ritsher & Phelan, 2004).

BOX 9.1
The Disclosure Dilemma

When a person with a psychiatric disability decides to seek employment, he or she may be faced with the question of whether or not to disclose the disability to the employer. The decision is often a difficult one.

On the one hand, the results of disclosure can be very negative. The applicant who discloses might not be hired. The employee who discloses might be discriminated against in explicit ways, such as not being considered for advancement, or more subtly, such as being treated as less capable or fragile. On the other hand, not disclosing may leave the individual feeling vulnerable about someone discovering the illness at a later time. Any supports the person may need would also be unavailable if the person had not disclosed the illness.

On the positive side, disclosure allows one the opportunity to request and gain accommodations that may be essential for the worker's success. Some workers feel more comfortable if their employer knows about the disability and they do not have to hide it. In some workplaces, informal support among coworkers on personal issues is common, and workers with psychiatric disabilities may benefit from accessing it.

How would you assist someone in deciding whether or not to disclose? What would be the important factors in deciding when, to whom and how much to disclose?

Misguided Services

Uninformed beliefs on the part of professionals about the abilities, desires, and needs of people with a psychiatric disability have resulted in both unnecessarily delayed access to vocational services and unnecessarily limited vocational options (Bond, Dietzen, McGrew, & Miller, 1995; *Rehab Brief*, 1993). Concerns about stress, symptomatology, medication compliance, and rehospitalization have caused providers to withhold access to vocational services until the client or member has demonstrated successful participation in a setting (such as a day program) that is segregated from the regular community. These policies persist even though research suggests that functioning in one setting is not predictive of functioning in other settings (Anthony & Jansen, 1984). Additionally, studies show that direct entry into competitive employment does not result in increased symptoms, rehospitalization, or homelessness, as has often been feared (Bond et al., 2001; McFarlane et al., 2000; Torrey, Becker, & Drake, 1995). Instead, direct entry may result in "increased involvement in other community activities; . . . increased general supports; and . . . increased independence of consumers" (Torrey et al., 1995, p. 72). Similarly, Bond and Dincin (1986) and Bond et al. (1995) found increased rates of full-time competitive employment as a result of "accelerated entry into community jobs" (Bond et al., 1995, p. 106). In this latter study, Bond and his colleagues also found that delayed entry into employment because of participation in prevocational (often shortened to "pre-voc") activities, including sheltered work, decreased one's likelihood of ever entering competitive employment and lowered the participant's self-expectations (p. 106). In a similar vain, Blankertz and Robinson (1996) point out that although wages are an important motivator, many programs expect people to demonstrate motivation prior to actually accessing paid employment opportunities.

Often the employment options offered by providers are restricted to low-skill jobs with little or no chance of advancement, even when the worker has advanced academic degrees, a strong work history, or simply greater aspirations.

Lack of Vocational Experience

Another barrier to employment for many people with a psychiatric disability is their limited experience and understanding of themselves as workers and of the world of work (Danley & Anthony, 1987). Early experiences in employment provide us with important information about our skills, preferences, interests, and aspirations. These experiences also help us learn about the expectations in the world of work. Over time, multiple experiences in employment contribute to our ability to make appropriate career choices and, ultimately, to be successful in a career. For people who experience a psychiatric disability, these employment experiences and the crucial vocational information they contain have oftentimes been missed (Danley & Anthony, 1987; Russert & Frey, 1991; Rehab Brief, 1993). People entering vocational services after long periods of psychiatric disability often have considerably less knowledge of their own skills, interests, and preferences than would be expected from comparable persons their own age. Typically, vocational service programs are evaluated by how many persons they place in jobs and how long the people hold these jobs. Because of this, they are usually neither able nor willing to provide the multiple employment experiences that may be needed to provide someone with the knowledge necessary to select a vocational direction that is appropriate for that person and provides advancement opportunities.

Lack of Education

In the same way that someone's psychiatric illness may have interfered with early work experiences, it may also have interfered with the completion of high school or college. The absence of education reduces the quantity and quality of jobs available whether an individual has a disability or not (Baron & Salzer, 2002). Support in acquiring education is discussed in Chapter 10.

Psychiatric Disability

Other barriers to employment may be the result of the mental illness itself—the impact of the mental illness on thought and affect as well as the episodic and cyclical nature of the disability (Russert & Frey, 1991; Rutman, 1994; Rehab Brief, 1993). This means that many people with serious mental illness experience difficulties with memory, concentration, organization, or even interpersonal interactions at least some of the time. Some effects of the mental illness may be what Jansen (1988) called "psychological problems," such as a lack of self-esteem and self-confidence, fear of failure, anxiety, and difficulty getting along with others (p. 36). Finally, the obvious physical side effects of medications can be severe and pose a significant barrier to employment (Braitman et al., 1995; Rutman, 1994).

Less obvious, but no less important, are the social side effects of medications. For example, a medication that increases one's sensitivity to the sun may also interfere with the user's ability to play on the company softball team and put the person in the uncomfortable position of having to disclose personal information or be seen as "not part of the gang." Similarly, someone who cannot drink alcohol because of his or her medication may feel awkward when invited to join coworkers for a beer after work. In fact, any medication side effect that has an impact on the person's social activities can increase the person's appearance of differentness and make it harder for the person to fit in (Roberts, 1997, p. 83).

Possible Loss of Benefits

For individuals in the United States who receive Supplemental Security Income (SSI) or Social Security Disability Insurance (SSDI), the Social Security Administration (SSA) regulations regarding the effect of earned income on benefits are often perceived as posing a substantial barrier to employment. Most people with mental illness are aware that their illness can flair up at any time. In the event of a relapse, Social Security may be the only source of income available. The fear of losing one's benefits, coupled with the fear that one may not be able to sustain employment, makes the perceived risk of attempting employment very great (Ford, 1995). In fact, the perceived risk is often much greater than the actual risk. The Social Security regulations regarding earned income and work incentives are discussed in Box 9.2.

BOX 9.2
Social Security Benefits and Earned Income

In 1999, President Clinton signed the Ticket to Work and Work Incentive Improvement Act (TWWIIA) into law. This law was designed to reduce the disincentives to employment for which the previous regulations were notorious. Following are general descriptions of the current SSI and SSDI regulations regarding earned income and the provisions of the TWWIIA that address the most common concerns of people considering employment.

The regulations for SSI employ a formula for determining specific reductions in cash benefits as a result of earned income. The person's cash benefit will be reduced by $1 for every $2 the person earns in excess of any exclusions to which the person is entitled. Those exclusions may include an earned income exclusion and a general income exclusion. These exclusions ($20 and $65, respectively) are earnings that Social Security allows without effect on benefits.

The SSDI recipient is entitled to a 9-month trial work period (TWP) during which his or her SSDI cash benefit is protected even though the person is earning wages. This period is followed by a 36-month extended period of eligibility (EPE) during which time the person's entitlement to the cash benefit will depend on whether or not the person's earnings exceed the amount that is considered to be substantial gainful activity (SGA). There is no formula to reduce the SSDI amount. Instead, it is an all-or-nothing proposition. The person either receives the SSDI cash benefit or he or she does not.

Both of these programs include work incentives that can be used to reduce the person's countable earned income and maintain some or all of the cash benefit at least for a time.

Provisions of TWWIIA

Ticket to Work

The Ticket to Work is a voluntary initiative. Each eligible SSI and SSDI recipient is issued a document called a *ticket to work*. The ticket holder can use the ticket to obtain employment services from any approved employment service provider known as an employment network (EN). An EN may be a public or private service provider, a state organization such as VR or One-Stop Centers, schools, employers, or others (Jensen & Silverstein, n.d.; Roessler, 2002). In principle, the ticket holder gains a measure of control and choice in selecting services because he or she can withdraw the ticket and reassign it to another EN if he or she is dissatisfied with the services being provided. An additional benefit to the ticket holder is that while using a ticket he or she will not be subject to continuing disability reviews by Social Security. Payments to the EN are based on the ticket holders' reduced cash benefits due to earned income.

Medical Insurance

For most recipients of Social Security benefits, the greater fear is the loss of medical coverage. SSI recipients are covered by Medicaid and may continue to be covered until their earnings reach a particular amount, even after their earnings have resulted in the cessation of their cash benefit. TWWIIA made it possible for states to allow working individuals with incomes greater than 250% of the federal poverty rate to purchase Medicaid coverage if it is needed to cover medical costs. SSDI recipients are eligible for Medicare. TWWIIA extended the period of Medicare coverage to 93 months after the trial work period (Jensen & Silverstein, n.d.; Roessler, 2002). This results in a total period of 102 months during which time a SSDI recipient can be working and still be covered by Medicare.

ESR and BPAO

TWWIIA addressed other common concerns of people with disabilities considering employment. To ensure that the regulations and work incentives are widely understood and administered in a consistent way, SSA established employment support representatives (ESRs) to train local SSA claims representatives and to provide outreach about work incentives. Further, TWWIIA provided funding for the establishment of community-based Benefits Planning, Assistance and Outreach (BPAO) projects. These projects are staffed with well-trained specialists to assist people who are receiving benefits to understand and use SSA work incentives.

Expedited Reinstatement of Benefits

As mentioned before, a major concern for people with psychiatric disabilities in becoming employed is the fear of losing benefits and then being unable to sustain employment. TWWIIA addressed this concern by establishing an expedited reinstatement of benefits process. If an individual becomes unemployed for reasons related to their disability within 60 months of termination of their benefits, they can request an expedited reinstatement of benefits. That is, they do not have to go through a new application process. During the period that SSA is reviewing their request the person may receive temporary benefits including health care coverage. If SSA determines the person to be ineligible for benefits, the temporary benefits will not have to be repaid.

Developing Vocational Services

Features of Effective Vocational Services

Several researchers have attempted to guide effective vocational services by identifying the characteristics, circumstances, or experiences related to or predictive of vocational success. This has proven to be a difficult task.

In an extensive review of the literature, Anthony and Jansen (1984) concluded that past work experience is the best predictor of employment success. They also found that, counter to what is often believed within the populations of persons with serious mental illness, factors such as diagnosis and level of symptomatology were not related to vocational success. This finding makes sense based on our previous discussion of how persons tend to prepare for making vocational choices. Employment success is influenced by learning from past experience. In a later review of the literature, Anthony (1994) found that past work history, number and length of hospitalizations, marital status, race, and previous occupational level all had been found to be correlated to vocational outcome. In addition, work adjustment skills (i.e., work readiness, attitudes, and quality and interpersonal relations) were associated with positive outcomes. Diagnosis, symptomatology, and functioning in other life domains did *not* correlate with vocational outcome with a few exceptions. Anthony, Rogers, Cohen, and Davies (1995) did find negative correlations between symptoms and work skills. People with severe and persistent mental illness who became employed had lower symptom scores and higher work skills than those who never became employed. Nevertheless, participation in the rehabilitation programs appeared to have a positive effect on symptoms and work skills.

A slightly different picture was revealed by a Boston University Center for Psychiatric Rehabilitation study in which all subjects were individuals who had identified a vocational goal. They found the predictors of vocational outcome to be symptomatology, criminal justice involvement, and marital status. Anthony suggested that the fact that the subjects had selected a vocational goal and were receiving a vocational intervention may distinguish this group from previous research groups. Furthermore, in at least a few studies, diagnosis has been found to be related to vocational outcome (Anthony, 1994; Mowbray, Bybee, Harris, & McCrohan, 1995). McGurk, Mueser, Harvey, LaPuglia, and Marder (2003) found higher levels of positive symptoms to be related to more frequent use of job site supports. Some studies suggest a possible relationship between medication and work performance in that medication appears to impair work performance. Receiving Social Security benefits has correlated with vocational outcome in some studies and not in others.

Blankertz and Robinson (1996) examined the integration of vocational rehabilitation services with typical mental health services, suggesting that predictors of positive vocational outcomes are not characteristics of individuals but characteristics of programs. These authors asserted that "vocational rehabilitation should be an integral part of the mental health rehabilitation process" (p. 1222). Gowdy, Carlson, and Rapp (2004) agreed. In a study comparing high-performance with low-performance employment programs, they found 10 organizational characteristics that differentiated the two groups. In high-performing programs, directors, supervisors, and staff were more likely to hold different viewpoints and engage in specific practices. Ten features of these programs are summarized in Table 9.1.

A growing number of studies have found that the specific model of service provided is an important contributor to employment success. Supported employment has consistently been shown to produce better employment outcomes than other vocational services and is now considered an evidence-based practice (Becker, Smith, Tanzman, Drake, & Tremblay, 2001; Bond, 2004; Bond et al., 2001; Drake, et al., 1996, 1999). Supported employment will be discussed later in this chapter. Box 9.3 discusses federal vocational rehabilitation initiatives.

CONTROVERSIAL ISSUE
Is "Pre-Voc" Really No Voc?

A week after an interesting class discussion about the future of vocational services in psychiatric rehabilitation (PsyR), one of our graduate students (with many years of PsyR experience) reported having an interesting dispute at work. It seems that during a staff meeting at the psychiatric day treatment program (Chapter 6) where he worked, he had questioned whether it was really helpful to work on prevocational (pre-voc) skills with the clients if the goal was to prepare them for regular jobs. Instead, he had suggested that maybe "pre-voc is really no voc." He was very surprised by how upset some of the staff became by his remark. Yet, today there is a growing body of research suggesting that he was correct.

The case for prevocational training is very straightforward. For a number of very sound reasons, many of the first vocational services, which were set up in response to the deinstitutionalization movement, focused on teaching prevocational skills. These programs were designed to help individuals entering the community after years of psychiatric institutionalization. Members of this institutionalized population had spent much of their adult lives in settings where even the simplest decisions were made for them. There was no question that many of them lacked the prevocational skills— such as grooming, punctuality, and socialization— that are necessary to function effectively in the

workplace. In addition, program staff could readily identify and work with the prevocational skill deficits of their clients, but had scant information about the more specific job skills they might need at particular jobs. A subtle, but possibly no less important, reason for the emphasis on prevocational training is how services have been reimbursed. In many places, programs could not bill for off-site services. That meant that any work the staff might do outside the center in the community would not be reimbursable. This created a barrier to the staff doing realistic kinds of skill training, job development, and follow-up support. Instead, given very realistic financial concerns many administrators and staff members focused on what they felt they could do best, prevocational skills training.

Since the advent of supported employment (SE), the idea of forgoing prevocational training in favor of direct placement and the provision of support services on the job has received increasing research support. As previously mentioned in this chapter, a number of studies (Bond & Dincin, 1986; Bond et al., 1995; Torrey, Becker, & Drake, 1995) have found that direct placement is superior to prevocational training with respect to vocational outcomes. In their 1995 study, Bond and his colleagues suggested that during the time the client spends in prevocational training he or she may become dependent on the program, develop a support network that he or she does not want to leave, and lose some of the motivation to work a regular job. This makes sense if we consider the recovery theories put forth by Pat Deegan (1988) and William Anthony (1993), which are discussed in detail in Chapter 4. These theories suggest that the recovery task involves creating a new self-image that incorporates the fact of the mental illness. Consider the development of this new self-image after spending a year at prevocational training versus spending a year at a regular job.

Opponents of direct placement SE still argue that this strategy causes higher stress and higher hospitalization rates. Research has not supported these claims. Clearly, this represents an area of PsyR where our knowledge may be moving faster than the attitudes of many staff and administrators about what constitutes good service.]

TABLE 9.1
High-Performing Employment Program Characteristics

Beliefs and Viewpoints
1. Emphasize the possibility and the value of work.
2. Do *not* view societal stigma as a major barrier to program performance.
3. View consumers as wanting to work and motivated to work.
4. The potential loss of benefits is seen as a need for information and negotiation rather than as a major barrier.

Practices
1. Employ strengths-based practices.
2. Use employment outcome data to improve services.
3. Share stories that reflect a belief in consumers' ability to succeed.
4. Conduct frequent and regular meetings between vocational and case management staff.
5. Case managers are proactive in their support of employment goals and efforts.
6. Therapists support of employment goals.

Source: Based on Gowdy, Carlson, and Rapp (2004).

BOX 9.3
Vocational Rehabilitation: The Federal Initiative in the United States

In 1918, the federal government established the Office of Vocational Rehabilitation to assist the returning veterans of World War I in finding employment. The scope of vocational rehabilitation has been expanded several times from its original mission to assist veterans. In 1920, Congress decided that civilians with physical disabilities should also be eligible for vocational rehabilitation services. In 1943, services were expanded again to include persons with mental retardation and mental illness (Ledbetter & Field, 1978; Neff, 1988; Roberts, 1996). During the Great Society instituted by President Johnson in the 1960s, services were expanded

to recipients of SSDI and later to "the disadvantaged or socially and culturally deprived" (Ledbetter and Field, 1978, p. 36).

Prior to the 1970s, vocational rehabilitation services were not readily accessible to people with a psychiatric disability (Anthony & Blanch, 1987). In 1973, Congress overrode a presidential veto and passed the Rehabilitation Act. This act established the Rehabilitation Services Administration (RSA) and authorized it to do several things including, but not limited to, providing vocational rehabilitation services to people with the most severe disabilities and to those people who had been underserved in the past and to "develop new and innovative methods" to achieve vocational rehabilitation (PL 93–112, p. 3) (Ledbetter & Field, 1978; McGurrin, 1994; Roberts, 1996). This new emphasis on serving people with the most severe disabilities helped to make services more accessible to people with a psychiatric disability. The Rehabilitation Act also allowed for funding to be allocated to states to provide vocational rehabilitation services. This funding is based on the per capita income of the state (PL 93–112). Each state has a state agency that corresponds to the federal RSA. This agency, named different things in different states (Division of Vocational Rehabilitation, Office of Vocational Rehabilitation, VESID, etc.), employs vocational rehabilitation counselors in local offices.

In addition, the 1973 act established the Individual Written Rehabilitation Plan (IWRP) (Ledbetter & Field, 1978). The IWRP (later changed to IPE, Individual Plan for Employment) identifies the desired rehabilitation outcome and the services and activities that will be provided to achieve it. Each vocational rehabilitation (VR) client is required to be actively involved in the development of his or her rehabilitation plan to ensure that it reflects the desires of the individual. The vocational rehabilitation counselor works with individuals with disabilities to establish the IWRP and then to access the needed services. In some states the vocational rehabilitation agency provides those services, and in other states the services are purchased from authorized VR vendors such as many psychiatric rehabilitation providers. These services include assessments of the worker's capacity, skills, and interests; work adjustment such as attendance, grooming, and productivity; education or training; job acquisition; and initial support. Once a VR client is employed and stable on the job, VR will continue to be involved for a brief period of time (currently 90 days) and then will close the person's case.

Access to services was further improved in the 1970s when the National Institute of Mental Health (NIMH) established the Community Support Program (CSP) initiative. The CSP stressed vocational rehabilitation services as an important element of support for deinstitutionalized psychiatric patients. In 1978, partly based on the CSP initiative, the NIMH entered into a collaborative agreement with RSA establishing two rehabilitation

research and training centers focused on psychiatric disability (Anthony & Blanch, 1987; McGurrin, 1994).

In 1980, NIMH, RSA, the National Institute on Handicapped Research, and the Council of State Administrators of Vocational Rehabilitation entered into a cooperative agreement that led to the development of a work group focused on improving services for people with a psychiatric disability. This work group was instrumental in bringing about the 1986 Amendments to the Rehabilitation Act (Anthony & Blanch, 1987). In response to strong advocacy efforts, the 1986 Amendments to the Rehabilitation Act defined supported employment (SE), a newly emerging vocational service of great promise, established a category of funds to pay for supported employment (Title VI(C)), and made it possible for vocational rehabilitation counselors to use regular case service funds to pay for supported employment (Roberts, 1996).

In 1992, the Rehabilitation Act was amended again. In response to testimony from people with disabilities and advocates, the 1992 Amendments to the Rehabilitation Act modified the definition of supported employment, increased the emphasis on consumer choice and mandated "a 'presumption of employability' for all people" (Roberts, 1996, p. 19).

In August 1998, the Workforce Investment Act (WIA) was signed into law (PL 105–220). This law established a one-stop workforce development system that brought together employment, education, and training programs for adults, dislocated workers, youth, veterans, and others. Specifically, Title IV of the WIA contains the amended Rehabilitation Act. The Workforce Investment System authorized by Title I of WIA is based on these elements: (1) the design and management of training and employment programs will be done on the local level; (2) customers will have access to education, training, employment, and information at one site; (3) customers will have choice in selecting the training program that best meets their needs; (4) customers will have information about the effectiveness of training providers in preparing trainees for jobs; and (5) businesses will play a key role in ensuring that the system prepares a viable workforce (Skiba, 2001; http://www.doleta.gov/usworkforce/wia).

Title IV of WIA (the Rehabilitation Act amendments of 1998) extended appropriations for supported employment until 2003 and specified that vocational rehabilitation is a component of the one-stop system and that people with disabilities should have access to all one-stop services including vocational rehabilitation and established funds to provide one-time, time-limited grants to create telecommuting and self-employment options for people with significant disabilities. The WIA expired in 2003 and has not as of this writing been reauthorized. Funds continue to be appropriated, however, to carry out the goals and activities specified, and reauthorization bills have been proposed in Congress (http://www.nationalrehab.org).

In spite of these developments, it appears that vocational rehabilitation services for people with a psychiatric disability in some places remain inadequate. Noble (1998), in a review of reports generated by the General Accounting Office of the federal government, reported that although the amount of money allocated to vocational rehabilitation has increased substantially since 1975, the percentage of that money being used to purchase services for clients has declined. Furthermore, vocational rehabilitation agencies repeatedly have been found to ignore recommendations of best practice by continuing to use tests and assessments that are not good measures of vocational capacity for people with mental illness, failing to develop a specialization in mental illness among vocational rehabilitation counselors, and continuing to use outdated diagnostic nomenclature and categories. Noble stated, "The traditional vocational rehabilitation process is insufficient and top-heavy with personnel who stubbornly adhere to outdated methods and a time orientation that is insensitive to the intermittent or ongoing needs of people with severe mental illnesses" (p. 778). Although these criticisms may be warranted in general, it is also true that in some places the vocational rehabilitation agency has been instrumental in the development of vocational services for people with mental illness.

BOX 9.4
Americans with Disabilities Act

The Americans with Disabilities Act (ADA) passed by the U.S. Congress in 1990 is designed to protect people with disabilities from discrimination, in five areas: employment, transportation, telecommunication, public accommodation, and the business of local and state government (Mancuso, 1990; National Alliance of Business, 1991; Roberts, 1996). The ADA is not the first law to prohibit discrimination in employment against people with disabilities nor to refer to reasonable accommodations. The Rehabilitation Act of 1973 prohibits discrimination by federal agencies or employers who receive federal funds. Additionally, all but a few states have laws protecting people with disabilities from discrimination as does the District of Columbia (Lee, n.d.)

In the area of employment, the ADA prohibits discrimination against any qualified person because of his or her disability in all areas of employment including hiring, firing, advancement, compensation, and training. The ADA requires that employers consider whether a qualified applicant is able to perform the "essential functions" of the job with or without accommodations. A "qualified applicant" is one who has the experience or credentials required for the job. For example, if a job requires that the worker have a certain number of years of experience or a particular academic degree or training and the applicant does not have those things, the employer does not have to consider that applicant because the person does not have the qualifications. The "essential functions" are tasks that are integral to the job. In deciding which tasks are integral, employers usually consider whether the job exists to perform those tasks, how many people are available to perform those tasks, or what the result would be if the tasks were not performed. Employers are required to make reasonable accommodations for applicants or employees with disabilities. An accommodation is considered "reasonable" if it is not an "undue burden"; that is, if the cost is not excessive given the business' resources and if the accommodation does not change the nature of the work performed (Jones, 1993; Lee, n.d.; National Alliance of Business, 1991; Roberts, 1996). The ADA holds employers to a higher standard than previous laws regarding the definition of "undue burden." According to Lee (n.d.), the ADA "requires the employer to prove that an accommodation would be significantly difficult or expensive" (p. 3).

The Job Accommodations Network (JAN) is a service of the President's Committee on Employment of People with Disabilities and is set up to provide technical assistance in selecting or designing accommodations (Jones, 1993). JAN reports that most accommodations cost less than $500. In fact, they estimate that the "average cost of accommodation is less than $100 per person" (Jones, 1993, p. 8).

Accommodations for people with psychiatric disabilities are usually not costly because they are not usually structural. These accommodations are sometimes referred to as "soft accommodations." Jacqueline Parrish and Laura Mancuso have identified accommodations that have been helpful to people with psychiatric disabilities (in Jones, 1993). They identify four categories of accommodation as follows:

- *Human assistance*, including a job coach, additional training, coworker support, or mentoring.
- *Changes in workplace policy*, such as allowing telephone calls for support, using sick leave for emotional illness, allowing someone to work at home, and setting up a quiet workplace for someone whose concentration is impacted by distractions. Other policy changes might include holding a job for someone who is out for an extended period because of the mental illness, advancing paid or unpaid sick leave, flexibility in scheduling due to medical appointments, job sharing (in which two people share one job), or allowing the worker to set his or her own work pace.
- *Supervision*, including providing training to supervisors on management skills and topics such as the ADA.
- *Shaping coworkers' attitudes*, including sensitivity training and information about mental illness.

Although the ADA is not the first law to prohibit employment discrimination, it is a far-reaching law and a strong statement about the rights of people with disabilities to be included in the community.

Vocational Service Modalities

Perhaps the first PsyR community services that included work as an integral component took place at Fountain House in New York City, one of the original psychosocial rehabilitation clubhouses (Fountain House is also discussed in Chapter 6 of this text). Established in the 1950s, Fountain House provides work units in which clubhouse members work alongside staff completing the tasks necessary to operate and maintain the clubhouse. These activities give members the opportunity to contribute, to build self-esteem and confidence, and to develop relationships (Beard, Propst, & Malamud, 1994). Partly through the efforts of Fountain House, the clubhouse and other versions of psychosocial rehabilitation services that incorporate the use of prevocational work units have been established throughout the world.

Although the purpose of the work unit activities is the benefit one derives from making an important contribution, some also thought that the activities of the work units would provide the skill development necessary for regular employment. This has not necessarily been the case. As Marrone (1993) stated:

> Work units are not volunteer work (any more than cooking for your family is), specific skills training (any more than cooking meals at home helps you learn to run a restaurant), or a means of assessing or achieving "generic" work adjustment. (p. 45)

Transitional Employment

Perhaps the greatest contribution Fountain House has made to the development of specific employment services for people with psychiatric disabilities is the development of *transitional employment* (TE). TE provides program members with experiences at real jobs, in real employment settings, earning competitive wages. A TE job is acquired from the employer by the vocational services agency. The agency takes full responsibility for the job, which is initially managed by agency staff. Once the staff members have learned the job, they are ready to place program members in the job and to provide them with the training and support they need to succeed. A program member works the job for a time-limited period (usually 3 to 9 months, but this varies) before being replaced by another program member. The agency continues to be responsible for the job at all times. In fact, if the program member is unable to work on a certain day, it is the staff member's responsibility to take his or her place on the job. Obviously, the staff members are very motivated to thoroughly train and provide all necessary supports so that the program member can do the job successfully.

TE jobs are typically part time and require minimal skills so that they can accommodate a variety of members with a wide range of skill levels. Members have the opportunity to develop real work skills, gain regular work experience, and earn a paycheck. The employer is assured that the job will be continuously filled with trained workers (or by staff members).

Program members may go though a series of TE jobs. In fact, the Fountain House philosophy is that members will experience as many transitional employment jobs as needed to eventually achieve permanent employment in jobs of their own (Beard et al., 1994). Transitional employment has been an important forerunner to supported employment.

Fairweather Lodges

A very different approach to employment services, Fairweather Lodges, was developed by George Fairweather in the 1950s. Fairweather Lodges are programs where people with a mental illness live together and work together operating a member-run business.

Fairweather observed that the only social status available to psychiatric patients who were leaving the hospital and entering the community was an inferior one. He believed that a new subsystem in which people with mental illness could occupy valued roles, advance in social status, and challenge the image of people with mental illness held by the larger society was necessary (Fairweather, 1980). The lodge community was organized around a set of principles that addressed issues such as the importance of meaningful work, autonomy, advancement, tolerance, support, and similarity to the larger society (Fairweather, 1980).

The lodge community offers its members the opportunity to access valued societal roles in a mutually supportive, albeit segregated, environment. Members of the lodge occupy positions of responsibility within the business. The amount of responsibility one assumes is commensurate with one's ability at that time. Experts, such as accountants, are hired from outside the lodge when needed on a temporary basis.

Historically, referrals for lodge membership came directly from psychiatric hospitals, and the training in preparation for entry into the lodge was provided by the hospital. This training included topics such as group decision making, problem solving, and conflict resolution. More recently, referrals are accepted from a variety of sources. Lodge members are allowed to continue to participate in the work program even after moving out of the residence and some members are accepted to the work program without ever being in the residence (Ford, 1995; Onaga, 1994; Toms-Barker, 1994).

Hospital-Based Work Programs

On-site vocational opportunities have been developed at some hospitals giving patients the chance to do work for pay within the hospital setting during periods of hospitalization. These programs have been less successful than anticipated in improving postdischarge employment outcomes for patients. In fact, there is evidence that such programs result in the development of dependency in some patients and a desire to stay in the hospital (Bond & Boyer, 1988). According to Bond and Boyer, "Most reviewers have concluded that there is no relationship between successful adjustment to work programs within the hospital and post hospital employment" (p. 235).

Job Clubs

A job club provides the structure and resources necessary to assist participants to conduct their own job search. The club provides training and resources, such as instruction in job-seeking skills (resume writing, interviewing, etc.), access to telephones to call employers, and clerical support (McGurrin, 1994). An important feature that the job club supplies its members is peer support. This unique approach to job development may be less successful for many people with severe mental illness. Many individuals need a greater level of support in accomplishing the tasks of job acquisition (Bond, Drake, Mueser, & Becker, 1997).

Sheltered Workshops

Sheltered workshops solicit manufacturing jobs from local business and industry and provide support and supervision to people with disabilities in a factory-like setting owned or operated by the agency. Workers in the shop are usually paid a piece rate based on their productivity. This piece rate is based on the number of pieces that a worker without a disability could produce in a given period of time.

For some, sheltered work is expected to be a step toward competitive employment, whereas others see it as permanent placement (Bond & Boyer, 1988). According to Bond and Boyer, even when sheltered employment is expected to be short term, "there is a tendency for clients to remain indefinitely" (p. 241). Sheltered workshops have come under much criticism in recent years as new vocational strategies such as supported employment have demonstrated that even people with the most severe disabilities can be successful in community employment. With competitive employment an individual is more likely to earn better wages, enjoy greater status in the community, develop relationships with nondisabled peers (Murphy & Rogan, 1995), and work for longer periods of time (Bond et al., 1997).

Affirmative Industries

Affirmative Industries represent another way agencies offer supervised employment opportunities to clients or members. These businesses are owned, managed, and operated by the agency. Affirmative Industries, which can range from commercial cleaning or landscape crews to bakeries and caterers, provide goods and services to the community at large. The mental health agency secures contracts with local citizens and businesses to provide products or services. The workers are clients who are supervised by agency staff and are paid by the agency. This strategy provides members with a mix of support and a regular work experience. There are, however, a number of disadvantages to this approach. Consumer choice is quite limited. Clients must work in the business the agency runs. People with disabilities, working as a group or "crew," tend to generate stigma. This may be particularly true if the work crew is used as an employment opportunity for people with severe and more obvious disabilities. Finally, crew members' wages tend to be very low (Marrone, 1993). Similar to Affirmative Industries are client-employing businesses (Marrone, 1993). These businesses employ workers without disabilities as well as people with psychiatric disabilities and may be profit generating.

Supported Employment

> Supported Employment is really part of a social movement. It represents inclusion [of people with disabilities] into the fabric of community settings. (DiLeo in Roberts, 1996, p. 12)

With the advent of supported employment, people with the most severe disabilities, who were thought to have no vocational potential and were therefore denied access to vocational services, were finally given a chance in the workplace. Initially designed for people with severe developmental disabilities, *supported employment* (SE) emerged in the early 1980s as a response to unsatisfactory employment opportunities (Anthony & Blanch, 1987; Bond, et al., 1997). A small number of university-based projects demonstrated that even people with the most severe disabilities could work successfully in community settings if they were placed in jobs and provided the necessary training and support (Roberts, 1996).

This new place–train approach reversed the traditional train–place approach whereby clients would attend day programs or simulated work settings, which were segregated from the regular community, to prepare for employment (Anthony & Blanch, 1987; Danley & Anthony, 1987). Although the vocational and skill deficits produced by severe psychiatric disability made the train–place strategy seem logical, it resulted in very little actual employment and tended to screen out people with the most severe disabilities who were considered too low functioning to be successful in the workplace (Ford, 1995).

SE gained a great deal of attention in the field of psychiatric rehabilitation as well. In 1987, Danley and Anthony articulated the *Choose-Get-Keep model* of supported employment for people with a psychiatric disability (see Box 9.5). Danley and Anthony asserted that rather than being placed in a job, people with a psychiatric disability needed to be involved in the process of achieving employment outcomes and that the process needed to include choosing a job that matched an individual's interests, preferences, and skills. Reviewing studies of supported employment, Bond and his colleagues (1997) found that when workers were in jobs that matched their preferences, they stayed twice as long as when the job did not match the worker's preferences. This combination of choice and support, available either on or off the job site for the duration of the person's employment tenure, has become the hallmark of quality-supported employment for all people with disabilities (Carling, 1995; Roberts, 1996; Rehab Brief, 1993).

BOX 9.5
Karen S. Danley, Ph.D.

Karen Danley, Ph.D., was one of the founding members of the Center for Psychiatric Rehabilitation at Sargent College of Health and Rehabilitation Sciences, Boston University. Focusing on vocational rehabilitation, Dr. Danley was largely responsible for the development of the Choose-Get-Keep model of supported employment, which set the tone and standard for this service for PsyR and ultimately the entire field of supported employment. As the first director of Career Achievement Services, she established many new program initiatives for the Center for Psychiatric Rehabilitation as well as many innovations for the field. An experienced and successful grant writer, Dr. Danley's efforts helped to fund much of the important research and training carried out at the center. Her work included outreach to the inner-city youth of Boston who experience serious mental illness and using the Choose-Get-Keep strategy with veterans who have psychiatric disabilities.

Sadly, Karen Danley passed away in April 1998, a great loss for psychiatric rehabilitation. Perhaps her most important legacy is all the individuals she has helped to achieve vocational and educational success.

A critical feature of SE is the underlying philosophy that given adequate supports everyone is capable of competitive employment (Anthony & Blanch, 1987; Ford, 1995; Roberts, 1996).

Carl's Story

Carl first attempts to get into the workforce are representative of some of the problems people face in pursuit of their working goals. His story also illustrates some of the differences between transitional employment and supported employment. As you read this case, consider the following questions:

1. Why did Carl's first attempts at employment fail?
2. What were the differences between Carl's TE and SE experiences?
3. Is SE the best strategy for every person like Carl?
4. What will be required for Carl to continue to succeed as he moves on to college and more demanding jobs?

Carl is a 32-year-old who has been diagnosed with schizophrenia. He experienced his first psychiatric hospitalization at age 18, during his senior year in high school. The first symptoms he was aware of were hearing voices and feeling depressed. Carl's involvement in school activities had been minimal but his grades were good and he was expecting to go to college. After being discharged from the hospital, he had to really struggle to finish high school, but did manage to graduate with his class.

A month after graduation Carl was hospitalized again. This time the voices were more persistent and his depression was more pervasive. When Carl returned home he still felt confused, unmotivated, and lethargic and spent a great deal of time either sleeping or watching television. His dream of going to college and becoming an art teacher seemed remote. His friends from high school had stopped calling; they were busy getting ready for college. During the next 4 years, Carl was hospitalized five times. At his mother's urging, he attempted to take an art class offered by the local YMCA on Saturday mornings, but he felt too groggy in the morning and ended up missing most of the classes.

After Carl's seventh hospitalization, and in response to his parents' complaints that all he did was hang out at home, Carl's psychiatrist recommended that he attend the local day treatment program, but the program did not seem right for Carl. He was usually late in the mornings and only participated minimally in the prevocational units and recreational activities. He thought he would like the arts and crafts group but complained that the projects were too childish.

When a position opened for the program's transitional employment job at the local Kmart, Carl's counselor asked him if he would like to try working. Carl lasted for 1 week at the Kmart. He was almost always late, the voices were making it hard for him to concentrate, and he was reprimanded by his supervisor when he failed to hear a customer ask for help. Carl's counselor said Carl would get another chance to try TE but first he needed to improve his punctuality within the program and learn to accept feedback from his supervisor.

Six months later, Carl was given another TE job. This time Carl worked as a dishwasher in the cafeteria at the local high school. Carl's counselor thought this would be a good job for him because his punctuality had not improved and he would not have to be at this job until 11 A.M. The counselor also thought that because Carl knew people at the school he would feel less stress. This had been Carl's high school. In reality, Carl felt defeated ending up back at his school as a dishwasher. He worked there for 2 weeks before he ran into his former art teacher. Her surprise at seeing him working in the cafeteria highlighted his own feelings of disappointment and failure, and he quit the job.

Carl's program received funding for a new employment strategy, supported employment (SE). Shortly after the program started, Sharon, the SE specialist, found Carl outside her office reading the program description on the bulletin board. When she asked Carl if he was interested in work, he told her that he was not able to work because he couldn't get to most jobs on time, couldn't get along with people, and couldn't concentrate on even the simplest things like stocking shelves. Undaunted, Sharon said she was willing to give it a try if he was, and they agreed to meet the next day.

Sharon started by asking Carl to describe his ideal job, and Carl talked about being an art teacher. He described his love for art and how important his high school art teacher had been to him. He talked about the lost opportunity for college and his present inability to succeed at anything. They researched the necessary credentials to be an art teacher and talked about the possibility of college. Carl insisted that he did not have the concentration necessary to pass college courses right now and he was not even confident about his artistic abilities anymore.

Sharon and Carl examined his past experiences. They discovered many examples of Carl's ability to help others use their artistic abilities both in high school, where he worked with younger students, and at the program, where he helped other members in the arts and crafts group. They saw that even when he had to meet deadlines for his art projects, Carl didn't experience the same kind of stress that made him lose concentration when doing simple tasks. They looked at his work history to figure out why he wasn't successful on his jobs and what kinds of supports might have helped him at the time.

Sharon suggested that they contact Carl's high school art teacher because he liked and trusted her and he had worked for her informally by helping other students when he was in school. Sharon thought the art teacher could give them some ideas about jobs that were related to art but that didn't require a college degree. Carl was a little embarrassed and nervous, but agreed to let Sharon set up the meeting.

The art teacher met with Carl and Sharon and told them that the after-school program at the elementary school was looking for someone to work part time. She thought that Carl would be allowed to start an art program for the kids and she would be willing to help him plan it. She also agreed to talk to the program director and recommend Carl.

For the first time in a long time, Carl felt hopeful. He knew the morning grogginess from his medication would not interfere because this job started late in the day. He was excited about being involved in art again and felt confident that he could do it. Sharon helped Carl prepare for the interview and select pieces of Carl's artwork that he could show the program director. They reviewed bus schedules and figured out what bus Carl should take. At the interview, Carl told the program director that he hadn't worked for a while and was hoping someone would be nearby at first in case he felt overwhelmed. Carl and Sharon had agreed that knowing who to go to for help might keep Carl from feeling like he had to quit if he was feeling stressed. They also agreed that at first Sharon would drive Carl to work and stay outside in the car in case he needed her.

Sharon drove Carl to work for the first 3 days. At the end of his third day, Carl told Sharon that he'd take the bus the next day and that he'd call her if he needed help or at the end of the day if he managed okay. During the first month Carl called Sharon several times to talk through his nervousness about work. He never missed a day. When the school year ended, the program director offered Carl a job working in the summer recreation program. Sharon was surprised when Carl reported that he was thinking of turning it down. He told her he wanted to talk to her about going to college.

The Role of the Job Coach

Regardless of the supported employment approach, the primary support person to the supported employee is the job coach. In the early days of SE, the job coach typically arranged for the worker to be placed in a job and then provided training and support to the worker at the job site. Today, supports that are provided off the job site are more common. Previously, the job coach often educated the employer about disabilities and effective ways to teach the new employee and also tried to facilitate the development of relationships between the new worker and his or her coworkers. Today, more typically, job coaches do not disclose the disability status of the consumer they work with unless directed by the consumer to do so. Job coaches continue to assist the supported employee with money management, transportation, Social Security benefits monitoring, and other needed supports.

Over the years, there has been increasing recognition of the highly professionalized role that the job coach plays. Usually working without direct supervision, the job coach must successfully accomplish many different tasks. With the emphasis on career choice, the job coach has to know about career planning and development. Taking a broad view of potential careers for people with a psychiatric disability, the job coach has to know about marketing, job development, and effectively interacting with the business community. The job coach has to understand the needs of the business community in general and the needs and work culture of specific work settings.

In some cases, the job coach or employment specialist will teach the skills of job acquisition and the clients will do the actual tasks of job development themselves. Many clients prefer not to disclose their disabilities to potential employers and so prefer to do their own job development. In other cases clients need more direct support in this area, and the job coach will be more directly involved in contacting the employer, presenting the candidate's qualifications, and perhaps even accompanying the client to the job interview. The job coach also assists in the other tasks of job acquisition such as resume preparation and practicing interviewing. According to Becker and Drake (1994), job development strategies include time spent on the part of the job coach; getting to know the particular operations, needs, and hiring practices of potential employers; tapping into personal networks for job leads; and creating jobs where a task and setting match the skills and interests of a client but the job doesn't currently exist. This is sometimes referred to as *job carving* (DiLeo & Langton, 1993) and is a strategy often used when the severity of a person's disability prohibits the individual from performing all of the duties associated with existing jobs.

Gervey and Kowal (1995) reported that it takes an average of 42 job development contacts to generate one job offer. Obviously, the job coach has to be persistent. The job coach may interact with family members, community members, doctors, and other service providers in assisting the supported employee to access needed supports. Perhaps the most important characteristic of a job coach is flexibility. An active job coach may have to provide these services in an executive office, on a loading dock, and in a restaurant kitchen all on the same day.

Reflecting the complex nature of the task, the *job coach* title has undergone some changes as well. Titles such as *employment specialist*, *employment consultant*, and *human resource consultant* reflect the sophistication and professional nature of the job and the person doing that job.

BOX 9.6
APSE: The Network on Employment

APSE: The Network on Employment (formerly the Association for Persons in Supported Employment) was formed in 1988. This grassroots organization, founded by early practitioners and leaders in supported employment for people with developmental disabilities, is committed to increasing integrated employment opportunities for people with severe disabilities. APSE: The Network on Employment has grown over the years to include practitioners serving people with all disabilities, their families, funders, and businesspeople. Chapters of APSE exist in many states. APSE: The Network on Employment defines its mission as follows: "to improve and expand integrated employment opportunities, services, and outcomes for persons experiencing disabilities" (APSE, 2006).

═══ *Models of Supported Employment*

In the relatively brief time that SE has been available to people with mental illness, a variety of approaches have emerged. In part, this is because one of the critical features of SE is the individualized nature of services. Some feared that premature standardization of SE would eliminate the innovative thinking that led to its initial development. Another complication is that SE is sometimes added on to more traditional vocational services already being offered by an agency. This may result in an uncomfortable mix of values and competition for resources. Geography may also play a part in the design of services because agencies in rural areas, where jobs are fewer, may be inclined to develop group employment models. Nevertheless, in an update on the status of SE for people with mental illness, Bond and colleagues (1997) identified features of SE that appear to be common across many programs. These include:

> . . . a goal of permanent competitive employment, minimal screening for employ-ability, avoidance of prevocational training, individualized placement instead of place-ment in enclaves or mobile work crews, time-unlimited support, and consideration of client preferences. (p. 336)

Some of the main forms SE programs have taken are described next: the individual place-ment model, the enclave or work crew model, and assertive community treatment.

Individual Placement Models

The individual placement model is the most individualized approach to SE. In this model, a job coach works with an individual to identify and achieve the person's vocational goal. The services used to achieve this goal will differ depending on the client's needs and wishes as well as the agencies' approach.

The best-defined examples of the individual placement model for people with mental illness are the individual placement and support approach (IPS) articulated by the New Hampshire-Dartmouth Psychiatric Research Center (Becker & Drake, 1994, 2003) and the Choose-Get-Keep approach articulated by Boston University Center for Psychiatric Rehabilitation (Danley & Anthony, 1987; Danley, Sciarappa, & MacDonald-Wilson, 1992; MacDonald-Wilson, Mancuso, Danley, & Anthony, 1989). Both of these approaches emphasize competitive employment based on the preferences of the individual and the importance of ongoing support. The IPS approach further emphasizes rapid job search and the integration of vocational and clinical services, whereas the Choose-Get-Keep approach provides skill development in career planning activities. Although the two approaches have many similarities, which are described here, research has consistently found the IPS approach to be superior in achieving employment outcomes (Bond, 2004).

Both IPS and Choose-Get-Keep engage the client and the significant people in the cli-ent's life in identifying the person's skills, preferences, interests, resources, and support needs and then match these to a job and work setting. In the Choose-Get-Keep approach, this is done in the choose phase. By examining past experiences, the person is helped to identify and objectify those personal values and skills that will impact on the person's success and satisfaction in employment. Clients are helped to identify the skills they have developed through previous experiences and also their reactions to those experiences to illuminate their likes and dislikes, preferences, interests, and support needs. This leads to the development of a career goal and a plan for developing or acquiring the skills and resources necessary for success. (In some cases, the chosen career requires more credentials than the person has and may lead the person to seek training or education. Supported education, a strategy to provide people with the educational background they need, is discussed in Chapter 10.) Job development, which also occurs in the choose phase, is based on the skills and values of the individual. Significant people in the client's life are engaged in supporting the goal that the client has articulated (MacDonald-Wilson et al., 1989).

In the IPS approach these tasks are accomplished in the engagement and vocational assessment stages. This approach emphasizes rapid entry into employment and the need to do continual assessment after the client has gotten her or his first job, using each job to gain new information about skills, preferences, and personal style. In both the get phase of the Choose-Get-Keep approach and the obtaining employment stage of the IPS approach, the client is given the support needed and desired to obtain a job.

The keep phase of the Choose-Get-Keep approach and the job support stage of the IPS approach involve activities that identify and ensure access to adequate and ongoing support to promote successful and satisfying employment. Some supports may be in the area of learning new skills, learning to use skills in a new setting, accessing needed services, or arranging for environmental modifications. Supports are available on or off the job site and address not only meeting the requirements of the new job or adjusting to the workplace but also coaching and support in the area of interpersonal interactions. In some cases the job coach accompanies the new worker to the job for a period of time. In this case, the job coach may be providing support in mastering the job, negotiating accommodations, and also in fitting into the workplace and developing relationships with coworkers.

If the job coach provides some of the job training for the worker, it is usually because the worker requires more training than the employer typically provides. It is least stigmatizing for the supported employee to access the same training that is available to all workers in that setting. Often the support is provided off the job site. This may include supportive counseling, problem solving, and even role-playing of difficult interactions. Support provided is not limited to work issues but will include any area of the person's life that affects successful employment. For example, a job coach may assist a supported employee in negotiating a different psychiatric appointment schedule if the current one conflicts with his or her work schedule.

Ideally the job coach is not the sole means of support but has worked with the supported employee to identify and develop a support network. The network may include family, friends, counselors, coworkers, or anyone the client chooses. In fact, there has recently been greater emphasis placed on using "natural supports"; that is, those people or things that are naturally present in the setting. Not only is this usually less stigmatizing, but it is also frequently more effective. Most workplaces and workers in that setting have developed ways of supporting each other. The supported employee should be assisted in accessing those supports and in contributing support to others. It is important that the supported employee hold a valued role as a participant and contributor in the work setting. The level, type, and frequency of support needed by the supported employee may change over time and the support provided should change accordingly.

The IPS approach emphasizes the integration of vocational services and clinical services. This means that the vocational counselor or job coach works as part of the clinical team. In this approach, the clinical team then becomes an important part of the supported employees' support network. In fact, studies show that this vocational/clinical integration is one of the critical factors in positive employment outcomes (Drake, Becker, Bond, & Mueser, 2003).

Recently the Choose-Get-Keep approach was changed to the Choose-Get-Keep-Leave approach, recognizing the importance of assisting people in leaving a job in a way that contributes to future successes (http://www.bu.edu/cpr).

The Enclave or Work Crew Model

Instead of focusing on an individual, the enclave model of SE places a small group of workers with disabilities in a community employment setting. The group usually works as a separate unit within the business or industry and is trained and supervised by a job coach who is present with the enclave or work crew for the entire workday. In some cases the workers who make up the enclave are dispersed throughout the business or industry. The Rehabilitation Act specifies that an enclave or work crew must include no more than eight individuals with disabilities in order to satisfy the definition of "integrated setting" (*Federal Register*, 1992). This part of the regulation reflects the PsyR principle of normalization. By keeping work crews or enclaves small, the opportunity for contact with workers who do not have disabilities increases.

As with other group models of employment services, however, this model of supported employment does have disadvantages. Although the enclave or work crew is located in a place of business, it is usually separate from the "regular" employees, which reduces chances for interaction and increases stigma. Furthermore, consumer choice is quite limited as consumers must be willing to do whatever work the enclave or work crew was hired to do.

Supported Employment in Assertive Community Treatment

Assertive community treatment (ACT) programs, which are described in depth in more detail in Chapter 7, often include a vocational component. This strategy combines vocational rehabilitation services with other treatment services provided by the ACT team. In this model, one of the ACT team members is a vocational specialist although, as is common in ACT, all team members contribute to employment outcomes. Using an individualized placement approach, the service is based on the belief that employment is both an outcome and a treatment. "A basic assumption is that a complex relationship exists between symptoms and vocational functioning; thus the ACT model of treatment views work as a critical competing process to symptoms" (Russert & Frey, 1991, p. 342). In other words, the person who is concentrating on performing work tasks is less likely to be preoccupied with his or her symptoms and may be better able to develop coping strategies for symptom management.

Other Vocational Preparation Services

Different program models, whether explicitly prevocational, vocational, or not, can use specific strategies to enhance the pursuit and attainment of employment goals.

Vocational Exploration Services

In addition to a review of past experiences, many programs utilize community experiences to improve one's knowledge of oneself as a worker or one's perception of the world of work. This knowledge can facilitate the career choice process. Some examples of these experiences are discussed in the following list:

- *Tours of businesses:* For someone with extremely limited knowledge of the world of work, sometimes just observing the variety of jobs that exist in the community can be the beginning of identifying preferences.
- *Volunteering:* For some individuals, paid employment seems too big a risk or responsibility at first. Volunteering for a short time may help to build self-confidence.
- *Job sampling:* Job sampling programs are usually very brief (a few hours to a few days) work experiences in a variety of real work settings. The person doing the sampling may or may not be paid. If the person is paid, it is usually by the rehabilitation agency rather than the employer. Job sampling may help someone with very limited knowledge of work begin to identify preferences.
- *Job shadowing:* Accompanying someone else as he or she does a job may give one a clearer idea of the tasks involved.
- *Informational interviews:* Interviewing someone who is currently employed in a job or field of interest may help one get a clearer picture of what that career is like.
- *Worksite interactive internships:* This innovative employment service is a comprehensive career education and planning strategy to assist consumers through an occupational self-discovery process. Based on the career planning curriculum from the Boston University Center for Psychiatric Rehabilitation, this service is designed for people who are interested in going beyond selecting a job and want to explore an occupational area. Consumers are assisted in exploring their own general occupational values and interests and nonvocational activities of interest, and they also complete a self-rating of aptitudes, abilities, and skills to produce a worker profile. A comparison of the person's profile with characteristics of occupational areas results in the selection of an occupation or field of interest. This interest is then field tested through an internship in that occupation. The internship

is arranged by the agency that is providing the service, and it may or may not be paid. At the end of the internship, a consumer may decide to pursue this occupation by looking for a job or accessing training or education as required or the person may decide that he or she is not interested and return to the exploration process (Fishbein, 1998).

Supported Employment: An Evidence-Based Practice

A growing number of studies comparing SE with other services has provided substantial evidence of the superiority of SE in achieving competitive employment outcomes (Bond, 2004; Bond et al., 2001; Twamley, Jeste, & Lehman, 2003). These studies have also contributed to the illumination of the critical principles and practices of SE. SE services that are based on these principles and practices have come to be known as the individual placement and support (IPS) model, which was described earlier in this chapter. SE has been studied in comparison to day treatment services (Bond, 2004; Drake et al., 1994; Lehman et al., 2002; Mueser et al., 2004), conventional or enhanced vocational services (Bond, 2004; Bond et al., 1995; Drake et al., 1996, 1999; McFarlane et al., 2000; Mueser et al., 2004), and other mental health services (Chandler, Meisel, Hu, McGowen, & Madison, 1997). In each case, SE has achieved significantly better employment-related outcomes. That is, persons receiving SE services were significantly more likely to become competitively employed, work more hours, and to earn better wages (Bond, 2004). These superior outcomes have been consistent regardless of geographical characteristics (i.e., rural or urban areas) or race/ethnicity (Bond, 2004). As with other evidence-based practices, fidelity to the model is significantly related to better outcomes (Becker et al., 2001; Drake et al., 1996, 1999; Lehman et al., 2002; McGrew & Griss, 2005; Mueser et al., 2004).

Critical Ingredients of Supported Employment

- Services are focused on competitive employment
- Nonexclusionary criteria
- Rapid job search
- Integration of vocational and mental health services
- Focus on consumer preferences
- Time-unlimited, individualized supports
- Benefits counseling.

Service Outcomes of Supported Employment

- Competitive employment
- Higher number of hours worked
- Higher wages earned.

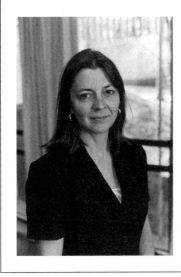

BOX 9.7
Deborah Becker

Deborah Becker, M.Ed., along with Robert Drake, has been one of the chief architects of the individual placement and support approach to supported employment. As the senior project director at the New Hampshire-Dartmouth Psychiatric Research Center, she has conducted critical research on employment for people with psychiatric disabilities. This research has helped to establish IPS as an evidence-based practice. Ms. Becker codeveloped the SAMHSA Evidence-Based Practice Supported Employment Resource Kit and works tirelessly to assist practitioners and agencies to develop and implement these services. Her extensive writing in the area of employment for people with psychiatric disabilities has helped significantly shape the field of supported employment, demonstrate the employability of people with psychiatric disabilities, and establish standards of supported employment services.

SE services, particularly those that adhere faithfully to these principles and practices, are far more successful than other services at achieving competitive employment outcomes. These programs have been shown to achieve 60% to 70% employment rates. However, there are still many unanswered questions. For example, what are the factors that inhibit successful employment for the 30% to 40% of people who are not becoming employed? What services or supports will improve job retention? What is the role of non-SE providers in promoting and supporting employment goals? Many more studies are needed to address these issues.

Summary

The barriers to employment for people with mental illness include stigma, the experience of the symptoms of mental illness, the disabilities brought about by the illness and its consequences, and concerns about the loss of government benefits.

Stigma reduces community acceptance of people with mental illness and results in discrimination. The stigma that exists among mental health professionals results in reduced quality services and fewer options offered to program clients. An individual's internalized stigma reduces the individual's belief in his or her potential and may be the hardest stigma to overcome.

Many people with mental illness have missed out on important vocational experiences. The illnesses themselves affect many areas such as memory, concentration, interpersonal interactions, self-esteem, and anxiety. Medication may have overt physical side effects and less obvious social side effects.

There is strong evidence that past work history is the best predictor of vocational or educational success. This research finding begs for individuals to begin to get some type of vocational experience as young adults.

Innovative vocational services were developed for people with psychiatric disabilities as early as the 1950s. Fountain House, one of the original clubhouses, introduced transitional employment, a program of real jobs in community settings. Fairweather Lodges provide a combination of residential and employment programs. Lodge members live together and work together running a small business. Services such as sheltered workshops and mobile work crews are more segregated and therefore more stigmatizing than regular community employment.

In the 1980s, supported employment was introduced for people with severe developmental disabilities, and it was adopted in the field of psychiatric rehabilitation as well. SE assists individuals to become employed in jobs that match their skills, interests, and preferences and provides whatever supports are needed to ensure success and satisfaction.

Research studies have found SE to be superior in achieving employment outcomes and is considered an evidence-based practice. A focus on competitive employment, nonexclusionary criteria, rapid job search, integration of vocational and mental health services, focus on consumer preference, time-unlimited supports, and benefits counseling are the critical ingredients of SE.

In the United States, the Rehabilitation Act of 1973, which established the Rehabilitation Services Administration, provides federal funding for vocational rehabilitation services. It also defines supported employment and emphasizes consumer choice and a presumption of employability for all people with disabilities. Furthermore, the Americans with Disabilities Act, passed in 1990, along with antidiscrimination laws in many states, protect people with disabilities from discrimination in a number of areas including employment. This act is a far-reaching statement about the right and ability of citizens with disabilities to be fully included in all aspects of community life.

Class Exercise

The clubhouse-type program where you have been a case manager for 3 years has just been notified that funding to develop supported employment (SE) services is going to be available soon. The director would like to apply for this funding and has brought together the staff members who are primarily responsible for the transitional employment (TE) program to design the SE program. It becomes evident immediately that there are many different opinions about how to structure the new SE program.

Scenario 1
Some think that SE should be completely separate from the rest of the program so that clients who want to can access SE without being involved or associated with the clubhouse

aspects of the program. Others want to use SE as the next step after TEP. Their reasoning is that people have to demonstrate commitment, motivation, and good work behavior before you can convince an employer to hire them.

Scenario 2

Still others want to develop a multistep program, in which clients spend 8 weeks in a work unit demonstrating attendance, punctuality, good grooming, adequate productivity, ability to work as a team member, and ability to accept feedback from a supervisor. At the same time, clients will attend a work-readiness group where they will discuss reasons for wanting to work. This will be followed by 3 months on a TE placement and then the individual can go into a SE job.

1. Considering what you have read about predictors of vocational success and quality vocational services, evaluate the ideas expressed in Scenarios 1 and 2.
2. Describe an SE program design that incorporates what you have learned about vocational issues and quality services.

References

Anthony, W. A. (1993). Editorial. *Psychosocial Rehabilitation Journal, 17*(1), 1.

Anthony, W. A. (1994). Characteristics of people with psychiatric disabilities that are predictive of entry into the rehabilitation process and successful employment. *Psychosocial Rehabilitation Journal, 17*(3), 3–13.

Anthony, W. A., & Blanch, A. (1987). Supported employment for persons who are psychiatrically disabled: An historical and conceptual perspective. *Psychosocial Rehabilitation Journal,* XI(2).

Anthony, W. A., Cohen, M. R., & Danley, K. S. (1988). The psychiatric rehabilitation model as applied to vocational rehabilitation. In J. A. Ciardiello & M. D. Bell (Eds.), *Vocational rehabilitation of persons with prolonged psychiatric disorders* (pp. 59–80). Baltimore, MD: Johns Hopkins University Press.

Anthony, W. A., Cohen, M., & Farkas, M. (2002). *Psychiatric rehabilitation.* Boston, MA: Center for Psychiatric Rehabilitation.

Anthony, W. A., & Jansen, M. A. (1984). Predicting the vocational capacity of the chronically mentally ill: Research and policy implications. *American Psychologist, 39,* 537–544.

Anthony, W. A., Rogers, E., Cohen, M., & Davies, R. R. (1995). Relationship between psychiatric symptomatology, work skills, and future vocational performance. *Psychiatric Services, 46*(4), 353–358.

APSE. (2006). About APSE. Retrieved February 8, 2006, from http://www.apse.org/aboutapsc.html

Arns, P. G., & Linney, J. A. (1993). Work, self, and life satisfaction for persons with severe and persistent mental disorders. *Psychosocial Rehabilitation Journal, 17*(2), 63–79.

Baron, R. C., & Salzer, M. S. (2002). Accounting for unemployment among people with mental illness. *Behavioral Sciences and the Law, 20,* 585–599.

Beard, J. H., Propst, R. N., & Malamud, T. J. (1994). The Fountain House model of psychiatric rehabilitation. In L. Spaniol et al. (Eds.), *An introduction to psychiatric rehabilitation* (pp. 42–52). Columbia, MD: IAPSRS.

Becker, D. R., & Drake, R. E. (1994). Individual placement and support: A community mental health center approach to vocational rehabilitation. *Community Mental Health Journal, 30*(2), 193–206.

Becker, D. R., & Drake, R. E. (2003). *A working life for people with severe mental illness.* New York: Oxford University Press.

Becker, D. R., Smith, J., Tanzman, B., Drake, R. E., & Tremblay, T. (2001). Fidelity of supported employment programs and employment outcomes. *Psychiatric Services, 52*(6), 834–836.

Bell, M. D., Milstein, R. M., & Lysaker, P. H. (1993). Pay and participation in work activity: clinical benefits for clients with schizophrenia. *Psychosocial Rehabilitation Journal, 17*(2), 173–176.

Blankertz, L., & Robinson, S. (1996). Adding a vocational focus to mental health rehabilitation. *Psychiatric Services, 47*(11), 1216–1222.

Bond, G. R. (2004). Supported employment: Evidence for an evidence-based practice. *Psychiatric Rehabilitation Journal, 27*(4), 345–359.

Bond, G. R., & Boyer, S. L. (1988). Rehabilitation programs and outcomes. In J. A. Ciardiello & M. D. Bell (Eds.), *Vocational rehabilitation of persons with prolonged psychiatric disorders* (pp. 231–263). Baltimore, MD: Johns Hopkins University Press.

Bond, G. R., Dietzen, L. L., McGrew, J. H., & Miller, L. D. (1995). Accelerating entry into supported employment for persons with severe psychiatric disabilities. *Rehabilitation Psychology, 40*(2), 91–111.

Bond, G. R., & Dincin, J. (1986). Accelerating entry into transitional employment in a psychosocial rehabilitation agency. *Rehabilitation Psychology, 31*, 143–155.

Bond, G. R., Drake, R. E., Mueser, K. T., & Becker, D. R. (1997). An update on supported employment for people with severe mental illness. *Psychiatric Services, 48*(3), 335–346.

Bond, G. R., Resnick, S. G., Drake, R. E., Xie, H., McHugo, G. J., & Bebout, R. R. (2001). Does competitive employment improve nonvocational outcomes for people with severe mental illness? *Journal of Consulting and Clinical Psychology, 69*(3), 489–501.

Braitman, A., Counts, P., Avenport, R., Zurbinden, B., Rogers, M., Clauss, J., et al. (1995). Comparison of barriers to employment for unemployed and employed clients in a case management program: An exploratory study. *Psychiatric Rehabilitation Journal, 19*(1), 3–8.

Carling, P. J. (1995). *Return to community: Building support systems for people with psychiatric disabilities.* New York: The Guilford Press.

Casper, E. S., & Fishbein, S. (2002). Job satisfaction and job success as moderators of the self-esteem of people with mental illnesses. *Psychiatric Rehabilitation Journal, 26*(1), 33–42.

Chandler, D., Meisel, J., Hu, T., McGowen, M., & Madison, K. (1997). A capitated model for a cross-section of severely mentally ill clients: Employment outcomes. *Community Mental Health Journal, 33*(6), 501–516.

Chapman, B. (1992). Poll shows support for disabled. *Orlando (Florida) Sentinel.*

Danley, K. S., & Anthony, W. A. (1987). The choose get keep approach to supported employment. *American Rehabilitation, 13*(4), 6–9, 27–29.

Danley, K. S., Sciarappa, K., & MacDonald-Wilson, K. (1992). Choose-get-keep: A psychiatric rehabilitation approach to supported employment. In R. P. Liberman (Ed.), *Effective psychiatric rehabilitation* (Vol. 53, New Directions in Mental Health Services, pp. 87–96). San Francisco: Jossey-Bass.

Deegan, P. E. (1988). Recovery: The lived experience of rehabilitation. *Psychosocial Rehabilitation Journal, 11*(4), 11–19.

DiLeo, D., & Langton, D. (1993). *Get the marketing edge.* St. Augustine, FL: TRN.

Drake, R. E., Becker, D. R., Biesanz, J. C., Torrey, W. C., McHugo, G. J., & Wyzik, P. F. (1994). Rehabilitative day treatment vs. supported employment: I, Vocational outcomes. *Community Mental Health Journal, 30*(5), 519–531.

Drake, R. E., Becker, D. R., Bond, G. R., & Mueser, K. T. (2003). A process analysis of integrated and non-integrated approaches to supported employment. *Journal of Vocational Rehabilitation, 18*, 51–58.

Drake, R. E., McHugo, G. J., Bebout, R. R., Becker, D. R., Harris, M., Bond, G. R., et al. (1999). A randomized clinical trial of supported employment for inner-city patients with severe mental illness. *Archives of General Psychiatry, 56*, 627–633.

Drake, R. E., McHugo, G. J., Becker, D. R., Anthony, W. A., & Clark, R. I. (1996). The New Hampshire study of supported employment for people with severe mental illness. *Journal of Consulting and Clinical Psychology, 64*(2), 391–399.

Fairweather, G. W. (Ed.). (1980). New Directions for Mental Health Services: No. 7. *The Fairweather Lodge: A twenty-five year retrospective.* San Francisco: Jossey-Bass.

Federal Register. (1992). Department of Education (pp. 28432–28442).

Fishbein, S., (1998, July 21). Director, Office of Human Resource and Rehabilitation Development, New Jersey Division of Mental Health Services. Personal Communication.

Ford, L. H. (1995). *Providing employment support for people with long-term mental illness.* Baltimore, MD: Brookes Publishing Company.

Gervey, R., & Kowal, H. (1995). Job development strategies for placing persons with psychiatric disabilities into supported employment jobs in a large city. *Psychosocial Rehabilitation Journal, 18*(4), 95–113.

Gowdy, E. A., Carlson, L. S., & Rapp, C. A. (2004). Organizational factors Differentiating high performing from low performing supported employment programs. *Psychiatric Rehabilitation Journal, 28*(2), 150–156.

Harris Interactive. (2002). Americans with disabilities still pervasively disadvantaged on a broad range of key indicators. Retrieved 2004 from http://www.harrisinteractive.com.

Jansen, M. A. (1988). The psychological and vocational problems of persons with chronic mental illness. In J. A. Ciardiello & M. D. Bell (Eds.), *Vocational rehabilitation of persons with prolonged psychiatric disorders* (pp. 35–46). Baltimore, MD: Johns Hopkins University Press.

Jensen, A., & Silverstein R. (n.d.). *Policy brief.* Washington, DC: Center for the Study and Advancement of Disability Policy.

Jones, T. L. (1993). *The Americans with Disabilities Act, a review of best practices.* New York: American Management Association.

Krupa, T. (2004). Employment, recovery, and schizophrenia; Integrating health and disorder at work. *Psychiatric Rehabilitation Journal, 28*(1), 8–14.

Ledbetter, J., & Field, T. F. (1978). A brief history of vocational rehabilitation legislation. *Psychosocial Rehabilitation Journal, II*(3), 35–42.

Lee, B. A. (n.d.). *Reasonable accommodation under the Americans with Disabilities Act.* New Brunswick, NJ: Bureau of Economic Research, Rutgers University.

Lehman, A. F., Goldberg, R., Dixon, L. B., McNary, S., Postrado, L., Hackman, A., et al. (2002). Improving employment outcomes for persons with severe mental illnesses. *Archives of General Psychiatry, 59*(2), 165–172.

Lysaker, P., & Bell, M. (1995). Work rehabilitation and improvements in insight in schizophrenia. *Journal of Nervous & Mental Disease, 183*(2), 103–106.

MacDonald-Wilson, K. L., Mancuso, L. L., Danley, K. S., & Anthony, W. A. (1989). Supported employment for people with psychiatric disability. *Journal of Applied Rehabilitation Counseling, 20*(3), 50–57.

Mancuso, L. L. (1990). Reasonable accommodations for workers with psychiatric disabilities. *Psychosocial Rehabilitation Journal, 14*(2), 3–19.

Marrone, J. (1993). Creating positive vocational outcomes for people with severe mental illness. *Psychosocial Rehabilitation Journal, 17*(2), 43–62.

McFarlane, W. R., Dushay, R. A., Deakins, S. M., Stastny, P., Lukens, E. P., Toran, J., et al. (2000). Employment outcomes in family-aided assertive community treatment. *American Journal of Orthopsychiatry, 70*(2), 203–214.

McGrew, J., & Griss, M. (2005). Concurrent and predictive validity of two scales to assess the fidelity of implementation of supported employment. *Psychiatric Rehabilitation Journal, 29*(1), 41–47.

McGurk, S. R., Mueser, K. T., Harvey, P. D., LaPuglia, R., & Marder, J. (2003). Cognitive and symptom predictors of work outcomes for clients with schizophrenia in supported employment. *Psychiatric Services, 54*(8), 1129–1135.

McGurrin, M. C. (1994). An overview of the effectiveness of traditional vocational rehabilitation services in the treatment of long-term mental illness. *Psychosocial Rehabilitation Journal, 17*(3), 37–54.

Mowbray, C. T., Bybee, D., Harris, S. N., & McCrohan, N. (1995). Predictors of work status and future work orientation in people with a psychiatric disability. *Psychiatric Rehabilitation Journal, 19*(2), 17–28.

Mueser, K. T., Becker, D. R., Torrey, W. C., Xie, H., Bond, G. R., Drake, R. E., et al. (1997). Work and nonvocational domains of functioning in persons with severe mental illness: A longitudinal analysis. *The Journal of Nervous and Mental Disease, 185*(7), 410–425.

Mueser, K. T., Clark, R. E., Haines, M., Drake, R. E., McHugo, G. J., Bond, G. R., et al. (2004). The Hartford study of supported employment for persons with severe mental illness. *Journal of Consulting and Clinical Psychology, 72.*

Murphy, S. T., & Rogan, P. M. (1995). *Closing the shop: Conversion from sheltered to integrated work.* Baltimore, MD: Brookes Publishing Company.

National Alliance of Business. (1991). ADA sourcebook, what you need to know about the Americans with Disabilities Act: A guide for small and medium-sized businesses. Washington, D.C.: author.

Neff, W. S. (1988). Vocational rehabilitation in perspective. In J. A. Ciardiello & M. D. Bell (Eds.), *Vocational rehabilitation of persons with prolonged psychiatric disorders* (pp. 5–18). Baltimore, MD: Johns Hopkins University Press.

Noble, J. H. (1998). Policy reform dilemmas in promoting employment of persons with severe mental illness. *Psychiatric Services, 49*(6), 775–781.

Onaga, E. E. (1994). The Fairweather Lodge as a psychosocial program in the 1990s. In L. Spaniol et al. (Eds.), *An introduction to psychiatric rehabilitation* (pp. 206–214). Columbia, MD: IAPSRS.

Rehab brief: Bringing research into effective focus. (1993), Vol. XV, No. 10, pp. 1–4. Washington, DC: U.S. Department of Education.

Ritsher, J. B., Otilingam, P. G., & Grajales, M. (2003). Internalized stigma of mental illness: Psychometric properties of a new measure. *Psychiatry Research, 121*(1), 31–49.

Ritsher, J. B., & Phelan, J. C. (2004). Internalized stigma predicts erosion of morale among psychiatric outpatients. *Psychiatry Research, 129*(3), 257–265.

Roberts, M. (Ed.). (1996). *Supported employment training: Competency-based instructional modules* (3rd ed.). Piscataway: University Affiliated Programs of New Jersey, University of Medicine and Dentistry of New Jersey.

Roberts, M. (1997). Supported/transitional employment program design and implementation. In *Integrated employment for persons with psychiatric disabilities: A rehabilitation and recovery-based approach, module II* (pp. 78–84). Ithaca, NY: Cornell University and Rehabilitation Support Services.

Roberts, M., & Rotteveel, J. (1995). Stigma in the workplace. Paper presented at the Sixth Annual APSE Conference, Denver, CO.

Roessler, R. T. (2002). TWWIIA initiatives and work incentives: Return-to-work implications. *Journal of Rehabilitation*, pp. 11–15.

Russert, M. G., & Frey, J. L. (1991). The PACT vocational model: A step into the future. *Psychosocial Rehabilitation Journal, 14*(4), 7–18.

Rutman, I. D. (1994). How psychiatric disability expresses itself as a barrier to employment. *Psychosocial Rehabilitation Journal, 17*(3), 15–35.

Skiba, J. A. (2001). Reaching the door to employment: Is it really open? *Journal of Vocational Rehabilitation, 16*(1), 39–46.

Toms-Barker, L. (1994). Community based models of employment services for people with long term mental illness. *Psychosocial Rehabilitation Journal, 17*(3), 55–65.

Torrey, W. C, Becker, D. R., & Drake, R. E. (1995). Rehabilitative day treatment vs. supported employment II: Consumer, family and staff reactions to a program change. *Psychosocial Rehabilitation Journal, 18*(3), 67–75.

Torrey, W. C., Mueser, K. T., McHugo, G. H., & Drake, R. E. (2000). Self-esteem as an outcome measure in studies of vocational rehabilitation for adults with severe mental illness. *Psychiatric Services, 51*(2), 229–233.

Twamley, E. W., Jeste, D. V., & Lehman, A. F. (2003). Vocational rehabilitation in schizophrenia and other psychotic disorders: A literature review and meta-analysis of randomized controlled trials. *The Journal of Nervous and Mental Disease, 191*(8), 515–523.

Chapter 10

Supported Education

Introduction 276

Benefits of Supported Education 276

Barriers to Education 277

   Unique Challenges for Persons with
   Psychiatric Disabilities 278

History of the Supported Employment
Model 280

   The Federal Response 282

Definition and Models of Supported
Education 283

   Unger's Three Models of Supported
   Education 283

   Other Models of Supported
   Education 284

   A Choose-Get-Keep Framework 286

Jose's Story 287

Applying Psychiatric Rehabilitation
Principles to Supported Education 289

Research in Supported Education 291

Dissemination of Supported
Education 295

Future Directions in Supported
Education 295

   Challenge 1: To Better Meet the Needs of
   Young Adults 296

   Challenge 2: Fostering More Freestanding
   Supported Education Programs 297

   Challenge 3: Integrating the Pursuit of
   Educational and Career Goals 297

Summary 298

Class Exercise 298

References 299

Successful achievement of educational goals, such as completion of an academic degree or a technical training program, helps many people achieve their long-term vocational goals and improves the quality of their lives. A psychiatric rehabilitation approach known as supported education has the capacity to help individuals coping with a psychiatric disability stay in school or return to complete their education. This chapter will explore the benefits of supported education for people with psychiatric disabilities, as well as the challenges encountered by these students and the programs that support them.

This chapter will answer the following questions:

1. Can people with severe and persistent mental illnesses successfully pursue postsecondary education?

2. What are the special needs of students with psychiatric disabilities? What types of special services and supports can be provided?

3. What does higher education offer persons with severe and persistent mental illnesses?
4. Are there supported education strategies that have been proven effective?
5. What is the future of supported education as a psychiatric rehabilitation service?

Introduction

A common consequence of schizophrenia and other severe mental illnesses is the interruption of postsecondary educational pursuits (Anthony & Unger, 1991; Unger, 1990). As you may recall from Chapter 1, Paul had his first acute episode of schizophrenia during his freshman year at college. Many adolescents and young adults have had similar experiences; in fact, it has been estimated that more than 4 million people would have completed their college education if they were not faced with the many challenges associated with having an early-onset psychiatric disorder (Kessler, Foster, Saunders, & Stang, 1995).

The inability to achieve an important personal goal such as successful completion of a college semester often results in feelings of failure, shame, and disappointment. In addition, many individuals are told by misguided mental health professionals that they will probably never be able to return to school and should settle for less stressful pursuits. Countless people diagnosed with severe mental illnesses have had their dreams shattered because they believed that college degrees and professional careers were out of their reach.

In addition to the psychological impact of an interrupted education, it is important to consider the socioeconomic implications for people with disabilities who do not acquire advanced education or training. People who lack further education have fewer employment opportunities and the jobs they do get are often on the lower end of the pay scale (Kessler et al., 1995; Megivern, Pellerito, & Mowbray 2003; Stodden & Conway, 2003).

Benefits of Supported Education

In the 21st century, a college education or advanced technical education has become a critical ingredient of success for the vast majority of persons seeking professional and semiprofessional employment. Most readers will be familiar with the potential benefits of a higher education including more opportunities for upward mobility, higher salaries, and increased career satisfaction (Megivern et al., 2003; Mowbray, 1999, 2004a; Moxley, Mowbray, & Brown, 1993). College campuses are also an important resource for developing social networks and business contacts (Murphy, Mullen, & Spagnolo, 2005). For people without disabilities these benefits are rarely questioned, but they are just as essential for persons with disabilities.

It is also important to consider a number of additional benefits that may be unique to people who are coping with severe mental illnesses. Mowbray (1997) identified five key benefits of supported education for people with psychiatric disabilities:

1. *New identity*: Moving from the role of psychiatric patient or mental health consumer to the socially valued role of student.

2. *New and normalized environment*: Moving from a psychiatric hospital or day treatment program to a classroom on a college campus.

3. *Structure*: Academic studies and other campus activities provide meaningful and productive ways to spend time.

4. *A clean slate*: Often in a bind when a potential employer asks what they have been doing in recent years, persons with psychiatric disabilities who are attending college classes can honestly say that they decided to pursue a new career and took time off to continue their education.

5. *Hope*: Enrollment in college classes and progress toward a degree are major steps toward the realization of goals and dreams that may have seemed impossible prior to involvement in supported education (pp. 67–68).

Thus, for many people, supported education can be an important step on their road to recovery. The following quotes, taken from various first-person accounts, emphasize the important benefits of postsecondary education for people who are recovering from severe mental illnesses.

> *Through this supported education program I have been given a most precious gift; the realization of my own potential. Regardless of my disabilities, both physical and mental, I am an asset to the very same society that I feared for so many years. (Mayer, 1993, pp. 39–40)*
>
> *In my current recovery process, I am doing better in my life than I have ever done before. My personal life has gotten better. I have married since being in this program. I am feeling more hopeful about what I can achieve for myself in life. I am having fun while learning and meeting new and interesting people. (Spencer-Watts, 2002, p. 100)*
>
> *I know that I have great potential and the Michigan Supported Education Program has given me back the confidence to believe in myself again as well as triggering in me courage, persistence and determination to continue to pursue my dreams and aspirations. They have alerted me of the fact that, although college is difficult, it is possible. (Ishmael, 2002, p. 32)*
>
> *While I was attending [the supported education program and college classes]—I was not manic. I was not homeless. I was not a mental patient or an ex-mental patient. I was a STUDENT! And it felt great! (Cloutier, 1997, p. 66)*

Barriers to Education

Clearly supported education (SEd) has the capacity to greatly enrich the lives of people with psychiatric disabilities. Why then are there still relatively few individuals pursuing educational goals? Why, as we will explore later in this chapter, are there so many communities in the United States that do not provide supported education services?

Some of the barriers to higher education are the same as those for people without disabilities, particularly persons in the lower socioeconomic classes. A major barrier to education for many Americans is *economic instability*. People who are struggling to pay housing and grocery bills are hard pressed to consider managing the rising costs of college tuition. Certainly financial aid can help; nevertheless, costs such as books, computers, supplies, and fees can make a college education unaffordable for many. Lack of affordable and accessible *transportation* is another major issue for people with limited incomes. In one study, transportation was cited as the number one barrier to attending college (Shearman, Hart-Katuin, & Hicks, 2002).

Many college students, particularly older students who are returning to school, struggle with *balancing schoolwork with other responsibilities*, such as jobs, children, and household chores. People on limited incomes often have fewer resources available to address these challenges, such as lack of funds to pay for child care. Among the general population, fewer than 50% of high school seniors entering college go on to complete a bachelor's degree, and overall community college dropout rates also exceed 50%. Clearly, postsecondary education can be a daunting task for many people, regardless of illness or disability (Adelman, 2004; Mowbray, 1999).

Unique Challenges for Persons with Psychiatric Disabilities

In addition to these barriers encountered by many college students, people with psychiatric disabilities face a number of unique challenges. Perhaps the most obvious challenge is the mental illness itself. The case of Paul, explored in Chapter 1, clearly illustrates how acute *psychiatric symptoms* such as hallucinations and delusions can interfere with one's ability to focus on course material or sometimes even get to class. However, even when major symptoms are in remission, many people continue to struggle with residual symptoms such as reduced ability to concentrate or process information. *Functional deficits* can also interfere with ability to perform well in academic settings. For example, a student who lacks appropriate social skills may monopolize class discussions or repeatedly ask the professor irrelevant questions and then be unaware that his behavior is disrupting the flow of the class. (*As university professors, however, we can attest that this deficit is not unique to persons with psychiatric illnesses.*) In addition, *side effects of psychotropic medications* can cause difficulties such as slowed movements and inability to stay alert in class due to sleepiness (Cooper, 1993; Dougherty et al., 1996; Frankie et al., 1996; Megivern et al., 2003; Mowbray, Moxley, & Brown, 1993).

The *stress* associated with final exams or major class projects is a challenge for most students. For those with a severe mental illness, stress may contribute to the recurrence or exacerbation of symptoms (see the discussion of the stress-vulnerability-coping-competence model in Chapter 2). At times, either because of stress-induced relapse or simply due to the episodic nature of a severe mental illness, *hospitalizations* occur that can interrupt a student's course of study. Not surprisingly, many students who have psychiatric disabilities become discouraged by the effects that even a brief hospital stay can have on missed work, poor grades, and incomplete semesters. For some people, it is not so much the psychiatric symptoms themselves, but the fear of recurring symptoms or hospitalizations that creates a barrier to the completion of educational goals.

Another challenge faced by people with psychiatric disabilities who are trying to return to school is *systems management*. Many people have already been frustrated by the mental health system, the vocational rehabilitation system, and the Social Security Administration. Taking on yet another bureaucracy such as a large university with its own complicated systems of admission, financial aid, and registration may be overwhelming. Some students give up before they start because the application process alone is so complex. Managing these systems often requires tenacity, creativity, flexibility, and support (Cooper, 1993; Dougherty et al., 1996, Frankie et al., 1996). Many schools fail to provide adequate services for students with disabilities, and are particularly ill equipped to serve students with psychiatric disabilities. Lack of coordination between campus-based student support services and community-based mental health services is yet another systems management failure (Megivern & Pellerito, 2002; Mowbray, Megivern, & Holter, 2003b).

As if the above-mentioned challenges were not enough, many people with psychiatric disabilities also must face *negative attitudes and stigma* while attempting to pursue an education (Mowbray, 1999; Unger, 1994). Sometimes, these come from otherwise well-meaning family members and friends who firmly believe that their loved one is too fragile to cope with the pressures of being in school. Unfortunately, many people are also discouraged by mental health and rehabilitation professionals who hold antiquated beliefs about the capabilities of persons who have severe mental illnesses, and are thus reluctant to support them in achieving their educational goals or to refer them to supported education programs (Cook & Solomon, 1993; Frankie et al., 1996; Mowbray et al., 1993). Although many current practitioners do embrace the concepts of recovery and empowerment, too many others still convey disheartening messages such as "College and competitive employment are not in your future. If you want to stay out of the hospital you should participate in less stressful activities."

Negative attitudes and misconceptions about people with psychiatric disabilities are also commonly held by the faculty, administrators, and staff of many postsecondary educational institutions (Becker, Martin, Wajeeh, Ward, & Shern, 2002; Mowbray, 1999; Unger, 1994). Most know very little about severe mental illnesses and how these illnesses may affect students in the classroom and in other areas of college life. Many academic personnel express concern that students who experience psychiatric symptoms will be disruptive, violent, dangerous, or unable to meet academic standards (Frankie et al., 1996; Housel & Hickey, 1993; Jasper, 2002; Unger, 1998). In fact, until the passage of the Americans with Disabilities Act in 1990, some colleges and universities had dismissal polices for those who were diagnosed with a severe mental illness, even if there was no evidence of poor academic performance or dangerous behaviors (Mowbray, 1999). Despite the fact that there is now evidence that many people with psychiatric disabilities can successfully complete degree requirements and that laws are in place that protect their right to do so, attitudes on many campuses have been slow to change. Mowbray (1999) reported that in her experience academic administrators were often reluctant to spend time discussing SEd strategies and were sometimes more interested in talking about keeping people with psychiatric disabilities out of the classroom.

As you will see later in this chapter, there are many supports and resources that can help students with psychiatric disabilities overcome what may seem like insurmountable barriers to education. However, sometimes the biggest challenge is the student's own belief that he or she will be unable to manage both a mental illness and a postsecondary education. Many people with a psychiatric disability have expressed fears of failure, discrimination, and isolation in academic settings (Cooper, 1993; Dougherty et al., 1996; Mowbray et al., 1993). In addition, being labeled with a psychiatric diagnosis, failing at attempts to achieve personal goals, and experiencing the stigmatizing attitudes of others can all contribute to the low self-esteem experienced by many people with psychiatric disabilities. This type of low self-esteem has been labeled "self-stigma" and may be the most daunting barrier to overcome.

History of the Supported Education Model

Services to help people with psychiatric disabilities access educational opportunities and overcome the many barriers to education addressed in the preceding section began to emerge in many places around the country in the 1980s. In 1981 the term *supported education* (SEd) was first used by psychiatric rehabilitation pioneers, such as Karen Unger at the Boston University Center for Psychiatric Rehabilitation. She recognized the importance of postsecondary education in enhancing quality of life, social mobility, career options, career advancement, and self-improvement for anyone, while also recognizing the supports that may be critical to success for persons with a psychiatric disability (Anthony, 1993a; Cook & Solomon, 1993; Dougherty, Hastie, Bernard, Broadhurst, & Marcus, 1992; Mowbray et al., 2003b; Unger, 1990, 1993; Wells-Moran & Gilmur, 2002). However, before the concept of SEd became widely known and implementation began, a number of related developments occurred that influenced mental health service systems.

The 1980s brought advances in the treatment and rehabilitation of severe mental illnesses. New medications were discovered. Effective skills training techniques, geared toward helping people learn the adaptive behaviors needed to live, learn, and work in normalized settings, were introduced. Research studies, such as the Harding, Brooks, Ashikaga, Strauss, and Brier (1987) longitudinal study that followed former patients of a Vermont state psychiatric hospital, showed that the abilities of persons with severe mental illnesses far exceeded earlier expectations of practitioners. All of these promising trends helped to change the attitudes and practices of mental health professionals who were beginning to develop more positive ideas about the outcome of severe mental illnesses. If people were able to cope with their symptoms, develop effective social support networks, and work, shouldn't they also be able to enroll in postsecondary academic and training programs?

Some of the initial efforts to support people with psychiatric disabilities in their pursuit of educational goals were not necessarily focused on postsecondary education. In the early 1980s, clubhouse model programs such as Fountain House in New York City and Thresholds in Chicago began offering classes and tutoring aimed at helping members obtain their high school equivalency certificate or pursue personal enrichment through subjects such as creative writing (Dougherty et al., 1992; Engelstein, Horowitz, & Romano, 2002; Kerouac & McCoy, 2002).

Also during the 1980s, many providers began to notice a shift in the demographics and characteristics of people receiving community-based services (Unger, 1998). In the early years of deinstitutionalization, many of the people being discharged were middle-aged and older adults who had spent a substantial portion of their lives in psychiatric hospitals. Due to this experience, many of them were passive and dependent and seemed to readily accept a marginalized existence, living in supervised group homes or boarding houses and spending their days in highly structured day treatment programs or sheltered workshops. Many providers serving this population were somewhat unprepared to deal with the younger cohort of consumers that followed. This new population between the ages of 18 and 35 had spent much less time in the hospital. Frustrated service providers, who viewed them as resistant and hard to work with, labeled them "young adult chronics" (Pepper, Ryglewicz, & Kirshner, 1981). These individuals tended to be dissatisfied with traditional services and did not want to spend their lives in stigmatizing treatment programs with older members who seemed to represent a bleak future. Instead they wanted to live, learn, work, and socialize in the same places as their healthy peers (Unger, 1998). They hoped for the brighter futures that postsecondary education and training promised, but in order to achieve their goals, they needed supports and services that most mental health systems did not yet provide (Anthony, 1993a; Unger, 1993).

To address the needs of this younger population, programs were developed to teach them the social, vocational, and independent living skills needed to function successfully in normalized community environments. Some of the more innovative programs were offered in nonstigmatizing settings such as an adult education center program at a high school or on a community college campus. The idea was that these settings would be more attractive to young people than mental health settings and would offer them opportunities to interact with the community at large. These programs were the precursor of today's SEd programs (Unger, 1998).

The Continuing Education Program, operated by the Boston University (BU) Center for Psychiatric Rehabilitation during the early 1980s, is probably the best-known example of these early educational programs. Students attended classes on the BU campus, a location that helped them develop a positive self-image. Students were assisted in identifying short- and long-term educational and vocational goals, and then learned the skills they would need to achieve these goals. They were also encouraged to utilize resources at BU such as the student center and athletic facilities. The program ran several hours per day over four semesters. Graduates had the opportunity to receive ongoing support from the staff of the BU center as they pursued educational and vocational goals (Sullivan-Soydan, 2004; Unger, 1998).

By the early 1990s, the emerging recovery vision (see Chapter 4) encouraged both consumers and providers to expand their notions of what was possible to achieve. Enlightened rehabilitation professionals no longer dissuaded people from pursuing ambitious goals and dreams. These new ideas were the catalyst for the development of new services that addressed the skills, supports, and resources needed by persons who wanted to pursue postsecondary educational goals (Anthony, 1993b; Sullivan-Soydan, 2002). Programs such as Threshold's Community Scholars Programs (Kerouac, 1997; Kerouac & McCoy, 2002) and the Michigan Supported Education Project (Carey, Duff, & Robertson-Kean, 2002; Collins, Bybee, & Mowbray, 1998; Mowbray, 1999; Mowbray, Collins, & Bybee, 1999) served as models for the development of SEd programs in many areas of the United States.

The Federal Response

It is also important to note that the advent of SEd programs beginning in the late 1980s was encouraged in part by the adoption of several federal laws intended to eliminate discrimination in educational settings against people with disabilities and mandate the development of services to help them succeed in school. Four landmark pieces of legislation were passed between the early 1970s and 1990:

1. Section 504 of the Rehabilitation Act of 1973 mandated that people with disabilities have equal access to institutions such as colleges and universities that receive federal funding.
2. The Carl Perkins Vocational Education Act of 1984 provided funding for the establishment of offices on college campuses that provide special services for students with disabilities (Brown, 2002). For example, the staff of a disability services office might assist students in obtaining reasonable accommodations from their professors.
3. The Individuals with Disabilities Education Act (IDEA) of 1990, which was reauthorized in 1997 and again in 2004, mandated that children with disabilities receive a free, appropriate public education designed to meet their unique needs and prepare them for employment and independent living. This includes the provision of transition services, which continue until the age of 21, and for some students includes assistance with the move from high school to a postsecondary education or training setting. While children with developmental disabilities most commonly have access to transition services, children and teenagers who have psychiatric disorders should also receive transition services to help them to maximize their chances for success in college and beyond.
4. The Americans with Disabilities Act (ADA) of 1990 both expanded the scope and clarified the intent of Section 504 of the Rehabilitation Act. According to Unger (1998), the intent of both Section 504 and the ADA was to make it illegal to deny admission to college programs and services to students with disabilities if they are otherwise qualified. The laws aimed to include people with psychiatric disabilities with other groups of individuals with disabilities (p. 61).

To summarize, the legislation described in the preceding list intends to ensure that all schools have nondiscriminatory admission polices and provide services, supports, and accommodations for students with disabilities. It is also important to note that the laws described here would not exist without the relentless advocacy efforts of people with disabilities. One such advocate was Ed Roberts who was motivated by his strong desire to attend college despite a severe physical disability; he pushed for the development of the very first program to support students with disabilities at the University of California at Berkeley in 1970. He went on to become a leader in the disability rights movement and fought for legislation such as the ADA until his death in 1995 (Independent Life USA, 2004).

Definition and Models of Supported Education

Borrowing from the definition of Supported Employment found in the 1992 Rehabilitation Act (see Chapter 9), Unger (1990) defines SEd as:

> Education in integrated settings for people with severe psychiatric disabilities for whom postsecondary education has not traditionally occurred or for people for whom postsecondary education has been interrupted or intermittent as a result of a severe psychiatric disability and who, because of their handicap, need ongoing support services to be successful in the educational environment. (p. 10)

SEd has taken many forms. Some programs are located on collage campuses; others are based in psychiatric rehabilitation programs or community mental health centers. Some models emphasize peer support groups or classes specifically for people with disabilities, while other models focus on quickly integrating students into campus life with an emphasis on natural supports. Some provide time-limited services, whereas others offer long-term supports. In 1990, Unger identified three distinct models of supported education, which are discussed in the following section:

1. The self-contained classroom
2. The on-site support model
3. The mobile support model.

Unger's Three Models of Supported Education

In the *self-contained classroom model*, classes of students, all of whom have a psychiatric disability, take a prescribed curriculum. The Boston University Continuing Education Program mentioned earlier is one example of this model. Another example of this model is Thresholds' Community Scholar's Program (CSP). Thresholds, located in Chicago, is a comprehensive psychiatric rehabilitation agency that began as one of the early clubhouse programs (for more on clubhouses, see Chapter 6). CSP offers a number of college preparatory classes at the clubhouse, for example, a class on study skills and another on research and writing skills. One-on-one educational counseling and tutoring are available and the use of peer (fellow consumers) tutors is encouraged. Members currently enrolled in a postsecondary school can attend a weekly school support group and some may receive tuition scholarships from Thresholds. CSP also provides training to college faculty in the Chicago area to help them work more effectively with students who have psychiatric disabilities (Kerouac & McCoy, 2002). While the self-contained classroom is the least integrated model of SEd, this approach is thought to provide an essential "confidence-building" step for individuals who do not feel ready to attend regular college classes.

The *on-site support model* assists students on a college campus and helps them to access resources that already exist within the college community. For example, the supported education staff may work to make regular campus resources such as Disabled Student Services or Student Counseling Services more relevant and accessible for students with psychiatric disabilities (Mowbray et al., 1993; Unger, 1990). A variety of supports and services can be provided on campus such as individual educational counseling, negotiating reasonable accommodations with a professor, and referrals to an academic tutor or a mental health agency. Another important service provided by campus-based SEd staff is assistance in documenting a disability so that a student becomes eligible to receive supports and accommodations. Note that in order to receive academic accommodations, students only need to disclose their disability to someone in the school's Disabled Student Services office. Professors and other college personnel may need to be aware that the student has a disability, and thus needs accommodations, but they do not need to be given details such as a specific diagnosis (Chmielewski, 2002).

The *mobile support model* provides individualized SEd services. In this model, SEd staff members, sometimes called *mobile education support workers* (Cook et al., 1993), provide support on campus and/or off campus as needed by the student (Cook, Yamaguchi, & Solomon, 1993; Mowbray et al., 1993; Unger, 1990). Laurel House, which is a clubhouse program in Stamford, Connecticut, has a SEd program that illustrates this model. At Laurel House, the supported education program (SEP) was conceived of as analogous to their transitional and supported employment programs. If members want to pursue education, the clubhouse will do everything it can to help them build confidence and overcome barriers. The main focus of the SEP is the coordination of the community-based and campus-based services that an individual student needs. The SEP also supplements these services when required, for example, providing individualized help with homework. In addition, existing clubhouse resources such as computers are available to members receiving SEP services (Dougherty, 2002).

While much of the SEd literature of the last 10 to 15 years reflects Unger's classification system, in practice, many programs modify or combine features of these models to form eclectic programs. Some of the SEd programs developed during the 1990s did not clearly fit any of the three models described by Unger. For example, the Michigan Supported Education Program, a federally funded demonstration project, piloted several approaches to providing supported education services. They labeled one of their most promising approaches the *group model*. Individuals assigned to this approach met in groups that were located on a college campus. Two support staff facilitated each group, one of which was a consumer-provider. Group members were empowered to create their own agenda and explore their academic and career goals via self-directed study projects. (Carey et al., 2002).

Other Models of Supported Education

Mowbray et al. (2003b) offer an updated classification system based on their survey of more than 100 supported education programs in the United States. The new classification system includes four models of supported education:

1. Full clubhouse model
2. Partial clubhouse model
3. On-site model
4. Freestanding model.

Many of today's SEd programs are located in psychiatric rehabilitation centers that define themselves as clubhouses. In fact, the majority (66%) of the SEd programs surveyed by Mowbray et al. (2003b) were located in clubhouses. To meet the criteria for the *full clubhouse model*, the program must have an educational unit in the clubhouse, commit at least half of a staff member's time to supporting members in their efforts to achieve postsecondary educational goals, and offer individual educational counseling. In addition, at least two other SEd services must be provided such as tutoring, scholarships, peer support, academic skill refresher classes, and liaisons with the faculty and staff of local colleges. Programs that have an educational unit in the clubhouse and also provide SEd services outside the facility, such as mobile support on a college campus, also meet the criteria for the full clubhouse model (Mowbray et al., 2003b).

The term *partial clubhouse model* refers to clubhouse-based SEd programs that assist members in pursuing postsecondary educational goals but do not meet all of the criteria for the full clubhouse model (Mowbray et al., 2003b). Such a program may have a staff member who spends about one full day a week providing educational counseling and coordinating a peer-run tutoring program. College catalogs and computer resources might also be available in the clubhouse to assist members who are thinking about enrolling in college.

The *on-site model*, which was also identified in the earlier classification system articulated by Unger, refers to supported education programs that are located on a college campus. Sometimes a program will have offices at several schools in a community. This type of SEd program may be located within a college counseling center, or in a disability services office, or may have its own space on campus. If the program shares an office that provides other student services, it should have at least one staff member who specializes in working with people who have psychiatric disabilities and it should provide at least one service that is specifically geared toward students with psychiatric disabilities, for example, a weekly support group (Mowbray et al., 2003b).

Supported education programs that utilize the *freestanding model* offer a variety of services at more than one location. A freestanding SEd program might be affiliated with a large psychiatric rehabilitation agency that provides comprehensive services, or it might be part of a vocational rehabilitation agency that offers both employment and educational services. Many freestanding programs are also affiliated with one or more colleges, or at least have the capacity to provide mobile support services to students on a variety of campuses. Mowbray and her colleagues noted that their survey of SEd programs revealed that a relatively small group of programs follow the freestanding model. This may be the most innovative and comprehensive of the SEd models, but unfortunately it may also be the most expensive to implement.

Freestanding programs offer an eclectic mix of services. For example, at a program's main office service recipients might have access to individual educational counseling, study skill seminars, and a weekly peer support group. Groups designed to help people determine their readiness to return to school might also be offered at several psychiatric rehabilitation programs in the community. In addition, individualized SEd services would be provided on one or more college campuses by program staff that had well-established relationships with key members of the college faculty and staff (e.g., staff in the disability services office). Program staff might also provide seminars to college faculty and staff designed to reduce stigmatizing attitudes and help faculty learn about reasonable accommodations that might be needed by students with psychiatric disabilities.

The Michigan Supported Education Program (MSEP) is an excellent example of the freestanding model. As mentioned earlier in the chapter, it began as a research demonstration project that piloted several innovative SEd approaches such as the group model. The current MSEP combines the best features of these SEd models, and offers individuals with educational goals a variety of services including a structured support group that is co-facilitated by a consumer-provider, an academic support curriculum that helps students hone their study skills, individualized one-on-one support services that last as long as a student needs them, and a resource/tutorial center (Carey et al., 2002).

A Choose-Get-Keep Framework

The Choose-Get-Keep approach described in Chapter 9 is also utilized when providing supported education services (Russell & Strauss, 2004; Sullivan, Nicolellis, Danley, & MacDonald-Wilson, 1993; Sullivan-Soydan, 2004). This approach can be thought of as a framework for conceptualizing the stages a person goes through when pursuing educational goals. During this process, people with a psychiatric disability need to access relevant information in order to make an informed choice about going to school. Then they need to develop or refresh the skills and secure the supports necessary to be admitted to school and maintain enrollment. This framework for providing services can be applied within any of the supported education models described earlier.

A psychiatric rehabilitation provider who works in a SEd program may also be thought of as an education coach, in that his or her approach is very similar to that of a job coach in a supported employment program. During the *choose phase* of the SEd process, a person works with his or her education coach deciding what type of academic or trade school program he or she wants to pursue. Visiting schools, looking at catalogs, and conducting informational interviews with students and/or professors are examples of some useful activities during this phase.

During the *get phase* the education coach assists an individual in locating and applying to a specific school. It might also be the time to assist the person in applying for financial aid or perhaps accessing a tuition stipend through their state's office of vocational rehabilitation services.

The *keep phase* focuses on the skills and resource development necessary to help the person succeed in school. Skills that may need to be developed include time and task management, maintaining concentration, taking notes, writing papers, and asking for assistance (Murphy et al., 2005). To address resource development, a visit to the school's office for students with disabilities is often a good idea. As mentioned earlier, federal law ensures access to a variety of reasonable accommodations, also known as academic adjustments, in the classroom. However, students may need assistance in determining which accommodations are most useful in each individual situation. Some examples include note-takers, modified testing environments, books on tape, and use of assistive technologies, such as computer programs that help students with learning disabilities compose papers (Murphy et al., 2005).

As in supported employment, it is also important to help students with disabilities gain access to *natural supports* during the keep phase of supported education. Examples of these include use of existing resources on campus (tutors, study skills seminars), and establishing relationships with classmates for emotional support, friendship, note sharing, and study groups. Some SEd programs also help facilitate ongoing peer support groups so that students with disabilities who have educational goals, as well as those who are currently enrolled in classes, can provide each other with support, encouragement, and relevant information.

Jose's Story

The experiences of a person receiving services from a SEd program are described next. When reading about Jose's experiences, think about the following questions:

1. What events led to the first episode of Jose's illness?
2. Why did his early experiences at college make it so difficult for him to return to school?
3. What features of the SEd program described were most helpful to Jose?

Jose is a 36-year-old man who has struggled with bipolar disorder for more than 10 years. After graduating from high school, Jose got a job selling office supplies and attended a community college at night. He obtained a certificate in computer programming that helped him to get a better job at a computer software company. After a few years in this job, Jose realized that if he wanted to move up the career ladder he would need more education. He decided to pursue a bachelor's degree in computer science. Jose found the ordeal of dealing with admissions, registering for classes, and securing financial aid to be frustrating and annoying but no more so than the other students did. However, attending classes at night after working all day was very difficult. Jose had trouble falling asleep at night, which meant he was tired the next day. He found himself making mistakes at work and he started to feel extremely anxious. He was not aware that these were "prodromal" signs of serious mental illness (see Chapters 2 and 3). Soon it became almost impossible to concentrate on what his teachers were saying in class. Jose began to think he wasn't smart enough to go to college and that he'd be stuck in his dead end job forever.

One night after class when he knew he wasn't going to be able to fall asleep, Jose decided to go to the library to study. But it was after eleven o'clock and the library was closed. Jose was so frustrated that he started pounding on the library door. He pounded harder and harder until his fist broke through the glass. The alarm brought the police who found Jose lying on the ground bleeding and sobbing uncontrollably. Jose was admitted to the psychiatric hospital where he stayed for a month. He lost his job and dropped out of school. During the next 10 years he held several jobs, and made three unsuccessful attempts to return to school, each of which was closely followed by a hospitalization.

Three years ago, after his most recent hospitalization, Jose was referred to a supported housing program where he met Luke, a case manager. After getting to know Luke, Jose began to talk about his dream of finishing college and having a good job with a future. To Jose's surprise Luke didn't laugh or point out all of Jose's failed attempts as so many others had. Instead Luke talked to Jose about a supported education program, North Shore Scholars, based on the freestanding model of SEd. Luke explained that the SEd program had education specialists who helped people deal with the stresses of school and helped to get accommodations if they were needed. Jose was interested but a little apprehensive. He doubted that any school would even accept him after failing so many times and he just couldn't forget that every attempt at school had ended with a stay in the hospital. Luke understood Jose's ambivalence and suggested that he talk to the program's education specialist, and possibly attend a four-session readiness group for people who are considering school but are not sure. Jose agreed to give it a try.

At the first group meeting Jose met Beth, a supported education specialist, and five other people who were thinking about going back to school. Group members spoke openly about their fears and concerns. Over the 4 weeks, Jose talked about his past failures, his difficulty concentrating, and the overwhelming anxiety he feels when he has to write a paper or take a test. He could really relate to some of the things the other group members described, like the young woman in the group who said, "I'm afraid that the other students will find out that I have a mental illness and will look at me like I'm a scary freak." Beth told the group members about some possible accommodations in the classroom for students who have psychiatric disabilities and described tutoring and study skill seminars that are available to all community college students. She also reassured members that if they chose to disclose to the college disabilities office that they have a mental illness (in order to receive accommodations), the nature of their disability would be kept confidential and would not be shared with faculty members or other college personnel.

During the last group session, a man who had been receiving services from the North Shore Scholars for about 2 years spoke to the group. He told the members about the challenges he had faced returning to school and how supported education services had helped him achieve success. Afterward, Jose approached Beth and said, "I'm still not sure that I'm ready, but I'm going to give it a try. Can you help me get registered for the fall semester?" Beth seemed pleased and Jose felt hopeful for the first time in a long time. Beth helped Jose prepare for an appointment with an admissions counselor at Middlefield Community College. She also helped him complete his financial aid forms and together they figured out how Jose would cover the tuition, books, and associated fees.

Jose was admitted to the school and assigned a regular advisor, but he checked in with Beth to get her perspective before registering for two computer science courses. Beth suggested that he consider taking one computer science course to begin with and a pass/fail course called "Reentry Seminar" that is offered to all beginning students over the age of 25. The seminar course focused on study skills and time management, and also helped students become familiar with college resources such as the library and computer lab. Beth told him that it was also a good place to meet other students his age who were probably also anxious about returning to school. Jose decided to follow Beth's advice.

Once the semester began, he met with Beth once a week to talk about his progress and he sometimes checked in with her by phone as well, for example, on the day before an exam. Beth helped Jose think of some specific ways to apply the study skills and time management skills he was learning about in the Reentry Seminar. Jose also found it helpful to talk with Beth when he felt anxious about things like upcoming assignments or approaching his computer science professor who intimidated him. When he decided he wanted to ask for an accommodation for his computer science class, she helped him get registered at the Office of Disabled Students Services. She explained that his professor would receive written notice that Jose required an alternate testing site for his exams, but that Jose might need to talk to the professor about the logistics. Beth offered to accompany him to meet with his professor, but Jose decided that he would do it himself. To prepare, they role-played the meeting and this helped reduce Jose's anxiety.

While studying for his final exam, Jose told Beth that he thought he was experiencing some early signs of a manic episode. Beth enlisted Luke's help in getting an emergency appointment for Jose with his psychiatrist. The doctor prescribed a slight increase in one of Jose's medications, which was enough to get him through the last few weeks of the semester. Jose got a C on the final exam and a B in the course. He had a very positive experience in the Reentry Seminar and befriended two students in the class with whom he started to socialize outside of school. When Jose received his grade report in the mail, he was flooded with a mixture of feelings. He was certainly relieved and proud of his accomplishment, grateful to Beth for her support, but also a little apprehensive about what his parents' reaction would be. For once he had tried and not failed, but it was a far cry from their expectations of him so many years ago. A few days after Christmas, Jose called Beth to tell her that he showed his grade report to his parents on Christmas day. He told her, "My parents were so proud of me! My father hugged me and looked at me the way he used to before I got sick. It felt so good!"

Applying Psychiatric Rehabilitation Principles to Supported Education

There are some key values and principles that should be inherent in all SEd programs. Note that these SEd principles correspond to the values and principles of PsyR outlined in Chapter 4:

- *Self-determination*: The educational goals, learning environments, and supports are selected by the student (Sullivan et al., 1993; Unger, 1990).
- *Individualization*: The supports and services provided are designed to meet the unique needs of each student (Sullivan ct al., 1993; Unger, 1990).
- *Normalization*: The services are integrated and "consistent with the routines of the setting" (Unger, 1990; pg.13). Attention is given to achieving a good match between the student and the setting (Sullivan et al., 1993), for example, providing SEd services at a campus-based Office of Disabled Students rather than at a mental health center.
- *Ongoing support*: Support is available indefinitely and is flexible to match the changing needs of the student (Unger, 1990).
- *Dignity*: Supports and services are provided in a manner that protects the privacy and dignity of the individual (Unger, 1990).
- *Hope*: There is obvious belief in the capability of the individual to grow and achieve academic and vocational goals (Unger, 1990).

More recently, Mowbray (2004b) expanded on these principles and developed specific criteria for implementing them in supported education programs. Her work in this area is summarized in Table 10.1.

TABLE 10.1
PsyR Principles Relevant to Supported Education and Associated Criteria

PsyR Principle	Criteria for Supported Education
1. Normalization	1-1: Supported education programs conduct comprehensive, individualized assessments of participants (including academic needs and skills, personal goals and preferences, recovery/wellness plans) and help students establish vocational/career objectives.
	1-2: SEd programs utilize a campus setting for at least some of the services provided.
	1-3: SEd services are provided in a manner and in an environment that protects privacy, enhances personal dignity, and respects cultural diversity.
	1-4: SEd services are evaluated on an ongoing basis so they can be revised, as needed, to keep them responsive to students' needs.
2. Self-determination	2-1: SEd programs provide knowledge of the postsecondary educational environment (demands and resources), and skills training and practice to survive in postsecondary education, including brushing up or acquiring needed academic skills, or coping and adaptation methods (e.g., how to access available resources).
	2-2: SEd programs assist students to use their knowledge and skills to set their own educational goals and objectives.
	2-3: In SEd programs, choice is fundamental. Choices are offered in terms of teaching strategies and learning topics, the amount and type of support provided, how services are provided (in terms of modality: group, individual, face to face, mail, phone, etc.), frequency, and intensity. Students can make choices about service provision, based on individual needs and preferences.
3. Support and relationships	3-1: SEd programs invest staff resources in outreach to and engagement of potential program participants; making presentations and/or having an ongoing presence at settings in which these individuals are likely to hear the message, such as self-help groups, consumer-operated programs, and clubhouses.
	3-2: SEd services have continuing availability; they can be accessed on an as-needed basis for as long as students want or need them.
	3-3: SEd staff establish individualized and personal relationships with students. One-on-one educational counseling is available, as needed.
	3-4: Students are encouraged, given skills or assistance in establishing their own support networks to continue beyond the SEd program.
	3-5: Resources are available, as needed, to assist with overcoming individual barriers to educational involvement, e.g., needs for transportation or child care expenses, scholarship and loan information, resolving prior educational debt, or applying to loan forgiveness/repayment programs.
4. Hope and recovery	4-1: The SEd program philosophy and service delivery methods emphasize participant strengths, encourage possibilities, foster hope, and promote rehabilitation.
	4-2: Exclusion based on participant diagnoses or mental health history is not appropriate because it contradicts SEd values and principles. However, inclusion criteria may specify needed basic academic skill and survival levels.

TABLE 10.1
Continued

PsyR Principle	Criteria for Supported Education
	4-3: SEd programs have a rehabilitation and recovery philosophy, rather than focusing on mental health treatment or clinical services.
	4-4: SEd programs involve students in all aspects of operations, including paid staff positions, so that role modeling and examples of success are available.
	4-5: SEd programs facilitate participants transforming their perceived identity from the stigmatized role of psychiatric patient to the valued and culturally acceptable role of college student.
5. Systems change	5-1: SEd programs incorporate *personal empowerment* strategies, such as promoting and teaching self-advocacy, providing shared access to valued resources, and promoting nonhierarchical thinking and open communication.
	5-2: SEd programs promote and model *group empowerment,* whereby the group advocates on behalf of the generic needs of its members.
	5-3: SEd programs cultivate and maintain stakeholder involvement and incorporate stakeholder perspectives, needs, and demands into their programming. Resources of an educational setting and the community are brought together to work for the benefit of the students.
	5-4: SEd programs have a structure and mechanisms to address systemic barriers to full inclusion of students with psychiatric disabilities. These should include formal involvement with mental health agencies and with higher education institutions.

Source: From Mowbray, C. T. (2004). Supported education: Diversity, critical ingredients and future directions. *American Journal of Psychiatric Rehabilitation, 7*(3), 355–356.

Research on Supported Education

Several studies have examined SEd outcomes and described the characteristics and experiences of college students with severe mental illnesses. Mowbray and Collins (2002) reviewed all of the published studies of supported education programs between 1991 and 1998. They found that the studies varied in methodology, some being descriptive and some using quasi-experimental designs. Only one study met the criteria for a true experimental design. The outcomes evaluated included educational attainment, employment, consumer self-perception, and consumer satisfaction.

In terms of educational attainment, most studies reported modest success in terms of enrollment in one or more college or vocational school courses. It is important to note that only a few of the studies reviewed reported on long-term outcomes, so very little is known about how effective supported education programs are in terms of helping participants complete academic degrees.

A study of the Michigan Supported Education Program, which is the only randomized controlled trial study in the SEd literature, found that 12 months after completion of a structured on-campus group support program, 24% of the service recipients were enrolled in postsecondary academic programs compared with 9% of participants who were enrolled

CONTROVERSIAL ISSUE
Do Some SEd Models Adhere to PsyR Values and Principles More Than Others?

Collectively, supported employment, supported housing, and supported education have been referred to as supported approaches or community-integrated services. They share a common philosophy and strongly emphasize normalization and full inclusion in the community. Full inclusion means that people with disabilities should have the same opportunities to live, learn, and work in their communities as people without disabilities. The role of community-integrated service providers is to ensure that individualized supports are available to people with disabilities in the environments where they are living, learning, and working.

Viewpoint 1:

> The self-contained classroom provides a supportive environment that helps students with psychiatric disabilities build self-esteem and develop academic skills.

Many of the supported education programs described in the literature emphasize using the self-contained classroom where students diagnosed with severe mental illnesses spend one or more semesters together attending noncredit classes either at a psychiatric rehabilitation program or on a college campus (Hain & Gioia, 2004; Gilbert, Heximer, Jaxon, & Bellamy, 2004; Unger, 1998; Weiss, Maddox, Vanderwaerden, & Szilvagyi, 2004). These classes typically focus on academic skill development and development of career goals. They operate on the premise that many people with psychiatric disabilities interested in returning to college are hesitant to enroll because they fear there are too many barriers to overcome. For example, they believe that psychiatric symptoms such as poor concentration will get in the way, or they are wary of encountering college faculty and students with stigmatizing attitudes.

For these individuals, the self-contained classroom provides a supportive environment where people can gradually develop academic skills and get used to the role of student while still having daily access to professionals who can assist in coping with stress, symptoms, and other concerns.

Although many self-contained classroom programs are located in normalized settings, such as community college campuses, participants in these programs spend most of their time with other "students" who have a mental illness and "teachers" who are trained mental health professionals. To summarize, these programs provide education, skills training, and group support to people with disabilities in a segregated classroom. The goal of the classes, which program members typically take over a period of months or even years, is to prepare people to enroll in regular college classes or pursue other rehabilitation goals such as employment.

Viewpoint 2:

> Supported education interventions should focus on rapid enrollment in normalized postsecondary college classes.

Although little research has been done comparing the efficacy of the various supported education models, it is possible that, similar to prevocational programs, long periods of preparation in precollege programs may inhibit successful transition into integrated educational settings. Programs in the various modalities that emphasize what has been called a "train and place" approach, such as prevocational psychiatric day treatment programs and transitional group homes, spend lots of time and effort preparing people to move on to independent jobs and apartments that never seem to materialize. In contrast, programs emphasizing a "place and train" approach start by rapidly mainstreaming people into integrated employment or housing settings, and then providing any needed skills training or supports in the place where the person is actually living or working. This strategy helps people to quickly begin working or living independently while accessing the supports needed to be successful. (See Chapters 9 and 11 for a thorough review of literature on this topic.)

A SEd program resembling best practice in supported employment or supported housing would emphasize individualized educational counseling. In such a program, an educational specialist would begin by helping individuals clarify their educational goals and then assist them in enrolling in the school of their choice. Needed supports are then provided where and when a person requires them to maximize academic success.

when the study began (Mowbray et al., 1999, in Mowbray & Collins, 2002). Cook and Solomon (1993) reported on 43 members of the Community Scholars Program based at Thresholds, a full clubhouse model program that was described earlier in the models section. Among the community scholars, 42% entered a postsecondary educational institution and 14% received an academic certificate or degree. Other positive outcomes found in the studies reviewed by Mowbray and Collins (2002) included increases in competitive employment, number of hours worked, and average hourly wages. Improvements in consumer self-esteem, self-efficacy, and empowerment were also reported.

To learn more about the characteristics and experiences of current college students who have a psychiatric disorder, Megivern (2001) conducted a series of studies involving approximately 300 college students with an average age of 19. About 200 of them had a serious mental illness with an average age of onset of 13. Megivern found that first-time college students with severe mental illnesses are capable of academic performance equivalent to that of students without mental illnesses, but they face significantly more challenges academically and socially than their peers. This is especially true if they are not receiving mental health services. Generally speaking, students were found to be motivated to seek mental health services to help them achieve their educational goals. Unfortunately, these services were not always readily accessible to students, leading the author to recommend closer links between higher education and community mental health.

Megivern (2001) also found that student interest or investment in academic activities or goals was positively related to higher grades, the quality of the student's interactions with faculty, and the quality of interactions with other students. However, the degree of psychiatric symptomatology experienced interfered with interactions with both faculty and students. Looking at a combination of factors, Megivern also found that academic and social integration were predicted by both grades and severity of symptoms. Students with higher GPAs and less severe symptoms were better integrated academically and socially. In addition, women were slightly better integrated than men.

In a study done to determine what variables are predictive of productive activity among SEd program participants, Collins, Mowbray, and Bybee (2000) studied 147 people enrolled in a freestanding SED model program. Productive activity was defined as involvement in vocational or college education (outside the basic SEd program) or employment. Not surprisingly, the best predictor of productive activity at 1-year follow-up was productive activity at baseline. Those who required more encouragement to pursue educational goals were *less* likely to be productive. In addition, individuals who were never married, as opposed to those currently married, divorced, widowed, or cohabiting, were less likely to be engaged in productive activity at follow-up. Better financial adjustment, perhaps as a consequence of a better work history, was also associated with productive activity. An interesting finding was that individuals who had more difficulty keeping up with housework were *more* productive, perhaps because they were too busy at work and school to do housework.

Shearman et al. (2002) did a number of surveys of consumers, mental health center staff, and postsecondary school staff in Indiana. In one survey, 159 people interested in pursuing education or training reported that the types of assistance they most needed included tutoring, academic counseling, and help with goal setting and college and financial aid applications. Only 12% of these individuals said they were actually receiving this assistance, and most of the time they said it came from a case manager or family member. In terms of the barriers they perceived, the most commonly mentioned were lack of transportation and lack of financial resources. Other common barriers were negotiating application processes, stigma or stereotyping, and defaulting on a previous loan. Least frequently mentioned were symptoms of mental illness and side effects of medication. Mental health center staff identified a similar profile for barriers perceived, with one significant exception: They mentioned symptoms or side effects more frequently than consumers. School personnel also emphasized symptoms and side effects as barriers.

A somewhat different picture emerged in a qualitative study that examined the experiences of 35 individuals with psychiatric disabilities who had attended college. The subjects mentioned psychiatric symptoms as the most common reason for leaving school. Lack of academic integration, financial problems, and family obligation were also frequently cited as barriers to completing their education (Megivern et al., 2003).

Supported Education: An Emerging Evidence-Based Practice?

The number of research studies examining the outcomes of specific supported education models is relatively limited. Nevertheless, the Center for Mental Health Services at the U.S. Substance Abuse and Mental Health Administration (CMHS/SAMSHA) has already endorsed supported education as an exemplary service (Mowbray, Bellamy, Megivern, & Szilvagyi, 2001; Mowbray & Collins, 2002). Moving a service approach from an "exemplary" or promising practice to one that meets the criteria for being evidence based can be a long journey. Carol Mowbray, who was a researcher at the University of Michigan School of Social Work and who is profiled in this chapter (see Box 10.1), undertook a first step in this process.

To demonstrate that a PsyR service consistently produces positive outcomes for consumers, researchers must first identify a set of essential ingredients that describe the model. These ingredients are known as *fidelity criteria* (Mowbray, Holter, Teague, & Bybee, 2003a). Establishing fidelity criteria for SEd is a particularly challenging task because a number of diverse models have been identified in the literature as being effective examples of SEd. To address the challenge, Mowbray based her SEd criteria on principles of psychiatric rehabilitation that should be present regardless of a program's approach to providing services. So, for example, based on the PsyR principle of self-determination, she identified one SEd criteria as "SEd programs assist students to use their knowledge and skills to set their own educational goals and objectives." Addressing PsyR's emphasis on hope and recovery, she arrived at the SEd criteria "SEd programs have a rehabilitation and recovery philosophy, rather than focusing on mental health treatment or clinical services." The complete set of SEd criteria developed by Mowbray was presented earlier in Table 10.1.

> Of course, there is still much work to be done from this initial starting point, including determining how to operationalize SEd fidelity criteria. Dr. Mowbray (2004b) urged researchers to conduct effectiveness studies to find out "What works for whom, under what circumstances, and in which settings (p. 360)?" This work has to be carried out in the form of controlled clinical trials conducted by different researchers at different sites. And that will be just the start. Will SEd eventually become an evidence-based practice? Much work remains to be done to determine the answer.

Dissemination of Supported Education

Despite the importance that education plays in helping people with psychiatric disabilities realize their hopes and dreams and the promise that SEd programs provide for helping people achieve their career goals, dissemination of SEd programs remains fairly limited. In 2001, Mowbray, Bellamy, Megivern, and Szilvagi found there were fewer than 30 SEd programs in North America. The majority of these programs were in just six states. A few years later a national survey with broader acceptance criteria identified more than 100 SEd programs (Mowbray et al., 2003b). Nearly two-thirds of these programs were located in clubhouses (described in Chapter 6). Although this number is more encouraging than what has been previously reported in the literature, it is clear that we have a long way to go before most people with psychiatric disabilities have ready access to educational supports. It is disappointing that such a promising model, which has been in existence for more than 20 years, is still a novelty in many parts of the United States.

Lack of funding has been a key barrier to SEd dissemination. Federal and state legislation ensures that some funding is available to provide mental health and vocational rehabilitation services, but there are no external mandates to promote the development of SEd services (Mowbray et al., 1993). In fact, historically, neither the vocational rehabilitation nor mental health systems have recognized educational attainment as an important outcome for people with psychiatric disabilities (Anthony, Furlong-Norman & Koehler, 2002; Mowbray, Verdejo, & Levine, 2002; Unger, 1994). Too many programs that provide employment services have not fully embraced the recovery movement. They tend to steer consumers toward low-skill jobs, with little opportunity to move up a career ladder. These programs and staff members do not recognize the potential that people have to pursue career goals that require higher education. Clearly attitudes and priorities need to change for widespread dissemination of SEd programs to occur.

Future Directions in Supported Education

Supported education is an important component of PsyR services that is still not readily available to people with psychiatric disabilities in many parts of the United States. To

BOX 10.1
Carol Mowbray

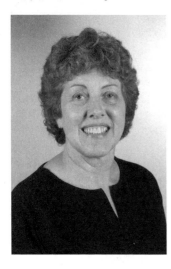

Carol Mowbray's career was devoted to reducing stigma and removing barriers to full community integration. Dr. Mowbray, who had a Ph.D. in developmental psychology from the University of Michigan, was one of the most highly respected researchers in the field of psychiatric rehabilitation. She began her career as a research analyst for the Michigan Department of Mental Health and eventually moved into an administrative position. Mid-career, she shifted into academia as an associate professor of social work at Wayne State University, and later as professor at the University of Michigan.

She also directed the Center for Research on Poverty, Risk, and Mental Health at the University of Michigan, School of Social Work.

An ongoing theme in all of Dr. Mowbray's studies is the involvement of people with psychiatric disabilities in their own recovery. She did research on a number of important issues such as women's mental health and consumer provided services, but is probably best known in the United States and abroad for her work on supported education for persons with psychiatric disabilities. She conducted the first evaluation of a supported education program using a randomized controlled trial, which led to the funding of the Michigan Supported Education Program and other model SEd programs in Michigan. Dr. Mowbray and her colleagues also hosted the first National Conference on Supported Education in 2002. She received much recognition for her efforts, including the prestigious Armin Loeb award given annually by U.S. Psychiatric Rehabilitation Association (USPRA, formerly known as IAPSRS) to an individual who has done significant research in the field of psychiatric rehabilitation.

Dr. Mowbray's prolific research, writing, and consultation efforts helped to define supported education and promote its dissemination worldwide. Sadly, Carol Mowbray passed away in August 2005. Her passing was a great loss for the field of psychiatric rehabilitation. Her outstanding contributions to the body of research will serve as an inspiration for researchers and practitioners for many years to come.

address this gap in services, resources to support the continuation and expansion of current programs as well as develop new programs need to be secured. Mowbray (2004b) suggested that programs seek funding from diverse sources such as state mental health and vocation rehabilitation offices, Medicaid, and postsecondary institutions. Research that provides mental health and vocational rehabilitation system administrators with a clearer sense of which models are most successful in helping people return to school and eventually to work is also likely to increase dissemination of this important service. As opportunities to develop additional programs present themselves, the authors hope the following challenges for SEd are addressed.

Challenge 1: To Better Meet the Needs of Young Adults

Currently, most SEd programs primarily serve adults who are at least in their late 20s, and have been out of school for many years (Megivern & Pellerito, 2002; Mowbray, 2004b). Early intervention services also need to be provided to help young people in the early stages of their illness stay in school or return to school quickly. Traditional college-age students who have a mental illness are a subgroup of consumers who face unique challenges and require individualized supports. SEd programs that target this population are probably best situated on college campuses and need to be proactive in educating students, faculty, and college administrators about the early signs of mental illness and the benefits of receiving treatment and supportive services as soon as possible (Megivern & Pellerito, 2002; Mowbray, 1999, 2004b). Many treatment and rehabilitation service providers also need to be better informed about the importance of SEd services for the young adult population. Individuals who are struggling with the early stages of mental illness often do not see the relevance of day programs and clubhouses. They feel more comfortable in normalized settings for people their age, such as a college campus (Anthony & Unger, 1991).

Because mental health systems and postsecondary educational institutions both struggle with the issue of adequately serving young adults with psychiatric disabilities, the opportunity for collaboration is rich with possibilities. For example, shared staffing and a cross-referral arrangement between a PsyR program and a campus-based office for students with disabilities could both assist PsyR program members with access to educational opportunities and help college students experiencing their first episode of mental illness get adequate treatment and rehabilitation services. The important topic of early intervention is also addressed in Chapters 7 and 14.

Challenge 2: Fostering More Freestanding Supported Education Programs

Currently a large majority of SEd programs most closely resemble the clubhouse or partial clubhouse model described by Mowbray et al. (2003b). While clubhouses are certainly an important access point for consumers with educational goals, additional dissemination of the other SEd models is needed in order to reach the many people with mental illness who are not clubhouse members. As mentioned earlier, campus-based services that follow the on-site SEd model are particularly important for reaching young adults. In addition the freestanding model of SEd, which has not yet been very widely disseminated, is a very promising approach. Freestanding programs, which offer a variety of educational support services at both a number of schools in the community and at community-based mental health and PsyR programs, are flexible enough to meet the needs of people who are at different ages and stages of their illness (Mowbray et al., 2003b).

Challenge 3: Integrating the Pursuit of Educational and Career Goals

More programs should be developed that offer both supported education and supported employment services, because these approaches complement each other. Even though these service approaches have much in common, they have historically been implemented in separate programs (Egnew, 1993). Individuals who only have access to supported employment services may lack the resources to access the additional training and education needed to move out of entry-level, low-paying jobs. Programs that integrate SEd and supported employment emphasize the concept of *career development*, as opposed to just job acquisition, and are essential to the recovery of many people striving to attain meaningful and productive roles in their communities (Murphy et al., 2005). In his description of an integrated program located in California, Egnew (1993) emphasizes the importance of helping individuals articulate both short- and long-term goals that link employment with education, and points out that "the integration of supported education/employment services results in a combined education and/or work experience typically found in society at large" (p. 127).

Russell and Strauss (2004) describe such an integrated program, Career Advancement Resources (CAR), located in Boston, Massachusetts. The program, which is part of the statewide Supported Employment and Education initiative, focuses on career exploration, assistance in gaining access to necessary education and training opportunities, ongoing support to maximize success in the classroom, and a variety of support services that assist in the transition from school to work. Murphy and her colleagues (2005) propose an enhanced individual placement and support model of supported employment, in which both supported education services and use of natural supports are emphasized. They hypothesize that this combination of services would help individuals find meaningful work and would ultimately increase job tenure. Widespread dissemination of PsyR programs that emphasize career development would go a long way toward helping people with psychiatric disabilities realize the goals of recovery, true community integration, and improved quality of life.

Summary

Education is an essential step toward the achievement of career goals for most people. People with psychiatric disabilities have the same dreams as everyone else, but often have their education interrupted by their illness and face many challenges when trying to return to school. A number of historical developments, including improved understanding of the service and support needs of people with psychiatric disabilities, led to the emergence of SEd programs. Currently, several diverse approaches are used to provide SEd, although some critical ingredients that are consistent with the principles and values of PsyR provide a common basis for implementing quality programs. To ensure that SEd services are made available to all people with psychiatric disabilities who want to achieve educational goals, mental health and vocational rehabilitation systems need to recognize the critically important role that education can play in recovery. Additional research also needs to be conducted so that we have a better understanding of which models of SEd produce the best outcomes for persons who are coping with severe mental illnesses.

Class Exercise

Read the two scenarios that follow and then answer the questions given below the scenarios.

Scenario 1

Jean is a 29-year-old woman who has a diagnosis of schizophrenia. Jean completed two semesters of college prior to the onset of her illness and is now returning to school after a decade-long interruption. She is taking a single psychology course. She is very anxious about being back in school but also very enthusiastic. Jean sometimes has difficulty focusing in class due to her thought disorder. There are times when her thoughts begin to wander and she suddenly feels lost in class. Her current response is to interrupt the class when this occurs and ask the teacher questions. Sometimes this happens several times during a class. Jean is beginning to feel that the teacher and other students are annoyed with her for being disruptive.

Scenario 2

Sam is a 25-year-old man who is in his second semester at a community college. He is currently enrolled in three courses. He has done pretty well on all his midterms and written assignments so far (his grades have been B's and C's). The semester ends in 3 weeks, and Sam is beginning to experience symptoms of a major depressive episode. He is having difficulty getting out of bed to get to his morning classes, and if he does get there he has trouble concentrating. Sam's psychiatrist wants to hospitalize him to try out a new medication. Sam thinks that if this happens he will fail his classes. He is already struggling to pay for tuition and books and worries that he cannot afford to re-take the classes. Worrying about school is exacerbating Sam's symptoms.

1. Can you identify some reasonable accommodations (also known as academic adjustments) that could be provided by the professor or the disability services office that may help these students?
2. Can you identify an individualized and nonstigmatizing support strategy that an educational support specialist could provide for these students?

References

Adelman, C. (2004). *Principal indicators of student academic histories in postsecondary education, 1972–2000.* Washington, DC: U.S. Department of Education.

Anthony, W. A. (1993a). Editorial. *Psychosocial Rehabilitation Journal, 17*(1), 1.

Anthony, W. A. (1993b). Recovery form mental illness: The guiding vision of the mental health service system in the 1990s. *Psychosocial Rehabilitation Journal, 16*(4), 11–23.

Anthony, W. A., Furlong-Norman, K., & Koehler, M. (2002). Shifting paradigms in mental health service systems: Supported education within the context of rehabilitation and recovery. In C. T. Mowbray, K. S. Brown, K. Furlong-Norman, & A. Sullivan-Soydan (Eds.), *Supported education and psychiatric rehabilitation: models and methods* (pp. 287–294). Linthicum, MD: International Association of Psychosocial Rehabilitation Services.

Anthony, W. A., & Unger, K. V. (1991). Supported education: An additional program resource for young adults with long-term mental illness. *Community Mental Health Journal, 27,* 145–156.

Becker, M., Martin, L., Wajeeh, E., Ward, J., & Shern, D. (2002). Students with mental illnesses in a university setting: Faculty and student attitudes, beliefs, knowledge, and experiences. *Psychiatric Rehabilitation Journal, 25*(4), 359–368.

Brown, K. S. (2002). Antecedents of psychiatric rehabilitation: The road to supported employment programs. In C. T. Mowbray, K. S. Brown, K. Furlong-Norman, & A. Sullivan-Soydan (Eds.), *Supported education and psychiatric rehabilitation: models and methods* (pp. 13–21). Linthicum, MD: International Association of Psychosocial Rehabilitation Services.

Carey, M., Duff, S., & Robertson-Kean, L. (2002). Michigan Supported Education Program. In C. T. Mowbray, K. S. Brown, K. Furlong-Norman, & A. Sullivan-Soydan (Eds.), *Supported education and psychiatric rehabilitation: models and methods* (pp. 89–98). Linthicum, MD: International Association of Psychosocial Rehabilitation Services.

Chmielewski, M. (2002). Serving student with psychiatric disabilities through the disability support services office. In C. T. Mowbray, K. S. Brown, K. Furlong-Norman, & A. Sullivan-Soydan (Eds.), *Supported education and psychiatric rehabilitation: models and methods* (pp. 253–261). Linthicum, MD: International Association of Psychosocial Rehabilitation Services.

Cloutier, G. (1997). Going sane: One man's battle with schizoaffective disorder. *Journal of the California Alliance for the Mentally Ill, 8*(2), 65–66.

Collins, M. E., Bybee, D., & Mowbray, C. T. (1998). Effectiveness of supported education for individuals with psychiatric disabilities: Results from an experimental study. *Community Mental Health Journal, 34*(6), 595–613.

Collins, M. E., Mowbray, C. T., & Bybee, D. (2000). Characteristics predicting successful outcomes of participants with severe mental illness in supported education. *Psychiatric Services, 51*(6), 774–780.

Cook, J. A., & Solomon, M. L. (1993). The community scholar program: An outcome study of supported education for students with severe mental illness. *Psychosocial Rehabilitation Journal, 17*(1), 83–97.

Cook, J. A., Yamaguchi, J., & Solomon, M. L. (1993). Field-testing a postsecondary faculty in-service training for working with students who have psychiatric disabilities. *Psychosocial Rehabilitation Journal, 17*(1), 157–70.

Cooper, L., (1993). Serving adults with psychiatric disabilities on campus: A mobile support approach. *Psychosocial Rehabilitation Journal, 17*(1), 25–38

Dougherty, S. (2002). Supported education in a clubhouse setting. In C. T. Mowbray, K. S. Brown, K. Furlong-Norman, & A. Sullivan-Soydan (Eds.), *Supported education and psychiatric rehabilitation: models and methods* (pp. 139–145). Linthicum, MD: International Association of Psychosocial Rehabilitation Services.

Dougherty, S., Hastie, C., Bernard, J., Broadhurst, S., & Marcus, L. (1992). Supported education: A clubhouse experience. *Psychosocial Rehabilitation Journal, 16*(2), 91–104.

Dougherty, S., Kampana, K., Kontos, R., Flores, M., Lockhart, R., & Shaw, D. (1996). Supported education: A qualitative study of the student experience. *Psychiatric Rehabilitation Journal, 19*(3), 59–70.

Egnew, R. C. (1993). Supported education and employment: An integrated approach. *Psychosocial Rehabilitation Journal, 17*(1), 121–127.

Engelstein, J., Horowitz, G., & Romano, J. (2002). The education mentoring program at Fountain House. In C. T. Mowbray, K. S. Brown, K. Furlong-Norman, & A. Sullivan-Soydan (Eds.), *Supported education and psychiatric rehabilitation: models and methods* (pp. 129–137). Linthicum, MD: International Association of Psychosocial Rehabilitation Services.

Frankie, P., Levine, P., Mowbray, C. T., Shriner, W., Conklin, C., & Thomas, E. (1996). Supported education for persons with psychiatric disabilities: Implementation in an urban environment. *Journal of Mental Health Administration, 23*(4), 406–417.

Gilbert, R., Heximer, S., Jaxon, D. & Bellamy, C.D. (2004). Redirection through education: Meeting the challenges. *American Journal of Psychiatric Rehabilitation, 7*(3), 329–345.

Hain, R., & Gioia, D. (2004). Supported Education Enhancing Rehabilitation (SEER): A community mental health and community college partnership for access and retention. *American Journal of Psychiatric Rehabilitation, 7*(3), 315–328.

Harding, C. M., Brooks, G. W., Ashikaga, T., Strauss, J. S., & Brier, A. (1987). The Vermont longitudinal study of persons with severe mental illness: II. Long-term outcome of subjects who retrospectively met DSM III criteria for schizophrenia. *American Journal of Psychiatry, 144*(6), 727–735.

Housel, D., & Hickey, D. (1993). Supported education in a community college for students with psychiatric disabilities: The Houston Community College model. *Psychosocial Rehabilitation Journal, 17*(1), 41–50.

Independent Life USA. (2004). *Ed Roberts, prophet of independence*. Retrieved November 11, 2004, from http://www.ilusa.com/links/ilcenters.htm

Ishmael, S. (2002). Out of the darkness and into the light. In C. T. Mowbray, K. S. Brown, K. Furlong-Norman, & A. Sullivan-Soydan (Eds.), *Supported education and psychiatric rehabilitation: models and methods* (pp. 31–32). Linthicum, MD: International Association of Psychosocial Rehabilitation Services.

Jasper, C. (2002). Life before supported education: The long journey. In C. T. Mowbray, K. S. Brown, K. Furlong-Norman, & A. Sullivan-Soydan (Eds.), *Supported education and psychiatric rehabilitation: models and methods* (pp. 23–30). Linthicum, MD: International Association of Psychosocial Rehabilitation Services.

Kerouac, J. W. (1997). Off the road: Supported education for college students with psychiatric disabilities. *Journal of the California Alliance for the Mentally Ill, 8*(2), 41–43.

Kerouac, J. W., & McCoy, M. L. (2002). The Thresholds Community Scholar Program. In C. T. Mowbray, K. S. Brown, K. Furlong-Norman, & A. Sullivan-Soydan (Eds.), *Supported education and psychiatric rehabilitation: models and methods* (pp. 147–153). Linthicum, MD: International Association of Psychosocial Rehabilitation Services.

Kessler, R., Foster, C., Saunders, W., & Stang, P. (1995). Social consequences of psychiatric disorders, I: Educational attainment. *American Journal of Psychiatry, 152*(7), 1026–1032.

Mayer, S. L. (1993). Coming over the rise. *Psychosocial Rehabilitation Journal, 17*(1), 39–40.

Megivern, D. M. (2001). *Educational functioning and college integration of students with mental illness: Examining the roles of psychiatric symptomatology and mental health service use*. Doctoral dissertation, University of Michigan, Ann Arbor.

Megivern, D., & Pellerito, S. (2002). Early intervention for students with psychiatric impairments. In C. T. Mowbray, K. S. Brown, K. Furlong-Norman, & A. Sullivan-Soydan (Eds.), *Supported education and psychiatric rehabilitation: models and methods* (pp. 279–284). Linthicum, MD: International Association of Psychosocial Rehabilitation Services.

Megivern, D., Pellerito, S., & Mowbray, C. (2003). Barriers to higher education for individuals with psychiatric disabilities. *Psychiatric Rehabilitation Journal, 26*(3), 217–231.

Mowbray, C. T. (1997). The future of supported education. *Journal of the California Alliance for Mental Illness, 8*(2), 67–69.

Mowbray, C. T. (1999). The benefits and challenges of supported education: A personal perspective. *Psychiatric Rehabilitation Journal, 22*(3), 248–254.

Mowbray, C. T. (2000). The Michigan Supported Education Program: Invited article for "Rehab Rounds" feature. *Psychiatric Services, 51*(11), 1355–1357.

Mowbray, C. T. (2004a). Overview of the special issue on supported education, *American Journal of Psychiatric Rehabilitation, 7*(3), 223–226.

Mowbray, C. T. (2004b). Supported education: Diversity, critical ingredients and future directions. *American Journal of Psychiatric Rehabilitation, 7*(3), 347–362.

Mowbray, C. T., Bellamy, C.D., Megivern, D., & Szilvagyi, S. (2001). Raising our sites: Dissemination of supported education. *Journal of Behavioral Health Services & Research, 28*(4), 484–491.

Mowbray, C. T., & Collins, M. E. (2002). The effectiveness of supported education: current research findings. In C. T. Mowbray, K. S. Brown, K. Furlong-Norman, & A. Sullivan-Soydan (Eds.), *Supported education and psychiatric rehabilitation: models and methods* (pp. 181–194). Linthicum, MD: International Association of Psychosocial Rehabilitation Services.

Mowbray, C. T., Collins, M., & Bybee, D. (1999). Supported education for individuals with psychiatric disabilities: Long-term outcomes from an experimental study. *Social Work Research, 23*(2), 89–100.

Mowbray, C. T., Holter, M. C., Teague, G. B., & Bybee, D. (2003a). Fidelity criteria: Development, measurement and validation. *American Journal of Evaluation, 24*(3), 315–340.

Mowbray, C. T., Megivern, D., & Holter, M. (2003b). Supported education programming for adults with psychiatric disabilities: Results from a national survey. *Psychiatric Rehabilitation Journal, 27*(2), 159–167.

Mowbray, C. T., Moxley, D. P., & Brown, K. S. (1993). A framework for initiating supported education programs. *Psychosocial Rehabilitation Journal, 17*(1), 129–149.

Mowbray, C. T., Verdejo, F., & Levine, P. (2002). The role of community mental health and vocational rehabilitation service systems in enhancing supported education services In C. T. Mowbray, K. S. Brown, K. Furlong-Norman, & A. Sullivan-Soydan (Eds.), *Supported education and psychiatric rehabilitation: models and methods* (pp. 199–213). Linthicum, MD: International Association of Psychosocial Rehabilitation Services.

Moxley, D. P., Mowbray, C. T. & Brown, K. S. (1993). Supported education. In P. W. Flexler & P. Solomon (Eds.), *Psychiatric rehabilitation in practice* (pp. 137–153). Boston, MA: Andover Medical Publishers.

Murphy, A. A., Mullen, M. G., & Spagnolo, A. B. (2005). Enhancing individual placement and support: Promoting job tenure by integrating natural supports and supported education. *American Journal of Psychiatric Rehabilitation, 8*(1), 37–61.

Pepper, B. Ryglewicz, H., & Kirshner, M. C. (1981). The young adult chronic patient: Overview of a population. *Hospital and Community Psychiatry, 32*, 463–469.

Russell, A. C., & Strauss, S. (2004). Career Advancement Resources (CAR): Supported education as a career development strategy. *American Journal of Psychiatric Rehabilitation, 7*(3), 249–264.

Shearman, K., Hart-Katuin, C., & Hicks (2002, April). *Postsecondary education for persons with mental illness: Exploring needs in Indiana*. Paper Presented at Supported Education Conference, Ann Arbor, MI.

Spencer-Watts, R. L. (2002). Supported education turned my life around. In C. T. Mowbray, K. S. Brown, K. Furlong-Norman, & A. Sullivan-Soydan (Eds.), *Supported education and psychiatric rehabilitation: models and methods* (pp. 99–100). Linthicum, MD: International Association of Psychosocial Rehabilitation Services.

Stodden, R. A., & Conway, M. A. (2003). Supporting individuals with disabilities in postsecondary education. *American Rehabilitation, 27*(1), 24–33.

Sullivan, A. P., Nicolellis, D. L., Danley, K. S., & Macdonald-Wilson, K. (1993). Choose-Get-Keep: A psychiatric rehabilitation approach to supported education. *Psychosocial Rehabilitation Journal, 17*(1). 55–68.

Sullivan-Soydan, A. (2004). Supported education: A portrait of a psychiatric rehabilitation intervention. *American Journal of Psychiatric Rehabilitation, 7*(3), 227–248.

Sullivan-Soydan, A. (2002). An overview of supported education. In C. T. Mowbray, K. S. Brown, K. Furlong-Norman, & A. Sullivan-Soydan (Eds.), *Supported education and psychiatric rehabilitation: models and methods* (pp. 3–10). Linthicum, MD: International Association of Psychosocial Rehabilitation Services.

Unger, K. V. (1990). Supported postsecondary education for people with mental illness. *American Rehabilitation, 14*(10), 10–14, 32–33.

Unger, K. V. (1993). Creating supported education programs utilizing existing community resources. *Psychosocial Rehabilitation Journal, 17*(1), 11–23.

Unger, K. V. (1994). Access to educational programs and its effect on employability. *Psychosocial Rehabilitation Journal, 17*(3), 117–126.

Unger, K. V. (1998). *Handbook on supported education: Providing services for students with psychiatric disabilities*. Baltimore, MD: Paul H. Brookes Publishing.

Weiss, J., Maddox, D., Vanderwaerden, M., & Szilvagyi, S. (2004). The Tri-County Scholars Program: Bridging the clubhouse and community college. *American Journal of Psychiatric Rehabilitation, 7*(3), 281–300.

Wells-Moran, J., & Gilmur, D. (2002). *Supported education for people with psychiatric disabilities*. Lanham, MD: University Press of America.

Chapter 11

Residential Services and Independent Living

Introduction 304

Barriers to Housing 304

Affordability 304

Stigma and Discrimination 305

Federal Response to Housing
Discrimination 306

Whose Responsibility Is Housing? 306

History of Residential Services 307

Boarding Homes and Single-Room-
Occupancy Residences 307

Family Foster Care 309

Fairweather Lodges 309

Residential Treatment Facilities 311

**Rehabilitation Treatment Facilities as
Residential Providers 312**

**Stigma and Residential Treatment
Programs 312**

**Emergence of the Linear Continuum
Paradigm 313**

**The Story of Joanna: An Experience of the
Linear Continuum Approach 315**

The Case against the Linear Continuum
Approach 316

**Supported Housing: A Better Approach to
Residential Services 318**

Implementing the Supported Housing
Approach 319

Outcomes of the Supported Housing
Approach 322

The Independent Living Movement 323

Housing First 326

Summary 330

Class Exercise 330

References 331

Helping people with psychiatric disabilities to choose and maintain safe and affordable housing is an important goal of psychiatric rehabilitation practitioners and one of its toughest challenges. Where we live is an integral part of our lives. Having a satisfactory home that we are generally content with and where we feel safe and secure has a positive impact on the quality of our lives. Residing in a place where we are uncomfortable and where our safety and security may be threatened is very stressful and has a negative impact on our sense of well-being and quality of life.

Many consumers reside in environments not of their own choosing. Those living in supervised residential programs may be uncomfortable with certain program policies such as curfews or mandatory attendance at day programs. Another source of discomfort may be sharing their living space with others who they do not know well and may not like. Some consumers live in substandard housing in neighborhoods characterized by poverty and high crime rates. In addition, a sizable percentage of people who have a severe mental illness are homeless for some period of their lives (Carling, 1994; Torrey, 2001). These and other difficult living arrangements are endured by a substantial number of consumers who do not have access to other options.

This chapter will answer the following questions:

1. *Why is it such a struggle for consumers to find a decent place to live in their communities?*
2. *Where did ex-psychiatric patients go once the era of deinstitutionalization began?*
3. *What are the current models of residential service provision?*
4. *Can people with severe functional deficits live in regular housing in the community?*
5. *How can people with psychiatric disabilities achieve the goal of independent living?*

Introduction

Before looking at current trends in residential services for persons diagnosed with severe mental illnesses we will examine some of the barriers to affordable housing and look at how residential services have evolved since the early years of deinstitutionalization. For many years transitional residential programs that required individuals to move gradually towards independent living dominated mental health systems. More recently there has been a move towards the supported housing model which is grounded in the PsyR principles of individualization, consumer choice and normalization.

Barriers to Housing

Although there are a number of barriers to decent housing for people who have severe mental illnesses, the main barriers to housing of their choice are affordability and discrimination.

Affordability

The primary barrier to acceptable housing is economic. As of 2006, the United States was undergoing a nationwide housing price boom affecting everyone with a limited income. This inflation in housing costs has been long term, but has particularly accelerated since 1999. Basically there are two reasons why safe, decent, and affordable housing is difficult to find. The first is the growing shortage of affordable housing. Part of the decline in low-income housing is due to the gentrification of many inner-city neighborhoods and expanding suburbs, with single professionals and couples with high incomes replacing individuals having middle or lower incomes. The second economic factor, which is reducing housing availability, is cuts in the funding earmarked for federally assisted low-income housing (Carling, 1993; Cooper, Herb, & O'Hara, 2003). Both of these factors are aggravated by the fact that the cost of both rent and home purchases has risen, while for many people incomes have not risen at a comparable rate. Many consumers rely on entitlements as their sole income, which typically keep them well below the poverty level and unable to afford most housing options. A study conducted by advocacy groups, *Priced Out in 2002* (Cooper & O'Hara, 2003), found that persons receiving federal disability benefits such as Supplemental Security Income (SSI) were unable to afford even modest rents anywhere in the nation. For the first time, the national average rent for a modest one-bedroom apartment was 105% of monthly SSI benefits. As rents rise the affordability crisis continues to deepen.

Stigma and Discrimination

The stigma associated with mental illness often results in housing discrimination for people with psychiatric disabilities. Many landlords refuse to rent to people with a known history of mental illness. Consider Ellen's experience:

> *After losing an apartment because her building was about to be demolished to make way for a mini-mall, Ellen finally located an apartment she could afford, a third-floor walk-up in a building in which the landlord also resided. Ellen made a good impression during her initial meeting with the landlord. He noticed she was a smoker, which wasn't a problem because he smoked cigarettes as well. However, when the landlord called one of her references and discovered her psychiatric history, he became wary. He discussed the situation with his wife, who was quite blunt in her assessment: "I don't want some crazy woman who smokes cigarettes in our building; she'll be sure to burn the place down!" When Ellen stopped by the next day she was told the apartment was already rented.*

Community opposition to living near mental health consumers is commonly referred to as the NIMBY ("Not in my backyard!") response. When community residents learn that people with psychiatric disabilities have moved in or are planning to move into their neighborhood they may have an overt negative reaction. This is particularly true with congregate care residences, where groups of people live together and receive support services from residential program staff. A typical concern, aggravated by the common myth portrayed in the media that mental illness equates with dangerousness, is for the safety of their children, family members, and themselves. Another common concern is that the presence of people with psychiatric disabilities will lower real estate values. Even though research suggests this is an unfounded assumption (Carling, 1995; Cook, 1997), it has been known to fuel organized efforts to rid a neighborhood of unwanted individuals.

The NIMBY attitude not only creates a barrier to housing, but can be hurtful in other ways as well. Negative actions taken by resistant community members include lawsuits, exclusion from community activities, and verbal and physical harassment. Housing advocates have cited examples of extreme reactions, such as group homes that were burned to the ground, allegedly by angry neighbors. All of these actions clearly convey to people with psychiatric disabilities that they are unwanted and undesirable.

Research suggests that residential stability may depend more on the characteristics of the community where a person resides than on the characteristics of the persons themselves (Carling, 1990). In fact Boydell, Gladstone, Crawford, and Trainor (1999) found that individuals were successful in coping with life in the community to the degree that they could "make do" and employ "passing strategies." "Making do" refers to the ability to tolerate other tenants and the noxious community elements that typically exist in the neighborhoods in which persons with mental illness must reside. The term "passing strategies" refers to the ability to blend in with the community and community members (Boydell et al., 1999).

Another factor that exacerbates stigma/discrimination problems is the fact that, often due to their illness, some persons with severe mental illness have criminal records. According to a 1999 U.S. Department of Justice report, 16% of adult inmates of the U.S. prison system have a mental illness. The President's New Freedom Commission on Mental Health found that a staggering 80% of youths entering the juvenile justice system have mental disorders (Honberg, 2004). A criminal record can have a very negative effect on a person's ability to obtain housing. A criminal record can prohibit someone from obtaining a rental subsidy from the state or federal government, such as a Section 8 Choice voucher from the U.S. Department of Housing and Urban Development. There can be problems even if financial considerations are not an issue. In some areas, landlords regularly require credit and criminal background checks before renting apartments. In response to this crisis, a nationwide advocacy group, The Bazelon Center for Mental Health Law "is committed to reducing the criminalization of people with mental illnesses" (http://www.bazelon.org).

Federal Response to Housing Discrimination

In 1988 the U.S. Congress amended the Fair Housing Act to add protections against discrimination for persons with disabilities and families with children. The act prohibits the use of local ordinances or zoning laws that discriminate against protected persons such as people with disabilities. However, it is not unusual for municipalities to attempt to challenge the Fair Housing Act. While residential programs that have good legal representation will eventually win such cases, the establishment of many programs have been delayed by community opposition.

Whose Responsibility is Housing?

Some advocates and researchers believe the social welfare and mental health systems may have inadvertently perpetuated the housing crisis for consumers because each group has attempted to "pass the buck" to the other (Carling, 1993; Hopper & Barrow, 2003). The mental health system has historically seen its role as providing residential treatment rather than permanent housing options. However, residential treatment programs, discussed later in the chapter, do not provide what many consumers want and need from a place of residence (Collaborative Support Programs of New Jersey, 1991, 1996; Tanzman, 1993; Yeich, Mowbray, Bybee, & Cohen, 1994). Also, because of their cost, residential service programs are available to only a small proportion of persons (Carling, 1993). On the other hand, from the social welfare system's point of view, public housing programs are not equipped to meet the special needs of people with disabilities (Carling, 1994; Hopper & Barrow, 2003).

As addressed earlier, the lack of decent and affordable housing has a negative effect on the quality of many consumers' lives. It has other negative effects as well (Carling, 1993). Families frequently take in relatives with psychiatric disabilities with nowhere else to go, despite being ill prepared for the emotional and financial burdens that may accompany such a living arrangement. Psychiatric institutions, in some places, often extend the stays of people ready for discharge simply because they have no place else to go. Considering the high costs of inpatient treatment, this is a huge waste of resources that could be used to support people in more productive ways. It also, of course, sends a very negative message to those persons who are retained in the hospital despite being ready for discharge: fostering passivity, prolonging dependency, and delaying recovery. As we will see, the field of psychiatric rehabilitation currently has a number of effective strategies to help people attain the type of housing that they want. However, the barriers just described continue to thwart efforts to provide many consumers with appropriate housing options.

History of Residential Services

From the mid-1950s to the mid-1970s, several hundred thousand people were discharged from psychiatric institutions throughout the United States (Torrey, 2001). Where did these people go after they were discharged? Unfortunately, the community mental health system did not create a clear plan, or allocate funding for housing after discharge. Some people went back to their families (for more on family involvement in the care of relatives who have a mental illness see Chapter 13), many went to live in boarding houses or single-room-occupancy hotels, and others were transferred to nursing homes. Increases in the numbers of homeless people were also associated with deinstitutionalization (Torrey, 2001).

Although some residential service models with rehabilitation goals were developed during this first phase of deinstitutionalization, implementation was scattered and reached only a small percentage of people. Among mental health professionals there was little agreement on what ideal residential services looked like and "the mental health system did not develop a coherent and widely accepted model for residential services in the first few decades of deinstitutionalization" (Ridgway & Zipple, 1990, p. 12).

Still, it is informative to examine some of these early residential options because many of them are still utilized today.

Boarding Homes and Single-Room-Occupancy Residences

A 1981 study done by Goldman, Gattozzi, and Taube estimated that at that time in the United States, 300,000 to 400,000 persons with severe mental illness were living in boarding homes, or what are also called *board and care facilities*. Boarding homes have existed in this country as a residential option for many kinds of people for hundreds of years. They generally involve provision of a room, meals, and other services such as laundry and housekeeping for a weekly or monthly fee. They are typically used by people on the lower levels of the socioeconomic scale, and often house those living a transient lifestyle. Some boarding home operators rent out a few rooms in their own homes; others own one or more large facilities each housing dozens of people.

It is not an accident that entrepreneurs throughout the United States responded to the deinstitutionalization movement by opening boarding homes, which exclusively catered to people discharged from psychiatric institutions. Some converted old hotels or apartment buildings into single-room-occupancy residences (commonly referred to as SROs) that housed 100 or more people. The financial incentive for these entrepreneurs was the establishment of Aid to the Disabled (ATD) in 1963, a monthly check provided by the federal government to people with disabilities who were not eligible for Social Security Disability (SSD) benefits due to lack of a substantial work history. ATD is now called Supplemental Security Income or SSI. Boarding home operators are able to establish themselves as payees for the people residing in their facilities. They are allowed to keep most of the money as payment for room and board, and give the remainder to residents in what amounts to a small monthly allowance—typically barely enough to buy coffee and cigarettes or a few personal items. While some boarding home operators viewed deinstitutionalization as an opportunity to make a decent living and to provide residents with a caring homelike environment, others focused solely on ways in which they could maximize their profits. Scandalous stories abound of residents subsisting on cold cereal and bologna sandwiches, sharing cramped quarters, filthy conditions, and dealing with physical and verbal abuse at the hands of operators, staff and roommates.

Many boarding homes are located in dangerous inner-city neighborhoods, where large old homes could be purchased inexpensively. It was not unusual, particularly for residents discharged directly to a boarding home after a lengthy hospital stay of 10 years or more, to rarely venture out in neighborhoods that were both unfamiliar and crime ridden. The result was a sort of "transinstitutionalization" (Carling, 1995, p. 33), since being discharged to what some referred to as "psychiatric ghettos" in no way resembled normalized community existence. Thus, for many consumers life in a boarding home was not much better and was, in some cases, worse than hospital life, particularly in terms of issues such as privacy and safety. In a 1982 study done by Lehman, Ward, and Linn, boarding home residents described a quality of life that was significantly less satisfying than the general population, and somewhat less satisfying than other socially disadvantaged groups.

Access to psychiatric treatment and rehabilitation for boarding home residents varies. Some operators contract with psychiatrists and other mental health professionals to provide services "in house," making these facilities even more like mini-institutions. Other operators establish a relationship with local community mental health centers or psychiatric rehabilitation (PsyR) programs. These situations typically involve sending residents, often "by the van load," to programs on a regular basis. In fact, sometimes boarding home operators require residents to attend psychiatric day treatment programs or to be away from the facility for significant portions of the day.

Family Foster Care

In some parts of the country, programs were developed that placed one or more consumers with a family other than their own. In the early 1980s it was estimated that the Veterans Administration, probably the largest utilizer of foster care for adults with disabilities, had approximately 11,000 ex-psychiatric patients in family foster care at any one time (Linn, Klett, & Caffey, 1980). Typically, families received payment and some level of professional support. The arrangement could either be transitional or long term. Family foster care in the United States has its roots in Geel, Belgium, where people with psychiatric disabilities have been cared for in private homes for centuries (Lamb, 1982; Linn et al., 1980). This approach was also probably influenced by foster care programs that target other disadvantaged populations such as those that serve children and elderly adults.

Ideally family foster care seeks to incorporate consumers in all aspects of family and community life. For consumers who desire an active family life, but are estranged from their own family of origin, this may be a viable residential option, if a mutually satisfying match can be made between the consumer and an interested family. Research suggests that several aspects of the family home environment may be associated with positive outcomes in the area of social functioning. Specifically, consumers may function better in foster families that care for fewer consumers, are not large in terms of total number of people residing in the home, and have more children living at home (Linn et al., 1980). When several consumers reside in a foster care setting, it is sometimes hard to distinguish it from a boarding home, and the potential benefits of the model are diminished.

Carling (1994) cautioned that in many family foster care settings only minimal supports are provided and true integration into the community is not realized. However, he cited the development of some creative ways to utilize family foster care. One development is as a short-term alternative to inpatient hospitalization. Such an arrangement is temporary, allowing an individual to stabilize during a period of crisis. Family foster care has also been used as a transition from the hospital to independent living. Such programs can "provide a caring home on a short term basis for individuals who are leaving a hospital, and who are trying to establish roots in a particular community" (Carling, 1994, p. 92).

Fairweather Lodges

During the early years of deinstitutionalization, a social scientist named George Fairweather recognized the difficulties that discharged people were having with community adjustment. In response he designed an experimental program to provide a long-term supportive residential environment that also addressed individuals' social and vocational issues. What began as a research study evolved into a distinct PsyR approach known as the *Fairweather Lodge model*. Fairweather began his research at a California Veterans Administration Hospital in the mid-1960s (Onaga, 1994; Onaga & Smith, 2000). Initially, he established small problem-solving groups of patients preparing for discharge. Each group was responsible for the individual progress of its members. These experimental groups were able to meet the criteria for discharge sooner than the control group that received traditional hospital treatment (Lamb, 1982). However, following discharge, recidivism rates were basically the same for both the experimental and the control groups. H. Richard Lamb (1982) discussed these programs:

> The crucial factor in remaining in the community was found to be the amount of support the patient received from the people with whom he or she lived. When these facts became clear, Fairweather's group decided to move these problem-solving patient groups as units from the hospital to the community. The new phase of the program involved setting up the Community Lodge program: a dormitory for patients and a sheltered workshop situation; a janitorial service owned and operated by the ex-patients themselves. (p. 50)

Professional staff acted as consultants to the lodge, initially providing a high level of support and assistance in dealing with both work and daily living issues. Eventually, the consultation needs of the lodge members decreased and they were able to maintain the lodge and the business with minimal staff assistance. Members received psychiatric care from a private physician. The original Fairweather Lodge was a resounding success in terms of recidivism rates and vocational outcomes (e.g., all of the lodge members were employed). Many members also reported an increase in self-esteem. The model was soon replicated in other parts of the United States, as well as in foreign countries (Lamb, 1982).

A number of essential principles guide the operation of community lodges. They were outlined by Fairweather, Saunders, Maynard, and Cressler (1969) in the book *Community Life for the Mentally Ill*. Onaga (1994) notes the similarity of these principles to some of the basic PsyR principles as stated by Cnaan, Blankertz, Messinger, and Gardner (1988). Some examples of Fairweather Lodge principles are as follows:

1. Lodge members must have meaningful roles in the lodge/business, and be given as much autonomy as possible. (These tenets are compatible with the PsyR principles of normalization and self-determination.)
2. Lodge members should have upward mobility within the lodge community. (This principle adheres to the PsyR value that people have the capacity to grow and change.)
3. The role of professional staff associated with Fairweather Lodges is that of a consultant who bases his or her level of involvement on the current needs and abilities of lodge members. Staff must be available to lodge members when they are having difficulties, yet be ready to step back when members are able to solve their own problems. (This approach is in agreement with PsyR attitudes about staff commitment and the deprofessionalization of the staff role.)

Evolution of the Lodge Approach

As PsyR ideas moved toward more integrated community living, the original Fair-weather Lodge approach became increasingly problematic. Essentially, the original lodges were subsocieties in which members spent most of their time living, working, and social-izing with other people with psychiatric disabilities. Today we recognize that given the right opportunities and continued support, community integration including regular employment is possible and a right (i.e., the *L.C. vs. Olmstead* decision) of people with psychiatric disabilities.

In response to these changes, Onaga and Smith (2000) described how lodges in Minnesota reinvented themselves to address the wishes of some lodge members for full-time integrated employment. This change necessitated lodge members working in regular settings rather than the lodge business. Members also had to accommodate 8-hour workdays. This change eventually led to the creation of a "full-time" workers lodge, since regular lodge members were on different schedules, which the 8-hour workers found disrupting.

Interestingly, Onaga and Smith (2000) credit three major events with spurring changes in the Fairweather Lodge model, rather than discrepancies between the lodge model and PsyR philosophy. The first change they note was the (nationwide) decline in state hospital admissions in response to the deinstitutionalization movement. This led to the creation of a "community training lodge," shifting the development of new lodges from the psychiatric institutions to the community. The second change they note was the passage of the Javits-Wagner-O'Day Act by Congress (1972). This act established NISH (National Industries for the Severely Handicapped), which consisted of set-asides for some government contracts for organizations employing people with disabilities. The advent of NISH created a situation in which it was beneficial for lodge members to own their own businesses and to hire people without disabilities to provide certain functions and services, both actions that initially were not sanctioned under original lodge rules. The final change they cite was passage of the Fair Housing Amendment Act of 1988. The protections afforded individuals by this act reduced the necessity for lodge members to live together to ensure housing stability.

The evolution of the Fairweather Lodge model may be instructive for understanding many early PsyR programmatic innovations. An effective innovation for meeting peoples' needs given the situation at the time it was developed, the lodge model had to evolve in response to environmental changes and changes in peoples' aspirations. As of 2006, 90 lodges were operating in 16 U.S. states (http://theccl.org/Fairweather.htm).

Residential Treatment Facilities

While boarding homes, SROs, and family foster care are typically nonprofessional ventures, a variety of residential programs run by mental health professionals emerged in the 1960s and in the 1970s during the early years of deinstitutionalization and they still exist today. Unlike Fairweather Lodges, most of these programs were not based on a clearly articulated model of service provision, but they did have a number of similarities. The most prolific approach to residential service provision has been segregated, congregate care facilities (Carling, 1994). These programs utilize various names, most commonly *group homes* and *halfway houses*. Like the partial care programs discussed in Chapter 6, most residential treatment facilities seek to establish a therapeutic milieu; in other words, an environment carefully crafted to encourage clinical and functional improvements (Ridgway & Zipple, 1990). Some of these programs have rehabilitation goals, striving to provide residents with independent living skills so that individuals can eventually move on to a less protected setting or into their own homes. Other programs focus on long-term care in a small homelike environment rather than a large institutional setting.

The number of consumers residing in a group home can vary. Many utilize typical single-family homes and house about 3 to 10 individuals. However, some professionally run programs may house large numbers of consumers and resemble SROs; and some may accommodate just a few individuals and resemble foster care settings. In most programs staff members are present, or readily available, 24 hours a day. Typical program activities may include staff-assisted group menu planning and meal preparation; individual or small-group activity of daily living (ADL) skills training (e.g., budgeting, hygiene, laundry); social and recreational activities; assistance in utilization of local transportation and other community resources; community meetings; individual and group counseling; and symptoms and medication education. In some programs residents spend weekdays outside of the residential facility either at day programs, workshops, school, or jobs. Other programs have on-site treatment and rehabilitation groups.

Rehabilitation Treatment Facilities as Residential Providers

When an agency provides both rehabilitation and residential services, housing problems may arise if treatment recommendations are not followed. In such situations there is often an explicit link between continuation in a residential setting and compliance with a treatment plan (Mize, Paolo-Calabrese, Williams, & Margolin, 1998). Sometimes such links are implicit but not articulated. An individual who may not be following treatment recommendations, for example, might be deemed not appropriate for a particular residence. Although this practice has been correctly labeled coercive (Chamberlin, 1978), it is not an uncommon policy of residential treatment facilities.

Mize and colleagues (1998) suggest a collaborative approach to developing a noncoercive situation. The collaborative approach addresses this problem by clearly separating the individuals' "tenant" and "consumer" roles and the provider's "landlord" and "worker" roles. This separation of roles is reinforced if the individual holds the lease to his or her living situation rather than the agency. They suggest that in a successful congregate setting, tenants must chose to live together, set their own rules, and be able to hold one another accountable for their actions.

Stigma and Residential Treatment Programs

Many residential treatment programs are located in urban and suburban residential neighborhoods. Ideally program residents become an integral part of the local community life (e.g., developing friendly relationships with neighbors, attending block parties, and joining religious congregations). Unfortunately, the NIMBY attitudes mentioned earlier often create barriers to true community integration. In fact, a key issue faced by residential treatment program administrators is whether or not to notify neighbors of their intention to open a group home. Some programs approach the issue collaboratively, notifying neighbors early on in an attempt to establish positive relationships. However, some studies have indicated that this approach can backfire and help fuel community opposition (Zippay, 1997). Other programs refrain from notifying neighbors in an effort to protect consumers' civil rights and avoid a stigmatizing confrontation. This latter strategy has been criticized due to its potential to create resentment and mistrust as neighbors begin to realize that a group home exists (Zippay, 1997). A third approach is to publicly announce intentions to open a residential facility, but rather than attempting to collaborate with a community that is expected to be resistant, some programs take a proactive stance and threaten to sue the community (Carling, 1995). How would you feel if a group home for people with severe mental illness opened in your neighborhood? If you were a consumer living in a group home, would you want neighbors to be notified before you moved in? What do you think would happen if neighbors were not notified beforehand or if a lawsuit were threatened?

Carling (1995) suggested that community members who oppose the presence of residential treatment facilities should not automatically be labeled as "the bad guys." Although people with disabilities should have the right to live wherever they choose, mental health professionals and consumer advocates must be sensitive to community members' concerns about having a group home in the neighborhood. Sometimes these concerns are based on lack of accurate information. However, one cannot ignore the fact that sometimes facility-based residential programs do alter the character of a neighborhood. In some cases, neighbors cite practical concerns such as parking and increased traffic problems (Cook, 1997). Carling stated that, in his experience, "most mental health professionals do not want a group home or other treatment program sited next to their own homes" (Carling, 1995, p. 116).

Despite the fact that numerous instances of community opposition to the establishment of residential treatment facilities have been reported, this is not the whole story. There are also many communities where group homes and single or multiple-family residences coexist peacefully. In some instances a substantial percentage of neighbors were not even aware that a group home for people with disabilities was in their neighborhood (Cook, 1997). Presumably this occurs most often when program staff and residents make an effort to keep a low profile. In other communities, positive relationships have developed between group home residents and their neighbors. One study found that neighbors cited the benefits associated with living near a group home (e.g., learning more about disabilities) about as often as they cited problems and concerns (Cook, 1997).

The Emergence of the Linear Continuum Paradigm

Many of the residential treatment programs were established to provide housing for persons being deinstitutionalized. Many of these individuals had spent considerable time in psychiatric hospitals and some had developed an "institutionalization syndrome" characterized by extreme dependence. Partly in response to the needs of this emerging population and to create an effective transition from the hospital to the community, many of these early programs devised a continuum of residential settings. This continuum was conceptualized as a series of residential steps to accomplish the transition between the hospital and independent living (Carling, 1994). In essence, the first step consisted of a living arrangement very similar to an inpatient setting: high amounts of structure and rules, 24-hour staff supervision, and few privileges. Subsequent steps, which usually meant moves to other residential settings, brought increasingly less structure, staff supervision, and rule restrictions. At the last step the individual was "transitioned" into the community at large. This approach to residential treatment has been called the linear continuum paradigm (Ridgway & Zipple, 1990).

Thus, the halfway house approach became augmented by the addition of different housing situations, each offering varying amounts of staff support, structure, and supervision. These steps might consist of quarter-way houses, typically located on the grounds of state psychiatric institutions (Carling, 1994); three-quarter-way houses, in which staff were no longer present around the clock (Campbell, 1981); and supervised apartments, semi-supervised apartments, and other residential options that represented steps toward the eventual goal of fully independent living. Some residential continua also include crisis alternative residences, also called *respite care,* designed to help acutely symptomatic consumers avoid a hospitalization (Carling, 1994).

Throughout the 1980s, and into the 1990s, in some places, the linear continuum paradigm dominated the field of residential services (Ridgway & Zipple, 1990). Although this conceptual framework is less favored today, the idea of transitional housing is still in evidence. It is important to examine how a linear continuum approach affects the consumers' adjustment to community living.

Exactly what is offered along a particular residential continuum varies, as do the names given to the different types of programming. It is therefore difficult to compare these residential approaches, and a clear idea of the ideal continuum has never emerged (Ridgway & Zipple, 1990). However, some basic assumptions characterize programs that adhere to this linear residential service continuum approach (Ridgway & Zipple, 1990):

1. Several residential settings are available that offer different levels of service provision, staff supervision, and restrictiveness.
2. Program participants are expected to move, in an orderly fashion, from the more restrictive level to a less restrictive level.
3. Participants in each setting are similar in terms of clinical stability and functional ability. They are expected to make progress before graduating to another level on the continuum.
4. If a program participant decompensates and returns to the hospital, he or she often reenters the continuum at the most restrictive level (i.e., he or she has to start over again at the bottom).
5. The ultimate goal is to move on to independent living and no longer require services from the program.

Research conducted on the efficacy of the residential continuum model is scant and inconclusive. As indicated earlier, it is hard to study an approach in which the nomenclature varies and clearly defined, consistent intervention strategies do not exist. In addition, most of the studies that have been done did not use rigorous experimental methods and thus are not very useful. The literature that is available on transitional residential treatment suggests that the approach is not particularly successful in helping people to achieve the PsyR goal of community integration (Carling, 1994).

It is also important to keep in mind that residential programs of this type only serve a small percentage of the people in need. In the early 1990s, the housing resources available in local mental health systems (such as money earmarked to buy houses, rent apartments, and staff residential continuum programs) provided services for fewer than 5% of the people with psychiatric disabilities (Carling, 1994). Identifying these governmental resources is somewhat difficult, however, because in many places the bulk of resources to support housing is not found in the mental health budgets.

While the linear continuum approach may seem to be a coherent strategy for helping consumers become gradually reintegrated into the community, we should question the use of this approach when 30 or more years later there are no strong research findings to back it up. At the same time, the monetary resources are not available to provide the service to the vast majority of consumers. In addition, consider some of the issues raised by Joanna's story.

The Story of Joanna: An Experience of the Linear Continuum Approach

Joanna is a 32-year-old woman who has never had a home of her own as an adult. She was diagnosed with a severe mental illness in her senior year of high school. She spent the next 10 years shuffling back and forth between psychiatric hospitals and her parents' home. When Joanna was 28 and residing at a state institution, her parents informed her and the hospital staff that when she was ready for discharge they could not take her back home. They were in the process of selling their house and moving to a retirement community and felt it was an appropriate time for Joanna to become less dependent on them. Joanna was put on a waiting list for a residential program that ran three types of facilities: group homes (with staff supervision 24 hours a day), a supervised apartment complex, and semi-supervised scattered site apartments.

Six months later Joanna moved into a group home where she was one of six residents and where she shared a bedroom with another woman. She liked the program better than being at the hospital, although she missed the privacy of her own room at home. She grew quite attached to some of the program staff who were supportive and seemed to truly care about her. However, her relationship with her roommate was not so good. They had little in common and some of the roommate's behaviors, such as pacing back and forth in the middle of the night, made Joanna uneasy.

After 10 months in the group home, the staff told Joanna she was ready to move to the next level in the agency's housing continuum: the supervised apartment complex where staff members were usually on site just a few hours a day. An opening was expected within a few months. Joanna had ambivalent feelings about the impending move. On the one hand, she was happy that the staff thought she had made progress and she liked the idea of having her own room. On the other hand she wasn't convinced she was ready to live more independently. She had learned to contribute to shopping and cooking for six people, although the staff was always on hand should something go wrong. Besides, in the new place she would be living with two other people. She wasn't sure if she would be cooking for herself or sharing meal preparation with roommates. What if she didn't like the roommates or got into an argument? The staff wouldn't be as available to intervene. She had many other concerns as well such as house cleaning routines, sticking to a budget, using public transportation instead of the agency van, and getting used to a new neighborhood. She also felt uneasy about the fact that her stay in the new apartment would also be temporary. She knew that one of the group home graduates, who lived for less than a year at the apartment complex where Joanna would be living, was already being pressured to move on to the semi-supervised apartments.

As the weeks went by and she came closer to her moving date, Joanna began to spend more and more time worrying about the impending changes. She began to get symptomatic again, but did not tell the staff because she feared they would be disappointed in her. One week before moving Joanna ended up back in the hospital. When a staff from the group home visited with her, several weeks later, Joanna said she was feeling better and would like to discuss some of her concerns about the new apartment. The staff told her not to worry about it. Another group home resident had been moved in her place. When she was ready for discharge she could come back to the group home again and work on her ADL (activities of daily living) skills so that she could be "ready" for the apartment the next time. Joanna felt both relieved and disappointed. She was back to square one again, as if the "progress" she had made in the group home had never happened.

The Case against the Linear Continuum Approach

Joanna's story illustrates a number of reasons why the linear continuum approach to residential treatment has been criticized in recent years. One inherent flaw in this approach is the requirement that consumers make frequent changes in their living situation. For most people, moving from one home to another is a stressful event. It means abandoning routines and settings that have become comfortable and getting used to a whole new place. Such changes are often hard to deal with for people without psychiatric disabilities. For people who have a severe mental illness, the stress involved with such a change can create real problems.

Think back to what you learned in Chapter 2. Mental illness is episodic in nature and stressful life events can exacerbate symptoms. Considering these facts, mental health professionals should not be surprised when people like Joanna end up back in the hospital just as they are about to make a major life transition. In this sense the linear continuum model and severe mental illness are not a good fit. Even if individuals are able to make it through all the levels of programming and graduate to independent living, they are often short changed by the program structure. With the linear continuum model, independent living typically means that consumers will have less access to program supports at a time when they may need them most. It is not uncommon for persons who have finally achieved their long sought-after goal of obtaining their own apartment to lose it when faced with a crisis situation because the needed supports were no longer available.

Another reason why the linear continuum approach may be ineffective was addressed in Chapter 5. Skills needed to function successfully in living, learning, working, and social environments are best learned in the specific settings where they will be used. It is hard for a person to generalize what they have learned in one setting (e.g., meal planning and preparation for the eight residents of a group home) to another setting (e.g., meal planning and preparation for oneself in an efficiency apartment). Thus, Joanna's concerns about how prepared she was to make a move may have been quite realistic.

Probably the best reason to question the linear continuum model, or any approach that utilizes facility-based congregate care settings, is that they do not provide the type of housing that most consumers want. Arguably, people with psychiatric disabilities may not always know what type of treatment is best suited to their particular illness. However, they certainly know a great deal about where they feel comfortable residing! In a society that places high value on personal freedom, everyone should have the right to pursue a home life of their own choosing. While prior to the mid-1980s the idea of asking consumers what kind of housing they wanted was not widely considered, more recently studies have been done that examine consumers' housing preferences (Goldfinger & Schutt, 1996; Tanzman, 1993). A literature review, which examined the results of 26 such studies, found that the majority of the people surveyed preferred living independently in either a house or an apartment. Not surprisingly, only a very small percentage of respondents in most of the studies had a preference for living in a residential treatment facility (Tanzman, 1993). Similar results were also found in subsequent studies (Collaborative Support Programs of New Jersey, 1996; Yeich et al., 1994).

Some housing preference studies have also explored the question of preferred housemates. In the preceding story, one of the things Joanna liked least about the group home was her roommate. Wondering who she would be "placed with" in the supervised apartment was one of her major concerns. Most of us can appreciate Joanna's apprehension about living with strangers. Imagine a living situation in which the only thing you know about your roommates is that they were all recently discharged from a psychiatric hospital. Even if you are an open-minded person, who does not buy into stigmatizing myths about mental illness, you would probably have some concerns about living with a person you had never met. Many consumers have these same concerns. Some find it hard to have to deal with both their own illness and the symptoms and problems experienced by roommates (Carling, 1994).

When given a choice, most consumers would rather live by themselves or with a spouse, friend, or family member (Tanzman, 1993). This is not a surprising finding. The vast majority of persons without disabilities would probably identify similar preferences. However, it is important to know that some consumers do choose to live with other people who have a mental illness. In 2 out of 16 studies that examined this issue, "more consumers preferred to live with other mental health consumers than with non-consumers" (Tanzman, 1993, p. 453). It may be that some people accustomed to living, learning, working, and socializing in facility-based programs feel most comfortable being with people who have had similar life experiences.

Considering the criticisms just outlined, there are strong reasons to question whether mental health systems should continue to allocate their limited resources to programs adhering to the linear continuum model. If true community integration is the goal, we must admit that thus far it has not been realized. Instead, Carling maintained that many residential treatment approaches "transinstitutionalize" consumers (Carling, 1995, p. 33), providing them with few opportunities to experience normalized community life. Likewise, in a system that currently professes to be consumer driven, neither residential continua nor long-term congregate care settings provide homes where most people want to live. Thus, the majority of residential service approaches that have been developed since deinstitutionalization began fall short on two key PsyR goals: community integration and improved quality of life.

Supported Housing: A Better Approach to Residential Services

In 1991 Paul Carling and Priscilla Ridgway (1991) identified a set of principles for community residential rehabilitation:

1. The rehabilitation approach avoids the notion of placement in favor of choice (p. 72).

2. Rehabilitation-oriented residential services seek to expand consumer control, minimize rules and external structuring (e.g., staff), and maximize active consumer responsibility for day-to-day problem solving and promoting mutual support, self-help, and consumer-operated services (p. 73).

3. Many consumers choose to live with family members, or live alone with considerable support from family members. These family members need to be involved in the rehabilitation process and should be given the support, information, and resources they need (p. 73).

4. Normalization, a guiding principle of PsyR, means a normal living environment, which is perhaps the most important environment in all of our lives. Normalization also means the recovery, creation, and maintenance of valued social roles (Wolfensberger, 1983), such as neighbor, tenant, and roommate, as opposed to group home or supervised apartment resident.

5. People with disabilities may need assistance in developing ADL skills. Skill development occurs most productively when it is specific to the environment in which the person plans to live on a long-term basis. Skills developed in a transitional group home may be of little use to someone planning to live independently.

6. Supports, both formal and informal, must be available and responsive to changing needs. Informal or natural supports include family members, neighbors, friends, peers, and other people in the community. Natural support systems are most easily fostered in normal housing situations (p. 73). Formal support services should also be accessible and well coordinated and should include crisis intervention and case management.

7. All needed supports should be flexible, individualized, and available for as long as an individual needs them. Many programs, while acknowledging the need for longer term support, in fact invest most of their staff resources in transitional living programs and significantly decrease support at precisely the time when the individual's needs may be the greatest (i.e., at the time of a move) (p. 74).

8. Advocacy is greatly needed to combat stigma, community resistance, and the lack of decent and affordable housing options for people with psychiatric disabilities.

These principles provide the basis for what has become the residential service model of choice in the field of PsyR, *supported housing* (Rog, 2004):

> Supported housing embraces a vision of people with severe mental disorders succeeding in the community living situation of their choice through access to flexible, individualized services and supports. (Parrish, 1990, p. 10)

Supported housing as an approach to residential service provision is a relatively new development. In 1987, a policy statement issued by the National Association of State Mental Health Program Directors (NASMHPD) recommended that states begin to move toward a more normalized model of residential services, which by the early 1990s was widely referred to as *supported housing* (Carling, 1990; Knisley & Fleming, 1993). Some state and local service systems have made significant progress in this area, while others have been slower to develop supported housing programs.

The essence of supported housing is that people reside in independent living situations of their choice in the community and receive support services to help them maintain those situations. Proponents of supported housing typically define independent living situations as permanent housing where the individual, rather than a program or agency, holds the lease. As discussed earlier, holding the lease helps to keep housing and services issues separate (Mize et al., 1998). In addition to the fact that consumers prefer to live independently or with loved ones, studies have found that people want supports to maintain their living situations (Tanzman, 1993; Yeich et al., 1994). According to the literature the most frequently mentioned supports include (1) availability of staff by phone 24 hours a day, 7 days a week for assistance in coping with crises; (2) financial resources; (3) assistance in budgeting money; and (4) house furnishings and supplies (Tanzman, 1993; Yeich et al., 1994). If a service system is truly responsive to consumer choice and committed to meaningful community integration, it should be helping people to attain independent housing and providing them with the supports to maintain that housing.

With regard to the PsyR literature on supported housing, there is strong agreement on key elements that define the approach (Ogilvie, 1997). Three essential elements are consistently mentioned: consumer choice; normal, integrated living sites; and provision of supports that are flexible and ongoing (Carling, 1990; Rog, 2004).

Implementing the Supported Housing Approach

Some PsyR residential services are in the process of completing a paradigm shift from the stepwise linear continuum approach to a supported housing approach (Ridgway & Zipple, 1990). This shift involves a number of changes, not only in the type of services that are provided, but also in staff attitudes and in how financial resources are structured.

Key changes in service provision strategies include a shift in staff responsibilities, which requires a different set of skills and attitudes. In the linear continuum model, staff members were expected to provide treatment and supervision in an effort to move residents to the next level of housing. Staff members who work in supported housing programs provide individualized, as-needed supports, teach skills to consumers in their homes, and assist people in acquiring resources. They need to be both flexible and creative in determining the most effective way to help consumers get what they need to live successfully in the community. Consider the following vignette:

Lisa used to live in a group home where staff supervised her in a number of ways. They watched her take her medication twice a day. They were always present when it was her turn to cook dinner. Staff reminded her (repeatedly if she procrastinated) to clean her room thoroughly every Saturday morning. Group home staff also provided psychiatric and mental health treatment. A psychiatric nurse met with her regularly to assess her current symptoms and monitor medications. Her case manager, a clinical social worker, met with her once a week to discuss any problems she was having.

Now Lisa has her own efficiency apartment and receives services from a supported housing program. Initially, she asked staff for a great deal of help in getting settled and learning new routines. For example, her laundry was building up because she wasn't sure how to get it to the laundromat and what to do once she got there. A staff member came over and showed her how to get her laundry done. Then the staff member helped her to write down a step-by-step procedure so Lisa could do it on her own. They then showed her how to fill a weekly medication dispenser and assisted her in establishing a routine for remembering to take her medication. The staff also helped her learn about social and recreational activities in the community that match her interests.

Lisa has now been in her apartment for 3 months and is doing well. Staff members check in with her regularly by phone, but only come over when she asks them to. However, she likes knowing that she can reach someone 24 hours a day, if needed. Lisa sees a psychiatrist once a month, and goes to a weekly support group at a local mental health center. She likes the fact that these treatment services are kept separate from her private home life.

Another important part of the paradigm shift is allowing consumers to take much more control over the services they receive. Supported housing promotes people making choices not only in terms of where they live, but also in terms of what supports are provided, when they are provided, and how they are provided. Consider a typical day at a facility-based program that requires all residents to be up and out of the house by 9:00 A.M., involved in a PsyR day treatment program, or otherwise productively engaged, and home by 4:00 P.M. to help cook dinner and then attend a community meeting. Contrast that picture with a supported housing program in which service recipients are not required to be accountable to support staff about how they spend their day, and where a consumer's preference for having staff visit, at a time convenient for the consumer, is respected. Such a program may support some people who only see staff members occasionally, when they call to request assistance; whereas others, who ask for it, are provided with a more intensive level of services. Notice that in order for a supported housing program to be successful, staff members must truly internalize the PsyR value of self-determination. For many practitioners this involves a shift from thinking that staff members always know what is best for the people they serve to building real partnerships with consumers (Pyke & Lowe, 1996).

PsyR practitioners involved in the provision of supported housing need to be much more active in both accessing and developing a range of community resources. For example, developing good relationships with potential or current landlords and affordable housing developers may increase consumer access to normal community housing. Finding out what supports and social opportunities are available at a local house of worship may provide consumers with information about potentially useful natural support systems. While group home staff may spend some time engaged in these types of activities, they must spend most of their time providing supports within their facilities. Supported housing interventions, on the other hand, provide more opportunities for people to live, work, and socialize with a range of people in their communities.

A number of supported housing programs have employed consumers in a variety of staff positions, including involvement in the provision of direct services and supports (Basto, Pratt, Gill, & Barrett, 2000; Besio & Mahler, 1993; Butler, 1993). Using consumers as staff has a number of benefits including a strong ability to empathize with the day-to-day concerns of other consumers, tolerance of unusual behaviors, and reduced likelihood of maintaining a professional distance in the helping relationship. Each of these benefits can contribute to more comfortable relationships between peer providers and the people they serve, ultimately resulting in superior outcomes. Peer providers have also been found to be highly skilled in obtaining necessary resources and advocacy (Besio & Mahler, 1993). Because of their own experiences, consumer-providers may be better attuned to what consumers need in order to accomplish independent living goals. They may also champion attitudes and behaviors that are respectful of consumers' right to privacy and need to be in control of their own home environment. More information about the use of psychiatric rehabilitation consumers as service providers can be found in Chapter 12.

Among the greatest challenges to the implementation of supported housing are (1) accessing housing that matches consumer preferences, (2) helping people to acquire rental or mortgage assistance, and (3) financing individualized support services. Shifting service provision paradigms not only involves changes in what is provided but also changes in how services are financed. Adopting a supported housing approach may initially seem very expensive because the provision of off-site, individualized services can be less efficient than the provision of standardized, facility-based services. However, when estimating the cost of a service, long-term outcomes must be considered. Consumers who initially require numerous staff hours to get the level of support they need may need very little in the way of staff resources once they have adjusted to their new home and neighborhood, and begin to make use of natural supports.

Accessing and financing enough decent and affordable housing for a local pool of consumers may present the biggest challenge to widespread implementation of supported housing services. As discussed earlier in the chapter, this is a problem throughout the

United States for people who have low incomes. Entitlements such as SSI are not enough to cover average rental costs in most areas. Historically, mental health system resources used for residential treatment have reached only a small percentage of people. So, the issue is not just reallocation of financial resources, it is facing the reality that we need to help consumers locate additional monies to rent or buy homes.

While this is certainly a large barrier to the provision of supported housing, it is not insurmountable. Some states, such as Ohio, have had real success in reallocating capital funding, previously used to build and maintain hospitals, CHMCs, and residential treatment facilities for use in developing integrated housing for consumers. Ohio also successfully used other strategies to increase funding for housing such as attracting federal grant monies and increasing access to federal rent subsidies (Knisley & Fleming, 1993).

Efforts of this type require a tremendous amount of time, energy, and commitment by state department of mental health officials and consumer and family advocates (Knisley & Fleming, 1993). Other states and local communities, including Rhode Island, western Massachusetts, and Madison, Wisconsin, have also successfully increased consumer access to integrated housing. They have done so through use of creative financing strategies such as housing cooperatives, assistance for first-time buyers, rental subsidies, and creative partnerships with state and local housing developers (Carling, 1995). Several states, including New Jersey, have set up *housing trust funds* in order to increase the amount of available and affordable housing for low-income persons with disabilities, including those with severe mental illness. These trust fund dollars are then used to leverage additional state and federal funding as matching funds (Holland, 2005).

Outcomes of the Supported Housing Approach

As mentioned earlier, supported housing is a relatively recent residential service strategy that is still being refined. A 1997 literature review on supported housing by Ogilvie concluded that there are still too few outcome studies on supported housing to draw firm conclusions about the efficacy of the approach. A more recent review of the supported housing literature by Debra Rog (2004) found that the evidence on supported housing is still insufficient. Rog identified, for example, only five studies that used "rigorous" scientific designs. Her review found convincing evidence that supported housing residents were less likely to become homeless, less likely to be hospitalized, and fared better than similar residents in other settings. The findings of three studies (Dickey et al., 1996; Dickey, Latimer, Powers, Gonzalez, & Goldfinger, 1997; Goldfinger et al., 1999;) suggest that housing stability is increased by providing supports rather than by a specific program model. Similarly, Tsemberis and Eisenberg (2000) found that the addition of the supports of an assertive community treatment (ACT) team (see Chapter 7) nearly doubled the rate of housing stability compared to typical residential treatment.

Earlier, supported housing demonstration projects in five states (Ohio, Oregon, Rhode Island, Washington, and Wisconsin) found that consumers reported a high level of satisfaction with their lives (Livingston, Gordon, King, & Srebnik, 1991). Although many of the people receiving services had a history of housing instability, most demonstrated a significant increase in stability once they became involved with the projects. Two critical factors were found to predict housing stability: symptoms and how much input a person had in choosing where he or she lived. The results of this study also suggest that along with providing consumers with opportunities to live in decent homes of their own choosing, communities need to focus on expanded social networks and employment opportunities.

Curtis, McCabe, Fleming, and Carling (1993) interviewed consumers, family members, agency staff, and administrators from seven supported housing demonstration projects in Texas. The most frequently mentioned outcomes were decreases in hospital use and increases in community tenure, access to housing, motivation, hope and empowerment, normal role functioning, and overall quality of life. Consumers also expressed a high level of satisfaction with the services they received.

A subsequent study of the Texas demonstration projects confirmed these initial findings (Texas Department of Mental Health and Mental Retardation, 1994). Utilizing participant data from the year prior to project involvement, and comparing these data to information gathered after 1 year in a supported housing program, this study found that there was an increase in housing stability, level of functioning, and quality of life, as well as a decrease in hospital usage.

A supported housing study by Brown, Ridgway, Anthony, and Rogers (1991) compared a group at high risk for rehospitalization and homelessness with a less disabled group that had requested supported housing services. Both groups significantly decreased their hospital usage in the 6 months following entry into the program, although as might be expected the former group utilized more support services. The authors concluded that the supported housing approach is a viable option even for persons who have severe disabilities.

Much more research needs to be done to determine the outcomes of supported housing services. Because there is still a lack of clear evidence for its efficacy, it is currently considered to be a promising practice (Rog, 2004). However, many consumers and providers believe that even without the research studies to back it up, supported housing programs are worthwhile endeavors because helping individuals find and maintain decent affordable housing is not a form of "treatment." It is a basic human need that profoundly affects the quality of a person's life.

The Independent Living Movement

The previously mentioned paradigm shift, from a linear continuum model of residential programming to a supported housing approach, was inspired in part by the efforts of people with physical disabilities to move away from institutionalized care and find innovative ways to live independently. Deegan (1992) describes the Independent Living (IL) Movement as comprised of three interrelated activities. The first is a grassroots advocacy movement led by people with physical disabilities who banded together and demanded civil rights and opportunities to live, work, and socialize in their communities.

The second piece of IL is a philosophy developed and lived by individuals who have physical disabilities. Some key principles of the IL philosophy follow:

1. Recognize that it is not something internal, such as a spinal cord injury, that prevents people with disabilities from living independently, although certainly these internal factors can make the day-to-day experience of living challenging. Rather, it is external barriers such as stairs, curbs, and stigmatizing attitudes that prevent people from getting places that they want to go.

2. People with disabilities have a right to self-determination. They also have a right to make mistakes and choices that others may identify as risky. Deegan (1992) described a young man with a spinal cord injury and his adjustment to independent living. In the early days he repeatedly tried to do things in his apartment that caused him to fall from a wheelchair and lie on the floor for hours until someone arrived to help. Many professionals would cite these incidents as proof that he could not live by himself. Eventually he learned his own limits and found the accommodations and supports to live more comfortably. Think about the many mistakes made, and risks taken, by people without disabilities as they first move away from the parental home. They may be criticized by their loved ones, but rarely are they threatened with professional interventions aimed at reducing their control over their lives.

3. "Integral to the philosophy of IL is the notion that people with disabilities can become experts in their own self-care. To live independently means to de-medicalize our lives by learning self-care techniques that minimize the medical presence in our daily lives" (Deegan, 1992, p. 16).

The third piece of IL is the existence of independent living centers that provide service delivery, coordinate advocacy efforts, and bring people with disabilities together to tackle mutual concerns. IL centers are primarily run by people with physical disabilities. Deegan (1992) describes her efforts to develop an IL center designed to meet the needs of people with psychiatric disabilities. She emphasizes the importance of establishing both a grassroots movement and a philosophy that are "similar in spirit to what people with physical disabilities discovered for themselves" (p. 17). She is cautious, however, about determining what services IL centers should provide. She does not recommend trying to duplicate what other disability groups have done, nor does she favor a peer-run version of what is offered by the mental health system. Instead, she envisions a new service approach that "will grow out of our emerging sense of what it is we need to regain control over our lives" (p. 17).

Farkas and Chamberlain (1998) have done work applying IL strategies to develop supports for people with psychiatric disabilities. Specifically, they taught consumers to hire, train, and manage personal assistants, in much the same way that people with physical disabilities have utilized personal care assistants. Personal assistance services (PAS) are tailored to meet the unique support needs of a consumer. Examples of services that could be provided include daily reminders about when to wake up and when to take medications, assistance with paying bills and maintaining a budget, and transportation to work. Basically PAS could involve assisting consumers with anything they have difficulty doing because of their illness. Services are provided by nonprofessionals who are hired by and work for the consumer, rather than for the mental health system. Farkas and Chamberlain have developed a curriculum for consumers that helps them to analyze what they need from PAS, hire and train a personal assistant, and manage the employer/employee relationship.

Consistent with the supported housing model, utilization of personal assistance services is a strategy that enables consumers to live independently. When evaluating whether a person with a psychiatric disability is capable of living in an unsupervised setting, it is important to remember that independent living does not necessarily mean going without supports or services. In the words of the late consumer advocate Howie the Harp (see Box 11.1):

> Independence involves freedom to choose, to choose whom to be independent with, for what purpose, and to what extent. Independence is one of this country's founding principles, and it should not be surprising that living independently is a goal of many disabled Americans. Inherent in their definition of independent living is the availability of support services. (Howie the Harp, 1993, p. 413)

BOX 11.1
Howie the Harp

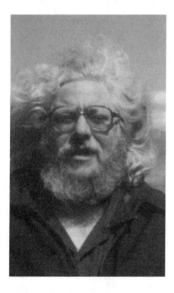

Photo taken by Moe Armstrong

Howie the Harp was a tireless advocate for the rights of people who have severe mental illnesses. His work spanned many areas of PsyR, including supported housing, self-help, and employment (particularly around the issue of reasonable accommodations). Howie was also remarkably effective in his work with individuals who were homeless and had a psychiatric disability. According to a former colleague, he had a unique ability to reach out and connect to people who came from the streets; to give them a voice, and to find ways to get them the things that they most wanted and needed (N. Thomas, personal communication, 1998).

Howie's motivation to help others was deeply rooted in his own experiences. In the words of his friend and colleague, Sally Zinman:

> Having experienced the horrors of being in a mental hospital and being homeless as a boy, he spent the rest of his life advocating for people with mental disabilities (his self definition), homeless and poor people. I don't know if many of us can trace so distinctly our life's pursuits to our childhood experiences. He never wavered in his direction, never took a detour. (Zinman, 1995, p. 1)

Howie became interested in patients' rights advocacy at the age of 16. At the time he had recently escaped from a psychiatric facility in New York City (NYC), following a 3-year involuntary hospitalization. He moved to Oregon, where he was exposed to an advocacy organization called the Insane Liberation Front. At 18 he moved back to NYC to start a local chapter of the advocacy group, the Mental Patients Liberation Project. This led to the opening of a crisis center, which assisted people who were trying to get out of psychiatric institutions.

While working with the Mental Patients Liberation Project, Howie became aware of the thousands of ex-patients enduring atrocious conditions at local SRO hotels. He organized Project Release, a tenant group dedicated to improving living conditions and advocating for residents' rights. Project Release was soon expanded to include a consumer-run drop-in center and a self-help group. The group also obtained several apartments where people could live temporarily while searching for decent housing. All of these accomplishments occurred in the early 1970s, at a time when the ex-patient movement and consumer-run services were still very new ideas. (Chapter 12 traces the history of these efforts.) Howie the Harp was one of the pioneers of PsyR.

When lack of funding opportunities in NYC became a major obstacle, Howie moved to California. There he became involved with supported housing services, working at the California Center for Independent Living (CIL). This was the first of the independent living centers for people with disabilities. He actually began his association with the CIL when he was homeless, and was helped to acquire and maintain housing. In addition to his psychiatric disability, Howie had a physical disability, and was thus uniquely qualified to understand the parallels in the service needs of both populations. One of his insights was that rather than treatment facilities, people with psychiatric disabilities needed access to individualized supports that would enable them to live independently. He was thus inspired to develop the Mental Disabilities Independent Living Program, which was a precursor to the Oakland Independence Support Center (OISC) and also led to other projects. The OISC, which is still flourishing, provides a variety of services to people with psychiatric disabilities who are homeless, or at risk for becoming homeless. Services include a drop-in center that provides a safe alternative to the streets, support services, and independent living services that utilize unique strategies to bring together homeless individuals and landlords who have vacancies (Howie the Harp, 1990). In 1993 Howie left a well-established OISC to return to his home town of NYC and work at a supported housing agency.

Howie had a way of describing himself and his viewpoint that was direct, easy to grasp, and often had a touch of humor:

> I am a former mental patient with a psychiatric disability. That does not describe who I am, but it identifies a profound aspect of my life. I am also a musician, a lover of nature, and a frustrated comedian. At one time I was considered to be "chronically mentally ill," and in need of "treatment" for the rest of my life, most likely never able to live independently, and certainly never able to hold down a full-time job. That was a load of crap. I consider myself to be psychiatrically disabled, but I define disability as the disability rights movement has re-defined the term. I have a condition that is neither positive nor negative—not an illness to be "cured", but a condition that can be accommodated in order to enable me to live the way I choose. (Howie the Harp, 1991, p. 1).

Howie the Harp passed away in 1995 at the age of 42. Though his life was short, his accomplishments were many. His efforts to improve the lives of people with psychiatric disabilities are greatly appreciated.

Housing First

Very much in line with PsyR values and principles, the Housing First strategy is based on consumer choice and harm reduction (see Chapter 8). As with supported employment, consumers are assisted in getting into housing of their choice first, not having to overcome unrelated prerequisites or obstacles first. For example, unlike many other residential services, Housing First does not require persons with a dual diagnosis of mental illness and substance abuse disorder to be substance free before obtaining housing. Instead, housing is obtained as soon as possible and then services are provided to deal with the mental illness and substance abuse.

Tsemberis, Gulcur, and Nakae (2004) tested the housing first strategy by randomly assigning 225 persons with a dual diagnosis to either receive housing contingent on prerequisites (e.g., sobriety) or receive housing without prerequisites. After 2 years it was determined that there were no differences in level of substance abuse between the two groups. Not surprisingly, the group without prerequisites obtained housing much more quickly and, being there longer, demonstrated greater housing stability. The group given prerequisites for housing did have higher substance abuse treatment utilization rates, but apparently did not benefit from the increased level of service.

These results strongly suggest that individuals respond favorably to harm reduction strategies and policies that respect and reinforce their rights as individual members of society. As the authors (Tsemberis et al., 2004) point out: "Consumers are allowed to make choices—to use alcohol or not, to take medication or not—and regardless of their choices they are not treated adversely, their housing status is not threatened, and help continues to be available to them" (p. 653) (see Box 11.2).

BOX 11.2
Sam J. Tsemberis, Ph.D.

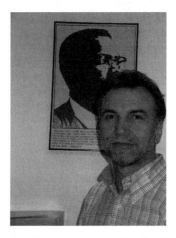

Sam Tsemberis, who founded *Pathways to Housing* in 1992, advocates for housing as a basic right for all people and is credited with establishing the Housing First movement. Pathways to Housing, which he directs, provides immediate access to independent permanent apartments to individuals who are homeless and who have psychiatric disabilities and substance use disorders. Dr. Tsemberis also assists agencies in cities around the nation to develop Housing First programs. These programs successfully demonstrate that providing persons with their own housing is a powerful first step toward recovery, rather than a distant goal to be achieved only after their psychiatric symptoms and addictions have been stabilized.

A faculty member of the Department of Psychiatry at New York University, Dr. Tsemberis' research and innovations have received wide recognition from sources including the Center for Mental Health Services, the National Alliance to End Homelessness, and the United States Interagency Council on Homelessness. In October 2005 Pathways received the American Psychiatric Association's Psychiatric Services Gold Award for first place in community mental health programs. *Pathways to Housing* has been profiled by National Public Radio's *All Things Considered*, the Public Broadcasting System's *Newshour with Jim Lehrer*, and written about in the *New York Times* and the *Christian Science Monitor*. There are currently more than 15 replications of the Pathways program across the country, each achieving remarkable success in ending homelessness for people with psychiatric disabilities. (For more information, see http:// www. pathwaystohousing.org.)

CONTROVERSIAL ISSUE
Is Supported Housing for Everyone? Should Facility-Based Residential Care Continue for People with the Most Severe Disabilities?

Despite the paradigm shift outlined in this chapter and evidence that consumers prefer to live as most people do, in houses or apartments with friends and family (Tanzman, 1993: Yeich et al., 1994), many people still reside in segregated facilities. Furthermore, in some parts of the United States, funding for community-based mental health services is still being channeled into the development of new facility-based residential programs, both transitional residential programs and long-term care facilities. If supported housing is an effective and philosophically sound model, why are many mental health administrators and providers passing it up in favor of outdated models of service? Does the supported housing approach have the capacity to support all people with psychiatric disabilities who need assistance maintaining their home life? Or should it be conceptualized as one option among a wider range of community based residential programs?

Supported Housing as an Option

Supported housing is an important component of a community support system. For many years a major gap in the transitional housing model was a lack of ongoing supports once people graduated from group homes or semi-supervised apartments into the community. The ongoing, as-needed supports provided by the supported housing model do a great deal to help people who are ready to live independently to maintain their community tenure. However, some people with severe mental illness are either not ready to live independently or prefer congregate living arrangements (Tanzman, 1993). For example, people who have spent many years in an institution, are accustomed to being extremely dependent on hospital staff, and may be reluctant to leave an institutionalized setting. For these individuals, a small (fewer than eight people) group home staffed by people who are familiar with the needs of people who have severe psychiatric disabilities can ease the stress of moving from an institution to the community. Some residents of such a facility may be ready to move on to independent living after a transition period. Others may desire long-term residency in a supervised setting.

People with more than one disability can benefit from around-the-clock supports and services that are more easily accessible in congregate settings than in independent housing. A good example is people who have a severe mental illness and a substance abuse disorder. A residential program that provides external controls and services specifically geared toward their needs can be a key to maintaining sobriety. A supported housing program might be hard pressed to provide the same level of support, which may be helpful during the early phases of recovery.

Individuals who have a disability that is severe enough to require extensive personal care services may benefit from the accessibility of supports and services available in small, congregate care settings. These may be people who have persistent psychotic symptoms that interfere markedly with their ability to care for themselves, or people with multiple disabilities including severe physical impairment (e.g., nonambulatory). While the Independent Living Movement (Deegan, 1992) and the experiences of supported living agencies that assist people with developmental disabilities (O'Brien & O'Brien, 1994) show that people with severe disabilities who need a high level of daily personal assistance can live independently, the current service structure can make it extremely difficult to do so. Hiring an around-the-clock personal care assistant or a home health aide for a single individual can be very costly. Many insurance plans do not cover such services. Skilled and reliable care may be hard to find. Group homes with 24-hour staff coverage might be better equipped to solve these problems and provide services more easily affordable to residents with limited resources.

Contrasting Viewpoint: Supported Housing Is Preferred for Everyone

Supported housing is a flexible, individualized model that can be adapted to the needs of everyone. It can be used by persons with varying levels of disability, but it is important to keep in mind that "the more severely disabled the client, the more critical the need for an individualized approach" (Carling & Ridgway, 1991, p. 71). Supported housing is really about finding solutions to everyday problems. Some of these problems are just tougher to solve than others.

A lesson can be learned from the field of developmental disabilities. This field has evolved from an era of lifetime institutionalization through a stage of deinstitutionalization, in which people were served in settings physically integrated into the community, but still fostered social segregation (i.e., group homes, sheltered workshops). The next stage in its evolution has been full community membership for individuals who have a developmental disability (Bradley, 1994). This approach stresses that community membership is everyone's right, not just a privilege reserved for people who are capable of a particular level of functioning. Keep in mind that some people with developmental disabilities have profound cognitive deficits and/or severe physical limitations. Nonetheless, local service systems have had real success in shifting from a residential treatment model to "supportive living," which is conceptually and practically similar to the supported housing approach (Carmody, 1994; O'Brien & O'Brien, 1994).

In Illinois, a project dubbed SPICE (Supported Placements in Integrated Community Environments) was created to help a group of people with severe cognitive and/or mobility impairments move from a nursing home into regular community housing (Carmody, 1994). The participants in the SPICE project were specifically selected because of the fact that they had severe and multiple disabilities, because the project sought to demonstrate that community integration could become a reality for the people considered to be the most disabled. From the very beginning of the project, the participants' input and involvement was sought. Some of them chose to live with families, others chose to live alone, still others opted for a roommate who was another project participant (such a decision had to be mutual). Participants helped interview and hire personal care assistants and other support staff. They were also assisted in accessing existing community resources (churches, community colleges, etc.). Outcome study results showed a significant gain in community living skills and a tremendous increase in satisfaction with their living arrangement. The project demonstrated "that anyone with disabilities can live in the community and that the community has the capacity to meet the needs of anyone, including people for whom nursing facilities had been thought the only 'appropriate' residential option" (Carmody, 1994, p. 479).

The history of service provision for people with psychiatric disabilities is clearly quite similar to that of people with developmental disabilities. However, the mental health system has not yet made as strong a commitment to the goal of community membership for all persons with psychiatric disabilities. The many obstacles include housing shortages, the high financial cost of providing in-home assistance (particularly to people who may need round-the-clock services), community opposition due to stigma, and the resistance of service providers who are reluctant to make major changes in how they think and operate. None of these obstacles is insurmountable, yet they often become excuses for maintaining the status quo. Supported housing is for everyone because all of us deserve the right to live in a place that is truly a home.

Summary

From the mid-19th century to the 1960s, most people who had a severe mental illness spent a good part of their lives residing in psychiatric institutions. Once deinstitutionalization began, a key question was "Where should consumers live?" Some consumers returned to their families, who were often ill prepared for their service and support needs. Other consumers were placed in boarding homes, nursing homes, and SROs where their quality of life was often little better and sometimes worse than what they left behind in the hospitals. A relatively small percentage of consumers were given residential treatment. Most of these housing options resulted in transinstitutionalization" (Carling, 1995, p. 33), meaning that true community integration was not realized.

By the 1980s the preferred model of residential treatment was the linear continuum, which moved consumers through a series of placements that became progressively less supervised and restrictive. The goal of this approach was graduation to independent living, typically without any ongoing support. Eventually it became clear that this model was not meeting the needs of most consumers. The field of PsyR now embraces a more normalized and individualized way to assist consumers in finding and maintaining homes. It is called *supported housing*. This approach seeks to support consumers in the home environments of their choice. Supported housing emphasizes integrated, long-term housing options. The philosophy of the supported housing approach is similar to the values and principles articulated by the Independent Living Movement begun by people who have physical disabilities.

PsyR practitioners who work in supported housing programs do not provide treatment, which is available elsewhere in the mental health system. Nor do they provide supervision, which is not wanted or needed by the vast majority of people with psychiatric disabilities. Instead, supported housing assists consumers in developing skills and obtaining the resources and supports that they want and need in their particular living situation. Supported housing is philosophically and practically similar to supported employment and supported education (see Chapters 9 and 10, respectively, for more on these approaches).

Finally, the success of new initiatives such as Housing First suggests that attending to the basic desire for a safe place of one's own is consistent with the values of PsyR such as self-determination and respect for the dignity and worth of each individual. Housing First has important implications for service design, particularly the lack of the need to make living arrangements dependent on treatment services. Given the complexities of housing, individualized services should be the rule rather than the exception.

Despite barriers such as stigma, community opposition, and lack of access to financial resources, supported housing brings real hope to consumers who want to live, learn, work, and socialize in the same ways as nondisabled members of their communities.

Class Exercise
Designing an Ideal Residential Services Program

Imagine that you serve on a newly formed board of directors for a new residential services program. Your target population is adults who have a long history of a severe mental illness and are currently at high risk for psychiatric hospitalization and/or homelessness. Thus, you can assume that the people you will be providing services for have had a great deal of difficulty residing in the community because they are psychiatrically unstable, have severe functional deficits, have other issues such as problems with substance abuse, or most likely some combination of these. Your task is to determine what type of residential services you want to provide and provide a clear rationale for your choices. Consider the following questions:

1. Do you want to establish group homes, develop a supervised or semi-supervised apartment complex, help individuals acquire regular homes in the community, or some combination of these?
2. If you choose to utilize facility-based housing, will it be transitional (i.e., residents must move on after a specified time period) or long term?
3. What types of services will the staff provide? How often will they be present in resident's living environments (e.g., 24-hour coverage? as-needed visits?)?

References

Basto, P. W., Pratt, C. W., Gill, K. J., & Barrett, N. M. (2000). The organizational assimilation of consumer providers: A quantitative assessment. *Psychiatric Rehabilitation Skills, 4*(1), 105–119.

Besio, S. W., & Mahler, J. (1993). Benefits and challenges of using consumer staff in supported housing services. *Hospital and Community Psychiatry, 44*(5), 490–491.

Boydell, K. M., Gladstone, B. M., Crawford, E., & Trainor, J. (1999). Making do on the outside: Everyday life in the neighborhoods of people with psychiatric disabilities. *Psychiatric Rehabilitation Journal, 23*(1), 11–17.

Bradley, V. J. (1994). Evolution of a new service paradigm. In V. J. Bradley, J. W. Ashbaugh, & B. C. Blaney (Eds.), *Creating individual supports for people with developmental disabilities.* Baltimore, MD: Paul H. Brookes Publishing.

Brown, M. A., Ridgway, P., Anthony, W. A., & Rogers, E. S. (1991). Comparison of outcomes for clients seeking and assigned to supported housing services. *Hospital and Community Psychiatry, 42*(11), 1150–1153.

Butler, W. (1993). The consumer supported housing model in New Jersey (the cornerstone to a new paradigm). *Innovations & Research, 2*(3), 73–75.

Campbell, M. E. (1981). The three-quarterway house: A step beyond halfway house toward independent living. *Hospital & Community Psychiatry, 32*(7), 500–501.

Carling, P. J. (1990). Supported housing: An evaluation agenda. *Psychosocial Rehabilitation Journal, 13*(4), 95–104.

Carling, P. J. (1993). Housing and supports for persons with mental illness: Emerging approaches to research and practice. *Hospital and Community Psychiatry, 44*(5), 439–449.

Carling, P. J. (1994). Supports and rehabilitation for housing and community living. In the Publication Committee of IAPSRS (Eds.), *An introduction to psychiatric rehabilitation.* Columbia MD: International Association of Psychosocial Rehabilitation Services.

Carling, P. J. (1995). *Return to community: Building support systems for people with psychiatric disabilities.* New York: The Guilford Press.

Carling, P. J., & Ridgway, P. (1991). A psychiatric rehabilitation approach to housing. In M. D. Farkas & W. A. Anthony (Eds.), *Psychiatric rehabilitation programs: Putting theory into practice.* Baltimore, MD: The Johns Hopkins University Press.

Carmody, K. (1994). Creating individual supports for people moving out of nursing facilities: supported placements in integrated community environments (SPICE). In V. J. Bradley, J. W. Ashbaugh, & B. C. Blaney (Eds.), *Creating individual supports for people with developmental disabilities*. Baltimore, MD: Paul H. Brookes Publishing.

Chamberlin, J. (1978). *On our own: Patient controlled alternatives to the mental health system*. New York; Hawthorne Press.

Cnaan, R. A., Blankertz, L., Messinger, K. W., & Gardner, J. R. (1988). Psychosocial rehabilitation: Toward a definition. *Psychosocial Rehabilitation Journal, 11*(4), 61–77.

Collaborative Support Programs of New Jersey (1991). *Consumer housing preference survey*. Freehold, NJ: Author.

Collaborative Support Programs of New Jersey (1996). *Boarding home resident survey for Monmouth and Ocean counties*. Freehold, NJ: Author.

Cook, J. R. (1997). Neighbors' perceptions of group homes. *Community Mental Health Journal, 33*(4), 287–299.

Cooper, E., Herb, M., & O'Hara, A. (2003). *Solutions that work: Innovative strategies to meeting the housing needs of people with disabilities* (Opening Doors: A Housing Publication for the Disability Community No. 23). A joint publication of The Technical Assistance Collaborative, Boston MA; and The Consortium for Citizens with Disabilities. Washington, D.C.

Cooper, E., & O'Hara, A. (2003). *Priced out in 2002: Housing crisis worsens for people with disabilities* (Opening Doors: A Housing Publication for the Disability Community No. 21). A joint publication of The Technical Assistance Collaborative, Boston MA; and The Consortium for Citizens with Disabilities. Washington, D.C.

Curtis, L. C., McCabe, S. S., Fleming, M., & Carling, P. J. (1993). *Implementing the supported housing approach: An impact evaluation of the Texas supported housing demonstration initiative*. Burlington, VT: Trinity College, Center for Community Change through Housing and Support.

Deegan, P. E. (1992). The Independent Living Movement and people with psychiatric disabilities: Taking back control over our own lives. *Psychosocial Rehabilitation Journal, 15*(3), 3–19.

Dickey, B., Gonzalez, O., Latimer, E., Powers, K., Schutt, R., & Goldfinger, S. M. (1996). Use of mental health services by formerly homeless adults residing in group and independent housing. *Psychiatric Services, 47*(2), 152–148.

Dickey, B., Latimer, E., Powers, K., Gonzalez, O., & Goldfinger, S. M. (1997). Housing costs for adults who are mentally ill and formerly homeless. *Journal of Mental Health Administration, 24*(3), 291–305.

Fairweather, G. W., Saunders, D. H., Maynard, H., & Cressler, D. L. (1969). *Community life for the mentally ill*. Chicago: Aldine.

Farkas, M., & Chamberlin, J. (1998, May). *Developing supports, not just skill, through personal assistance services*. Paper presented at the VI World Congress, World Association for Psychosocial Rehabilitation, Hamburg, Germany.

Goldfinger, S. M., & Schutt, R. K. (1996). Comparison of clinicians' housing recommendations and preferences of homeless mentally ill persons. *Psychiatric Services, 47*(4), 413–415.

Goldfinger, S. M., Schutt, R. K., Tolomiczenko, G. S., Seidman, L., Penk, W. E., Turner, W., & Caplan, B. (1999). Housing placement and subsequent days homeless among formerly homeless adults with mental illness. *Psychiatric Services, 50*(5), 674–679.

Goldman, H. H., Gattozzi, A. A., & Taube, C. A. (1981). Defining and counting the chronically mentally ill. *Hospital and Community Psychiatry, 32*(1), 22–27.

Holland P. (2005). Personal communication.

Honberg, R. (2004). *Advocates praise efforts to address criminalization of people with mental illness* (Campaign for Mental Health Reform press release). National Alliance on Mental Illness, Arlington, VA.

Hopper, K., & Barrow, S. M. (2003). Two genealogies of supported housing and their implications for outcome assessment. *Psychiatric Services, 54*(1), 50–54.

Howie the Harp. (1990). Independent living with support services: The goal and future for mental health consumers. *Psychosocial Rehabilitation Journal, 13*(4), 85–89.

Howie the Harp. (1991). *A crazy folks guide to reasonable accommodation and "psychiatric disability."* Burlington, VT: Trinity College, Center for Community Change through Housing and Support.

Howie the Harp. (1993). Taking a new approach to independent living. *Hospital and Community Psychiatry, 44*(5), 413.

Knisley, M. B., & Fleming, M. (1993). Implementing supported housing in state and local mental health systems. *Hospital & Community Psychiatry, 44*(5), 456–461.

Lamb, H. R. (1982). *Treating the long-term mentally ill.* San Francisco: Jossey-Bass.

Lehman, A. F., Ward, N. C., & Linn, L. S. (1982). Chronic mental patients: The quality of life issue. *American Journal of Psychiatry, 139*(10), 1271–1276.

Linn, M. W., Klett, C. J., & Caffey, E. M. (1980). Foster home characteristics and psychiatric patient outcome. *Archives of General Psychiatry, 37*(2), 129–132.

Livingston, J. A., Gordon, L. R., King, D. A., & Srebnik, D. S. (1991). *Implementing the supported housing approach: a national evaluation of NIMH supported housing demonstration projects.* Burlington, VT: Trinity College, Center for Community Change through Housing and Support.

Mize, T. I., Paolo-Calabrese, M. A., Williams, T. J., & Margolin, H. K. (1998). Managing the landlord role: How can one agency provide both rehabilitation services and housing collaboration. *Psychiatric Rehabilitation Journal, 22*(2), 117–122.

O'Brien, J., & O'Brien, C. L. (1994). More than just a new address: Images of organization for supported living agencies. In V. J. Bradley, J. W. Ashbaugh, & B. C. Blaney (Eds.), *Creating individual supports for people with developmental disabilities.* Baltimore, MD: Paul H. Brookes Publishing.

Ogilvie, R. J. (1997). The state of supported housing for mental health consumers: A literature review. *Psychiatric Rehabilitation Journal, 21*(2), 122–131.

Onaga, E. E. (1994). The Fairweather lodge as a psychosocial program in the 1990s. In the Publication Committee of IAPSRS (Eds.), *An introduction to psychiatric rehabilitation.* Columbia MD: International Association of Psychosocial Rehabilitation Services.

Onaga, E. E., & Smith, B. A.(2000). Reinvention of the lodge program: A case study of program changes to promote full-time employment. *Psychiatric Rehabilitation Skills, 4*(1), 41–60.

Parrish, J. (1990). Supported housing: A critical component of effective community support. *Psychosocial Rehabilitation Journal, 13*(4), 9–10.

Pyke, J., & Lowe, J. (1996) Supporting people, not structures: Changes in the provision of supportive housing. *Psychiatric Rehabilitation Journal, 19*(3), 5–12.

Ridgway, P., & Zipple, A. M. (1990). The paradigm shift in residential services: From the linear continuum to supported housing approaches. *Psychosocial Rehabilitation Journal, 13*(4), 11–31.

Rog, D. J. (2004). The evidence on supported housing. *Psychiatric Rehabilitation Journal, 27*(4), 334–344.

Tanzman, B. (1993). An overview of surveys of mental health consumers' preferences for housing and support services. *Hospital and Community Psychiatry, 44*(5), 450–455.

Texas Department of Mental Health and Mental Retardation, Research and Special Projects (1994, January). *TXMHMR supported housing program evaluation: Year one findings.* Austin, TX: Author.

Tsemberis, S., & Eisenberg, R. F. (2000). Pathways to housing: Supported housing for street-dwelling homeless individuals with psychiatric disabilities. *Psychiatric Services, 51*(4), 487–493.

Tsemberis, S., Gulcur, L., & Nakae, M. (2004). Housing first, consumer choice, and harm reduction for homeless individuals with a dual diagnosis. *American Journal of Public Health, 94*(4), 651–656.

Torrey, E. F. (2001). *Surviving schizophrenia.* New York: HarperCollins.

Wolfensberger, W. (1983). Social role valorization: A proposed new term for the principle of normalization. *Mental Retardation, 21*(6), 235–239.

Yeich, S., Mowbray, C. T., Bybee, D., & Cohen, E. (1994). The case for a "supported housing" approach: A study of consumer housing and support preferences. *Psychosocial Rehabilitation Journal, 18*(2), 75–86.

Zinman, S. (1995, Spring/Summer). The legacy of Howie the Harp lives on. *National Empowerment Center Newsletter*, pp. 1–9.

Zippay, A. (1997). Trends in siting strategies. *Community Mental Health Journal, 33*(4), 301–310.

Chapter 12

Self-Help and Peer-Delivered Services

Introduction *336*

Defining Self-Help and Peer Support *336*

The History of the Self-Help Movement *338*

Self-Advocacy and the Ex-Patient/ Consumer/Survivor Movement *339*

Collaboration between Consumers and Providers *342*

Self-Help for Persons with Dual Diagnoses *345*

Access to Self-Help *346*

The Story of David *347*

Beyond Self-Help: Categories of Peer-Provided Services *349*

Peer-Operated Services 349

Peer Partnerships 351

Peer Employees 352

Research on the Effectiveness of Self-Help and Peer-Delivered Services *352*

Research on Self-Help Groups 353

Peer-Provided Services: Feasibility and Perceived Benefits 353

Are Peer Providers as Effective as Other Providers? 354

Are Peer-Delivered Services Better Than Other Services? 355

Benefits to Peer Providers and Mental Health Systems 356

Limitations of the Studies and Ongoing Research Challenges 357

Challenges for Peer Providers *358*

Relationships with Nonconsumer Providers 359

The Issue of Disclosure 360

Supports and Professional Development *362*

Other Influential Roles for Consumers *364*

Summary *366*

Class Exercises *367*

References *367*

This chapter outlines the important contributions that people who have been diagnosed with a psychiatric disability make to their own rehabilitation and the rehabilitation of others. Like the field of alcoholism and drug addiction treatment, there is a long tradition of mutual self-help among persons who have severe mental illnesses. Today, consumers are also moving into professional psychiatric rehabilitation service provider positions in larger numbers. They are involved in operating peer support agencies, participating on boards of directors, and conducting sophisticated research. Consumer involvement in all aspects of the rehabilitation process is a fundamental principle of psychiatric rehabilitation (PsyR) that is being increasingly achieved.

This chapter will answer the following questions:

1. *How have self-help groups and the self-advocacy movement influenced PsyR?*
2. *What types of PsyR services are provided by people in recovery?*
3. *What are some of the important issues related to peer-provided services?*
4. *What are some of the benefits and challenges of peer-provided services?*
5. *Should a practitioner who has a mental illness diagnosis disclose his or her condition to other professionals?*

Introduction

People who are diagnosed with severe mental illnesses have a long tradition of participating in *self-help* and mutual support initiatives. Despite the history of stigma associated with these illnesses, consumers of psychiatric rehabilitation services, like their counterparts in alcohol and drug rehabilitation, are moving into professional service provider roles in larger numbers. The issues they face as they take on these new challenges are both complex and exciting. As many who have studied peer support and peer-delivered services have pointed out, these developments potentially represent real empowerment and an affirmation of the principles of psychiatric rehabilitation as described in Chapter 4.

This chapter will explore the concepts of self-help and peer-provided services. It will also review research findings regarding the benefits of peer-provided services, explore the various roles in the service delivery system that are filled by peer employees and volunteers, and examine the effect of being a consumer-provider on one's own recovery—including the positive impact and the challenges that must be faced.

Defining Self-Help and Peer Support

Persons who have severe mental illnesses can both help themselves and assist others in coping with the symptoms and challenges of severe mental illnesses.

> Self-help is an attempt by people with a mutual problem to take control over the circumstances of their lives. Founded on the principle that people who share a disability have something to offer each other that professionals cannot provide, self-help efforts take many forms. (Segal, Silverman, & Temkin, 1993, p. 705)

Most forms of self-help emphasize the benefits of mutual support among a group of people dealing with similar concerns. Some of these benefits can also be found in traditional therapy and counseling groups and include the experience of commonality (i.e., recognizing that you are not the only one experiencing difficulties), a sense of belonging, sharing of ideas and resources, opportunities to develop social skills, and increased opportunities to receive constructive feedback (Jacobs, Masson, & Harvill, 2005). Self-help groups have unique benefits as well, including the promotion of empowerment and a chance to establish ongoing friendships, which may be discouraged in professionally run groups. Many people who have a mental illness participate in self-help groups in part because they feel they can be more open and honest with their peers than with professionals. Exposure to role models who are managing their illnesses and leading satisfying lives is also an important benefit (Davidson et al., 1999; Deegan, 1993).

Peer support is a term commonly used in the PsyR literature to describe self-help initiatives. Mead, Hilton, and Curtis (2001) offer an insightful definition of peer support:

> Peer support is a system of giving and receiving help founded on key principles of respect, shared responsibility and mutual agreement of what is helpful. Peer support is not based on psychiatric models and diagnostic criteria. It is about understanding another's situation empathically through the shared experience of emotional and psychological pain. When people identify with others who they feel are "like" them, they feel a connection. This connection, or affiliation, is a deep, holistic understanding based on mutual experience where people are able to "be" with each other without the constraints of traditional (expert/patient) relationships. Further, as trust in the relationship builds, both people are able to respectfully challenge each other when they find themselves in conflict. This allows members of the peer community to try out new behaviors with one another and move beyond previously held self concepts built on disability and diagnosis. (p. 135)

This definition helps explain why peer support can be an essential resource in the recovery process for many individuals who are trying to reestablish a positive self-concept while struggling with a mental illness.

Experts in field of PsyR have identified a number of well-accepted theories that explain why peer support has the potential to provide many unique benefits (Salzer et al., 2002; Solomon, 2004). These include the following:

- *Social learning theory* (Bandura, 1977) emphasizing the importance of modeling of desirable actions
- *Social comparison theory* (Festinger, 1954), which says that people like to develop relationships with those who have had similar experiences
- *Experiential knowledge* (Borkman, 1999), which states that learning from personal experience adds a level of understanding beyond what can be gained from observation and research.
- *Helper-therapy principle* (Reissman, 1965; Skovholt, 1974) discusses the benefits for the helper attained by helping others
- *Social support theory* (Sarason, Levine, Basham, & Sarason, 1983) focuses on the various types of support that people rely on including emotional, instrumental, informational, companionship, and validation.

Some self-help strategies can be undertaken by individuals without the assistance of their peers. These approaches utilize written materials and structured tools to help individuals learn to cope with their illness and lead healthy, satisfying lives. The *Wellness and*

Recovery Action Plan, commonly referred to as *WRAP,* is probably the best known example of this type of self-help and will be explored later in this chapter (Copeland, 1997).

The History of the Self-Help Movement

Self-help and mutual support among persons coping with severe mental illnesses has been an important part of psychiatric rehabilitation since the field's beginning. In fact, there are some peer support initiatives that predate the establishment of PsyR as a distinct practice. For example, the group of ex-psychiatric patients described in Chapter 6, who dubbed themselves WANA (We Are Not Alone) in the 1940s, and then went on to establish Fountain House, began as a self-help group.

Alcoholics Anonymous (AA), founded in 1935, is the oldest self-help organization in the United States (Robertson, 1988). Another early self-help initiative was started by a psychiatrist named Abraham Low. In the 1930s Low developed a treatment method similar to what is now known as cognitive-behavioral therapy. He worked with people who suffered from a wide range of mental and emotional disorders, teaching them to control their symptoms and take responsibility for their lives. His methods are outlined in *Mental Health through Will Training* (Low, 1950). In 1952, two years before his death, he founded Recovery Inc., the second oldest self-help organization in the United States, which concentrated on the self-help aspect of his treatment.

Over the years, Recovery Inc. has grown into an international organization totally run by its members. In meetings, members share examples of everyday life situations where they have applied Recovery Inc. principles. They share their stories in four steps. In the first step the members summarize situations that trigger emotional distress. In the second step members specify symptoms that they experienced. The third step involves relabeling diagnoses, symptoms, and stressful situations using Recovery Inc. terminology. For example, a person diagnosed with bipolar disorder might stop referring to himself as a "manic-depressive" and instead say, "I am an average nervous person." This part of the process helps members to cognitively reframe symptoms and situations that they previously experienced as devastating into manageable aspects of their day-to-day functioning. The last step involves members speculating on how they would have handled the situation before they learned self-help techniques (Ackerman, 1997). Recovery Inc. is an important resource for people who are recovering from a variety of mental illnesses (Lee, 1995).

A number of successful self-help initiatives have developed outside of the United States. In 1957, a mutual support organization dubbed GROW was established in Australia by ex-patients (Finn & Bishop, 2001). GROW groups are similar to Recovery Inc. and AA groups in that they are highly structured, offer members a strong sense of community, encourage the sharing of personal stories, and utilize materials developed by the members of the organization. GROW, Inc., like AA, has a *Blue Book* that helps members apply personal growth and problem-solving strategies. There are now more than 300 mutual support groups operated by GROW in Australia, and more than 200 GROW groups in other countries, including the United States (Finn & Bishop, 2001). Other well known self-help initiatives include Schizophrenics Anonymous, which has been in existence for more than 20 years and includes at least 70 groups in the United States and Canada (http://www.schizophrenia.com) and the Depressive and Bipolar Support Alliance, which consists of more than 1,000 consumer-run support groups (http://www. dbsalliance.org).

In the mid-1970s peer support initiatives got a boost when the National Institute of Mental Health (NIMH) sponsored a conference focused on the identification of essential supports and services needed by people being discharged from psychiatric hospitals. It was one of the first times that consumers of mental health services were invited to the table to participate in discussions about mental health systems. At the conference, and in subsequent publications, peer support was identified as one of the 10 essential ingredients of an ideal community support system (Stroul, 1989, 1993; Turner, 1977). Community support systems are described in Chapter 7.

Throughout the 1980s federal funding supported the expansion of self-help initiatives throughout the United States. The Substance Abuse and Mental Health Services Administration's Center for Mental Health Services' (SAMHSA/CMHS') Community Support Program provided technical assistance to a number of consumer-run programs and also funded various demonstration projects in order to promote the development of self-help groups and other innovative peer support programs (Brown & Parrish, 1995; Schmidt, 2005; Van Tosh & Del Vecchio, 2000). State mental health authorities also began to support the development of self-help initiatives. For example, in the early 1980s, the New Jersey Division of Mental Health Services provided funding needed to open and operate drop-in centers, now called *self-help centers,* throughout the State (Barrett, Pratt, Basto, & Gill, 2000). Self-help centers are alternative programs that offer a variety of mutual support, social, and advocacy activities. Based on the original drop-in center model, these initiatives now have an expanded focus on wellness, recovery, and employment (Swarbrick, 2005). We will look more closely at self-help centers later in the chapter.

Today peer support initiatives are prominent components of most U.S. state mental health systems. The federal government continues to emphasize the importance of peer support as an adjunct to the conventional mental health system. Two major federal reports, *Mental Health: A Report of the Surgeon General* (U.S. Department of Health and Human Services, 1999) and the final report of the President's New Freedom Commission on Mental Health (2003), recommend the use of peer support to promote recovery-oriented services.

Self-Advocacy and the Ex-Patient/Consumer/Survivor Movement

Self-advocacy can be defined on two levels. When an individual stands up to defend one's own personal or civil rights, including the right to receive high-quality treatment and rehabilitation services, he or she is involved in a form of self-advocacy. The other type of self-advocacy is when people band together to rally support for a common cause. The history of self-advocacy among people coping with severe mental illnesses dates back to mid-19th century England and the formation of the Alleged Lunatic's Friend Society, the first known organization to protest deplorable conditions in psychiatric institutions. Two decades later in the United States, a woman named Elizabeth Packard established the Anti-Insane Asylum Society to protest her forced commitment (Chamberlin, 1990; Frese & Davis, 1997; Van Tosh, Ralph, & Campbell, 2000).

At the beginning of the 20th century, a man named Clifford Beers was hospitalized for treatment of a mental illness and was so dissatisfied with the care he received that he became a lifelong advocate for mental health system reform. In 1909, he helped to establish the National Committee on Mental Hygiene. This organization later became known as the National Mental Health Association, which is still one of the leading advocacy organizations in the United States (Beers, 1923; Schmidt, 2005; Van Tosh et al., 2000).

The civil rights movement of the 1960s helped give rise to the concepts of consumerism and empowerment for persons diagnosed with a mental illness. While this movement may have begun as an effort to combat racism and sexism, it soon spread to other disadvantaged populations such as those confined indefinitely to psychiatric institutions. It was during the height of the civil rights movement that deinstitutionalization was bolstered by the reform of antiquated commitment laws throughout the United States. Many people who were released after long, sometimes abusive, hospital stays found that the services being offered in outpatient settings were not meeting their needs. Problems such as overmedication, the stigmatizing attitudes of mental health professionals, diagnoses that became negative labels, and limited treatment options undermined their efforts to adjust to the community and lead successful, satisfying lives.

Increasing numbers of ex-patients began to search for alternatives, and by the early 1970s the *ex-patient movement*, also referred to as the *survivor movement,* had begun (Rogers, 1996). Early on, some of the names of local grassroots organizations included the Mental Patients' Liberation Front, the Alliance for the Liberation of Mental Patients, and the Network against Psychiatric Assault (Chamberlin, 1984). These names give us a clear sense of the members' attitudes toward the mental health system and their need to regain control over their lives.

In contrast to the ex-patient groups that adamantly opposed existing mental health systems, some self-help and self-advocacy organizations developed with support from mental health professionals and administrators. Some peer-run initiatives operated groups in conjunction with traditional mental health services sharing space, resources, and mutual referrals. However, some people involved in the ex-patient movement continued to maintain that separation from the mental health system was essential. Judi Chamberlin (1984), a well-known activist for more than 30 years, stated "Many of us in the ex-patient movement believe that it is only outside the mental health system that self-help and mutual support can flourish" (p. 56).

In her book *On Our Own*, Chamberlin (1988) described both her personal experiences as a psychiatric inpatient and her involvement in some of these early self-advocacy initiatives. She described how "consciousness-raising" groups, which were not unlike those inspired by the women's movement, helped people labeled as mentally ill recognize the negative effects that the mental health system had on their self-image. Such groups helped ex-patients rebuild their self-esteem and inspired action such as the development and publication of a patients' rights handbook. Other groups led to the development of peer-run drop-in centers, communal residences, and projects focused on publicizing the deplorable conditions of mental institutions (Chamberlin, 1988).

The ex-patient's movement has continued to make progress in its quest to provide people coping with mental illnesses and emotional problems with support and service options that are separate from the professionally driven mental health system. While self-help group opportunities had flourished for many years, alternative programs, such as drop-in centers and peer-run residential programs, were very difficult to start up and maintain without reliable funding sources. In many places, "mental health departments were highly skeptical of the ability of ex-patients to run their own projects" (Chamberlin, 1990, p. 326). In other places where state mental health departments became interested in funding these services, the funding source became a controversial issue for many ex-patient groups. Some people objected, in principle, to establishing relationships with traditional funding sources because of the associated accountability and the possibility of being co-opted. Another concern was the creation of salaried staff positions in peer-run organizations where previously members had all shared the same status as peer volunteers.

By the early 1980s, however, people involved in the ex-patient movement began to establish greater credibility as presenters at national conferences, articulate participants in legislative hearings, and as members of key boards and committees throughout the United States. Gradually, funding opportunities such as Community Support Program grants from NIMH (later from CMHS) to fund demonstration projects, as well as funding from state mental health or vocational rehabilitation departments, became available.

Several prominent consumer-run organizations have been supported by CMHS funding. One of these, the National Empowerment Center (NEC) is a nonprofit organization located in Lawrence, Massachusetts, that was founded by and is primarily run by consumer/survivors. Its mission is to carry a message of recovery, empowerment, hope, and healing to people with psychiatric disabilities, their friends and family members, professionals, and the general public (http://www.Power2u.org). There are now five consumer-run advocacy and technical assistance centers that are supported by CMHS funding. These are the other four:

- National Mental Health Consumers' Self-Help Clearinghouse in Philadelphia, Pennsylvania
- Consumer Organization and Networking Technical Assistance Center (CONTAC) in Charleston, West Virginia
- Peer-to-Peer Resource Center in Chicago, which is part of the Depression and Bipolar Support Alliance (DBSA)
- Support Technical Assistance Resource Center, known as the STAR Center in Arlington, Virginia.

These organizations are involved in national and local advocacy efforts. They provide consumers with information and access to peer support and offer technical assistance to peer support initiatives. These centers also rotate the sponsorship of the annual *Alternatives Conference*. Since 1985, the Alternatives Conference has been bringing together consumers from all over the United States who are involved in a variety of peer support initiatives, thus giving them a chance to network and share innovative ideas.

Early mutual support/self-help initiatives and self-advocacy organizations started independently of each other, but they have since grown together and become intertwined. With increased funding and partnerships, the ex-patient movement has been able to involve itself in the provision of a wide array of services and supports (Chamberlin, 1990; Chamberlin, Rogers, & Ellison, 1996). Today, many peer support initiatives combine mutual support activities and peer-provided services, which we will explore later in this chapter, with advocacy activities. Thus consumers are not only strengthening their own personal support systems and assisting their peers, they are also helping to create stronger mental health systems by advocating for additional resources, rehabilitation and recovery-oriented services, and the protection of their civil rights. In recent years, key advocacy issues have included opposition to involuntary treatment, use of restraints and seclusion in psychiatric hospitals, and housing and employment discrimination. The motto "Nothing about us, without us" is often used by members of the consumer/survivor movement to emphasize the importance of consumer empowerment (Campbell, 2005).

Collaboration between Consumers and Providers

Self-help initiatives have gained both momentum and credibility in recent years, and have become essential elements in the recovery of many people who have severe mental illnesses. For some, self-help groups and other peer support services are an important adjunct to the professional psychiatric and rehabilitation services that they receive. For others, peer support initiatives represent a true alternative to the mental health system.

PsyR providers and mental health administrators refer people to peer support services and collaborate with consumers in developing such services for two important reasons: (1) They recognize that supports outside the mental health system are essential to the recovery process, and (2) they see it as a cost-effective way to provide people with additional supports, particularly during an era of dwindling mental health dollars (Kaufman, Freund, & Wilson, 1989). According to Joseph A. Rogers (1996), executive director of the National Mental Health Consumers' Self-Help Clearinghouse, "Consumer-run services are perfectly positioned to fill the service gap resulting from state and local cost-control measures such as managed care if consumers are educated and supported in their efforts to expand existing consumer-run projects, launch new ones, and test new models" (p. 22). However, it is important to keep in mind that there is a danger in promoting peer-delivered services primarily as a cost-cutting strategy. There is the potential to take advantage of and exploit peer providers. If consumers are providing the same types of services as other professionals, they should receive comparable compensation for their efforts (Lundin, 2005; Solomon, 2004).

Despite a trend toward increased acceptance of peer support initiatives, sometimes the attitudes of mental health professionals interfere with both the utilization and further development of self-help efforts. Some of the concerns that professionals may have about self-help efforts may stem from the following:

- A lack of information about key self-help initiatives (Lee, 1995) and the efficacy of such services
- Underestimation of the abilities of consumers as service providers, for example, dismissing them as second-class workers (Solomon & Draine, 1996; Mowbray et al., 1996)
- Negative reactions to efforts associated with the ex-patient movement, such as concern that rebellion and noncompliance with treatment will be promoted (Kaufman et al., 1989; Mowbray, Wellwood & Chamberlain, 1988).

BOX 12.1
Patricia Deegan

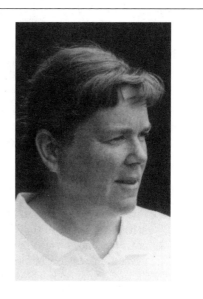

Dr. Patricia Deegan is an independent consultant who specializes in recovery and the empowerment of individuals diagnosed with mental illness. She is affiliated with the Boston University Institute for the Study of Human Resilience, the University of Kansas School of Welfare, and Advocates for Human Potential, Inc. She received her doctorate in clinical psychology from Duquesne University. She also established an award-winning program for people with psychiatric disabilities within the Northeast Independent Living Center (see Chapter 11 for more on the Independent Living Movement). Dr. Deegan is an activist in the ex-patient movement and cofounder of the National Empowerment Center (NEC), Inc. Between 1992 and 2001, she held the position of director of training at the NEC. Dr. Deegan has also published numerous journal articles and is a much sought-after consultant and lecturer. She has inspired thousands of mental health professionals, students, consumers, and family members in her speaking engagements throughout the United States, Canada, Europe, Israel, New Zealand, and Australia. Dr. Deegan has also lived her own journey of recovery from schizophrenia.

Deegan was first diagnosed with schizophrenia as a teenager and was hospitalized on several occasions. In her writing, she describes her experiences as dehumanizing, and the initial stages of her recovery as fraught with long periods of hopelessness and despair. Deegan's experiences, and the stories of other people with disabilities, led her to the realization that recovery is often impeded by mental health professionals whose low expectations and well-meaning but coercive interventions prevent people from achieving true independence.

Deegan initially chose to work in a traditional mental health program and tried to change the system from within. She decided, at that time, not to disclose her illness to her colleagues. Eventually, she became frustrated with both her attempts to help consumers within a system that frequently disempowered and stigmatized consumers, and with efforts to keep her struggle with her illness concealed. She began to speak at conferences about her experiences as a provider—and a consumer.

Deegan left traditional practice and became active in the consumer/survivor movement, becoming a founding member of M-POWER (Massachusetts People/Patients Organized for Wellness, Empowerment and Rights). At the same time she began writing articles and conducting speaking engagements to promote consumer's rights and her vision of recovery. In her own words:

> My real hope for re-humanizing the human services rests with people with disabilities as we begin learning that we can organize, that we have power in our numbers, and that we can overcome oppression through expression. The days of silence are over. As professionals and as fellow human beings, we have a great deal to learn from the people we seek to serve. It is important to listen to people with disabilities. (Deegan, 1990, p. 310)

One of Dr. Deegan's accomplishments was the publication of *Coping with Voices: Self-Help Strategies for People Who Hear Voices That Are Distressing.* While Deegan does not take an antimedication stance, she does object to mental health professionals who push consumers to become "medication compliant." Deegan's preference is to encourage people to use medications as "one tool among many tools that a person may choose to use in their recovery process" (Deegan, 1996, p. 1). Her most recent projects include the development of the Intentional Care approach to building recovery-oriented skills and competencies in direct services staff, a film about transitioning from institutions to the community, and research into ex-patient perspectives on the history of mental health services.

Despite these potential barriers, consumers and providers can and do work together effectively to develop self-help initiatives. One model for collaboration focuses on the changing roles of providers and consumers as a result of evolving mental health systems. As empowerment and self-help become more accepted, consumers increasingly take on more responsibility for supporting both themselves and their peers. In response to the same issues, the staff may begin to move away from the role of caretaker and adopt a more professional, consultative approach (Kaufman et al., 1989). A model that represents these changes is described as a five-stage process:

1. *Investment/nurturance:* Staff promote increased social interaction between members of a psychiatric rehabilitation program, while members become more invested in the well-being of their peers.
2. *Initiative/delegation:* Consumers assume greater responsibility in planning program activities. Some program members begin to emerge as leaders. Staff support these changes by delegating some of their responsibilities and teaching/modeling leadership skills.
3. *Rebellion/dialogue:* Members openly express dissatisfaction with both their role as a passive recipient of services and the control exerted by the mental health system; staff recognize the validity of their concerns and promote open discussions about stigma and consumer rights. During this stage work begins in the development of a self-help initiative. Staff work towards reducing administrative resistance to the initiative and provide consumers with access to information about self-help organizations.

4. *Accommodation/collaboration:* Members deal with role shift issues and may begin to adopt new labels such as *peer advocate*. It is also typical in this stage for members to begin to meet informally outside of the program. Staff can serve as important resources during this period of increased consumer autonomy.
5. *Self-help/consultation:* Consumers establish a formal self-help initiative. Staff are utilized in an as-needed consultant role (Kaufman et al., 1989, p. 10).

Self-Help for Persons with Dual Diagnoses

Participating in self-help groups may be even more important for people dealing with the dual diagnoses of both a mental illness and a substance abuse disorder. Historically, individuals with dual disorders were the first to be referred to self-help groups focused on recovery from substance abuse. Sadly, these referrals were more often caused by an inability or unwillingness of mental health professionals to deal with the substance abuse problem than an appreciation of the benefits of self-help. Still, professionals were aware that attendance at these substance abuse–related self-help groups was often helpful in the recovery process. For many professionals this knowledge led to an appreciation of the contributions self-help could make for persons with psychiatric disabilities.

Individuals who have both a mental illness and a substance abuse disorder are still the consumers most likely to be referred to self-help groups. As discussed in Chapter 8, people with a dual diagnosis require specialized programs and supports. These individuals are often encouraged by their caseworkers to utilize self-help groups to supplement the professional supports and services that they receive. Alcoholics Anonymous and Narcotics Anonymous (NA) are the most commonly utilized mutual support groups for persons recovering from alcoholism and other substance abuse disorders. Unfortunately, some people have not felt welcome in these groups when they disclosed they had a diagnosis of mental illness and take medication. Apparently, the stigma associated with severe mental illness exists even within groups such as AA and NA. In addition, AA and NA groups often discourage the use of psychotropic medications because they are viewed as obstacles to recovery from addiction. Partly in response to this resistance, many consumers have been receiving help in mutual support groups known as "double trouble" or *dual recovery* groups (Vogel, Knight, Laudet, & Magura, 1998). Note that the term *double trouble* was used for many years, but dual recovery, a more hopeful term, is currently preferred (Magura et al., 2003). Dual recovery groups are specifically geared to meet the needs of individuals who are coping with the symptoms and challenges of both a mental illness and a substance abuse disorder. Even so, they are very similar to AA and NA groups. Like AA and NA groups, these groups utilize a 12-step process of recovery and are run by persons who have substance abuse problems themselves (Alcoholics Anonymous World Services, 1981). In contrast, dual recovery groups have two important differences from AA and NA groups: (1) acceptance of the importance of psychiatric medications, and (2) a high tolerance of psychiatric symptomatology (Magura, et al., 2003).

Sometimes circumstances arise that require a variation of the traditional self-help model. For example, in certain inpatient settings or community-based agencies where regulations or insurance requirements necessitated staff involvement, consumer-run dual recovery groups have been developed that include the presence of professional staff at meetings or in proximity. Another variation of the dual recovery support group has been used in situations where acute symptoms interfered with group leadership. In this version, staff members, who have received training and information from an experienced dual recovery group member, provide interim leadership (Caldwell & White, 1991).

Access to Self-Help

Some people interested in self-help have difficulty accessing or interacting with a traditional face-to-face group. This may occur for a number of reasons, including lack of transportation, residency in a rural area with few resources, or because a person is not currently comfortable sharing his or her experiences in a face-to-face situation. Fortunately, a number of options are available for these individuals. Some peer support programs offer assistance via the telephone. This service is sometimes referred to as *warm lines*—in contrast to "hot lines," which are used to respond to crisis situations (Solomon, 2004). A number of Internet online support groups have been established in recent years. These groups utilize chat rooms and/or bulletin boards and sometimes, if the technology is available, live audio or video interaction with other group members. With the growing trend toward communication online via e-mail, chat rooms, bulletin boards, and instant messaging, it should not be surprising that some individuals prefer the convenience and anonymity of Internet support groups (Perron, 2002; Solomon, 2004). The Depression and Bipolar Support Alliance (DBSA) is a peer support organization that has emphasized the online support group option in recent years. A number of groups meet each week using a live chat format (http://www.dbsalliance.org/Info/OnlineSupport.html).

Another self-help approach that has grown in popularity during the last decade does not necessarily require any interaction with peers. These self-directed programs can be completed by an individual with the help of workbooks, audiotapes, or videotapes. Mary Ellen Copeland's Wellness and Recovery Action Plan (WRAP) is probably the best known example of this self-help approach (Copeland Center for Wellness and Recovery, n.d.; http://www.copelandcenter.com/whatiswrap.html):

> WRAP is a self-management and recovery system developed by a group of people who had mental health difficulties and who were struggling to incorporate wellness tools and strategies into their lives. WRAP is designed to:
>
> • *Decrease and prevent intrusive or troubling feelings and behaviors.*
> • *Increase personal empowerment.*
> • *Improve quality of life.*
> • *Assist people in achieving their own life goals and dreams.*

The WRAP process begins with the development of a daily plan of activities that promote wellness. Identification of circumstances that trigger symptoms, being aware of early warning signs of symptoms, and developing a plan to deal with personal crises are also essential parts of WRAP. While WRAP can be a completely self-directed process, individuals can choose to have family members, friends, and professionals assist them (Copeland, 1997). Copeland has also proposed that combining WRAP and peer support groups is a very effective way to promote recovery (Copeland & Mead, 2004).

As you can see, self-help has become a widely accepted component of mental health services throughout the country. Numerous organizations throughout the United States provide information, referrals, and easy access to existing groups that offer support to people with a variety of psychiatric and medical disorders as well as other problems and issues (New Jersey Self-Help Clearinghouse, 2005). The National Mental Health Consumers' Self-Help Clearinghouse is a noteworthy organization that provides a number of important services. It provides up-to-date information and resources relevant to peer support and advocacy initiatives, such as technical assistance to help people organize coalitions and establish self-help groups and other peer-run programs (http://www.mhselfhelp.org/about.php).

The Story of David

Whether it is encouraged by professionals or generated entirely by consumers, peer support is used by many people as an adjunct to professionally delivered treatment and rehabilitation services. As you read about David, consider the role that peer support plays in his rehabilitation and recovery process.

David is a 32-year-old man who has been coping with a severe mental illness since he was 19 years old. During the last 13 years, he has been in a variety of inpatient and outpatient mental health services. David is currently attending a PsyR day program where, because of his interest in computers, he spends most of his time working in the prevocational clerical unit. His goal is to enroll in a computer training program and eventually get a full-time job using computers. However, his caseworkers have told him that he is not ready for training or work yet. They feel he needs to be more compliant with his medication regimen and improve both his punctuality and concentration in the clerical unit. David has tried to explain that he occasionally neglects to take his medication because he doesn't like to feel lethargic all the time. This lethargy is also the reason he frequently gets to the program late. He thinks his "concentration problems" have more to do with the boredom he experiences while working on tedious clerical tasks than with his symptoms.

Lately, David is feeling increasingly discouraged and frustrated. He feels that the treatment he is receiving at the program isn't getting him anywhere, but he doesn't know where else to turn. David is familiar with the various mental health treatment and rehabilitation programs offered in his county and has been involved with many of them. In fact, he likes his current program better than the others he has been to, mostly because he likes some of the staff members, and because he has made some close friendships with other program members. One of these friends is Jean, who has been attending the program for several years herself. Jean tells David that while she finds the structure and support offered by the day program helpful in coping with her illness, she sometimes finds the groups to be boring and irrelevant. She wishes she had more control over what kinds of group activities are offered. They joke about starting their own program called CONTROL (Consumer Operated Network to Recover Our Lives).

One day Jean calls David and asks him if he wants to attend a conference she heard about that has been organized by a local chapter of a statewide consumer advocacy group. David is excited about the idea and the following week they attend the conference. While there, they meet a number of people who are involved in self-help and self-advocacy initiatives and they find out that there are plans to open a new self-help center not far from where they live. One of the conference organizers asks if anyone is interested in volunteering to help get the new self-help center started. He explains that, like the other self-help centers that have opened in the last few years in other parts of their state, the new center will be run by consumers and provide a variety of activities such as peer-run support groups, social activities, and information sessions. State grant money will be provided to rent space and to fund several part-time positions to be filled by consumers who are interested in helping to facilitate the self-help center. David enthusiastically volunteers to help out.

About a month later, David begins attending a series of organizational meetings. The meetings are led by some people who have been running a self-help center for a few years in another county. A variety of issues are discussed such as location, hours of operation, center activities, hiring part-time staff, and the roles the staff will play. David is a little hesitant to participate in the first meeting, but soon finds himself offering ideas and volunteering to help with a number of tasks such as moving furniture and helping to set up a computer. During a discussion about choosing a name for the center, David mentions the name that he and Jean had discussed. Several weeks later they acquire space in a local community center for two afternoons and one evening a week, and soon, CONTROL, a peer-operated self-help center, becomes a reality.

David continues to receive services at the day program, but because he is busy with activities at CONTROL he reduces his schedule to just 1 or 2 days a week. He shares his positive impressions of CONTROL with other program members and encourages them to come to the new center. The reactions of the day program staff are mixed. Some of the older, more traditional staff members are suspicious of CONTROL and are concerned that the group will spark a "revolution" among program members who may abandon needed professional services in favor of this radical new group. The director of the program privately speculates that a reduction in attendance could mean a substantial loss of revenue for the program. Other staff members recognize positive changes in David and are optimistic that this new self-help initiative will complement their efforts to support program members' recovery.

David begins running a weekly computer class at CONTROL to help some of his peers at the self-help center learn to use the computer to explore the Internet and send and receive e-mail. He also participates in a twice weekly peer support group and attends social activities. He likes the relaxed atmosphere of the center and the feeling that he gets when he knows he has helped one of his peers. He finds that his contribution to the development and running of CONTROL has given him more self-confidence. After a few months he is offered a part-time paid position at the center. The enthusiastic encouragement and support he receives from his peers has also helped him decide to start taking computer science classes two mornings a week at the community college.

Beyond Self-Help: Categories of Peer-Provided Services

Self-help groups are just one way that persons who have severe mental illnesses help others who are coping with similar challenges. There are also other categories of *peer-delivered services*, which have been defined as services provided by individuals who identify themselves as having a mental illness who are specifically employed to help other consumers (Solomon, 2004; Solomon & Draine, 2001). Almost from its inception, the field of substance abuse counseling recognized the benefits of utilizing individuals recovering from alcoholism and other substance abuse disorders as regular service providers (Moxley & Mowbray, 1997). An obvious benefit of this strategy is the ability of an individual who is in recovery to truly empathize with the experiences of the persons to whom he or she is providing services. Providers who share the experience of coping with a similar illness or disability may also have an advantage over other professional providers in the length of time it takes to establish trusting relationships with service recipients. The field of mental health has been much slower to recognize these benefits, perhaps because there is greater stigma attached to having a mental illness than to a substance abuse disorder. It is interesting to note that in some substance abuse treatment settings, traditionally, counselors who are in recovery have a higher status than those who have not struggled with an addiction. By contrast, in the mental health field, peer providers have frequently been given job titles such as peer advocate that indicate their consumer status and are often relegated to paraprofessional or counselor aide roles.

Three distinct categories of peer-delivered services have been identified by Solomon (2004):

1. Peer-run or operated services (also referred to in the literature as consumer-run, consumer-operated, or consumer-delivered services)
2. Peer partnerships
3. Peer employees.

We will look closely at each of these categories in the following subsections, as well as some illustrative examples of peer-delivered service programs. Note that the types of PsyR services and supports that these programs provide are quite varied. Persons who have severe mental illnesses are involved in the implementation of the full range of PsyR models described in this textbook, including employment services, residential programs, case management, and assertive community treatment.

Peer-Operated Services

A *peer-operated* initiative is developed, controlled, and operated by individuals who identify themselves as having a diagnosis of a mental illness. Nonconsumers may also be employed to contribute to service delivery and/or the administration of the program, but consumers clearly direct the entire service delivery process including planning, policy development, direct service provision, and program evaluation. These programs, which address the social and emotional needs of consumers, are considered both a complement to and an alternative to traditional mental health services (Chamberlin, 1990; Davidson et al., 1999; Petr, Holtquist, & Martin, 2000; Salzer & Shear, 2002; Solomon, 2004; Solomon & Draine, 2001; Van Tosh & del Vecchio, 2000; Zinman, Harp, & Budd, 1987). Peer-operated initiatives come in all shapes and sizes. There are relatively small programs such as the self-help center described earlier in David's story, as well as large peer-operated agencies that run a variety of programs such as Collaborative Support Programs of New Jersey (CSP-NJ), described in Box 12.2.

A study by Chamberlin and colleagues (1996) reviewed 64 programs that were administratively operated by consumers. They found a wide array of services being provided, including social/recreational activities, individual and system level advocacy, assistance with housing and employment, transportation, and assistance with activities of daily living. This study also found that the majority of people who utilized these programs were very involved, spending an average of 15.3 hours a week at the program (Chamberlin et al., 1996). The programs studied also received very positive ratings on a variety of program satisfaction measures. Most of the service recipients surveyed also utilized some type of professional mental health service in addition to utilizing peer-delivered services.

Clay (2005) identified three distinct types of consumer-operated programs:

1. *Drop-in centers* provide consumers with a place to connect and socialize, as well as an array of supports and services such as meals and assistance finding jobs or housing. The CONTROL self-help center described earlier is a good illustration of this type of program.
2. *Peer support and mentoring programs* emphasize one-to-one relationships, and outreach to consumers in their homes or in other natural community settings. The Friends Connection in Philadelphia, Pennsylvania, targets individuals who are coping with both a mental illness and substance abuse disorder. Consumers are matched with peer support providers who visit them regularly and help them identify and achieve recovery-oriented goals. Group social and recreational activities are also provided to help consumers decrease their isolation and build a supportive social network (Whitecraft et al., 2005).
3. *Education and advocacy programs* offer consumers peer-run skill training classes focused on recovery and self-advocacy. A good example of this type of program is BRIDGES, an innovative program that began in Tennessee and has spread to other parts of the United States and Canada. BRIDGES, which stands for Building Recovery of Individual Dreams and Goals through Education and Support, offers consumers a 15-week course on mental illness and recovery followed by ongoing peer-run support groups (Hix, 2005).

BOX 12.2

A Peer-Operated Agency:
Collaborative Support Programs of
New Jersey

Collaborative Support Programs of New Jersey (CSP-NJ), provides a good example of the kinds of peer-delivered supports and services that PsyR agencies can offer. In terms of Solomon's categories of peer-provided services, CSP-NJ would be considered to be a peer-operated agency. CSP-NJ started as a grassroots agency in 1985 with a budget of $65,000 and by 2006 was operating with a budget of more than $8.5 million. The agency is directed and managed by a consumer-driven board (more than 66% of the board members are consumers) and a vast majority of the staff of CSP-NJ are past or current recipients of mental health services.

The development and provision of supported housing is one of CSP-NJ's key missions. Staff (both consumer and nonconsumer staff) assist consumers in obtaining decent, safe and affordable housing in apartments and homes. They provide supports to the residents of this housing on an as-needed basis, including a strong focus on financial services encour-

aging financial literacy and economic self-sufficiency. The agency has a subsidiary organization, Community Enterprise Corporation, which helps with the physical maintenance of the homes.

Another key CSP-NJ activity is the development and support of consumer-run self-help centers. CSP-NJ has developed 21 self-help centers throughout the state. CSP-NJ provides a number of technical assistance services to the self-help centers. CSP-NJ recently developed the Institute for Wellness and Recovery Initiatives, which provides training, education, and technical assistance to mental health providers, agencies, and consumers. Another innovative project is the Recovery Network. Peer facilitators conduct weekly wellness and recovery groups at the state psychiatric hospitals (Swarbrick & Brice, 2006).

CSP-NJ encourages and supports the professional development of all of its staff members, and has encouraged many consumers to prepare for the Certified Psychiatric Rehabilitation Practitioner examination (see Chapter 1 for details on this credential) and to pursue psychiatric rehabilitation education at all levels (certificate, bachelor's, master's, and doctoral degrees).

Peer Partnerships

In a *peer partnership* program, consumers collaborate with nonconsumer providers to operate a program that emphasizes peer-delivered services. In a peer partnership, the direct services providers are people who identify themselves as consumers, and consumers also have substantial input into the operation of the program, but the program is closely affiliated with a traditional (i.e., nonconsumer) human service agency that provides administrative support. For example, a large comprehensive PsyR provider offering a full range of services and supports including case management, vocational, and residential services may have a peer-provided supported education program under its umbrella. The director of the program and all of the service providers are individuals who identify themselves as consumers, but the fiscal management of the program and some of the administrative responsibilities are handled by a traditionally run umbrella agency.

In both peer-operated programs and peer partnerships, the consumers who are delivering supports and services may be either paid employees or volunteers. Often, programs utilize both types of resources, for example, a large self-help center may hire several consumers in either part-time or full-time positions to take responsibility for the overall operation of the center. Other functions, such as facilitating social events or providing outreach to local mental health agencies, may be carried out by volunteers.

Peer Employees

Growing numbers of PsyR and mental health agencies purposefully employ individuals who have experienced a severe and persistent mental illness (Davidson et al., 1999; Moxley & Mowbray, 1997; Salzer et al., 2002; Solomon, 2004). Some of these individuals act as service providers in peer-operated initiatives and peer partnerships. They are also hired to provide a wide range of psychiatric rehabilitation and mental health services in the traditional mental health delivery system. Mowbray and colleagues (1996) examined this trend toward consumers working as service providers. Their work identified four principal reasons for this trend:

1. *Consistent with a rehabilitation philosophy, productive and important work is made available and accessible to consumers.*
2. *Inclusion of consumers as mental health workers can increase the sensitivity of programs and services about recipients.*
3. *[Consumers] can serve as effective role models for clients.*
4. *The inclusion of consumers is an expression of affirmative action and is consistent with contemporary civil and disability rights policies. (Mowbray et al., 1996, p. 48)*

There is a great deal of variation in the level of professionalism attached to the peer employee or consumer/provider role. There are many individuals who identify themselves as having a mental illness working as professionals on staff teams. Some rehabilitation counselors, social workers, nurses, psychologists, psychiatrists, and other credentialed PsyR and mental health service providers are also consumers of mental health services.

On the other hand, some agencies have designated peer employee positions that are meant to be an adjunct to professionally provided services. For example, an assertive community treatment team that consists primarily of professionals with degrees and credentials may include two peer employees who serve as community resource aides. Positions that are specifically developed for peer providers have been given a number of labels including *peer counselor, peer advocate, peer specialist,* and *consumer case manager* (Solomon, 2004). Peer employees have been referred to at times as "prosumers." Manos (1993) stated that:

Prosumers are former mental patients, graduates of various forms of living hell, transformed into consumers and now activated toward a wide variety of work roles to help others who are still in the first stages of defining their selves and their beings. (p. 117)

Research on the Effectiveness of Self-Help and Peer-Delivered Services

To understand and support the ongoing development of self-help and peer-delivered services, a body of research examining the benefits and limitations of these services is emerging. This research examines the outcomes of peer support initiatives, as well as their feasibility and impact.

Research on Self-Help Groups

There has not been a great deal of research focusing on the outcomes of self-help groups for persons diagnosed with a mental illness. Most of the current research has examined two specific approaches: Recovery Inc. and GROW (Davidson et al., 1999; Rappaport et al., 1985; Van Tosh et al., 2000). Studies that looked at the impact of self-help groups have found evidence that over time consumers who stay involved in mutual support groups have lower levels of symptomatology (Davidson et al., 1999; Finn & Bishop, 2001; Galanter, 1988; Luke, 1989). There is also some evidence that the duration of hospital stays is reduced for GROW members (Davidson et al., 1999; Finn & Bishop, 2001; Kennedy, 1989; Rappaport, 1993; Rappaport et al., 1985). In addition, self-help can improve both daily functioning and a person's ability to manage his or her illness (Powell, Yeaton, Hill, & Silk, 2001). A study of Recovery Inc. found similar benefits including improved coping skills, acceptance of the illness, and willingness to take medications (Raiff, 1984).

Long-term participants in self-help groups have larger social networks and are more likely to pursue educational and employment opportunities (Carpinello, Knight, & Janis, 1991; Davidson et al., 1999). GROW members also showed improvements in psychological well-being such as increased autonomy and personal growth (Finn & Bishop, 2001). Both the length and level of involvement with a self-help group were positively correlated with improved outcomes.

Peer-Provided Services: Feasibility and Perceived Benefits

In the late 1980s and early 1990s, a number of descriptive studies were conducted that explored the feasibility of employing peers as service providers and reported on some of the potential benefits of offering peer-provided services (Kaufman, Ward-Colasante, & Farmer, 1993; Lyons, Cook, Ruth, Karver, & Slagg, 1996; Mowbray, Chamberlain, Jennings, & Reed, 1988; Mowbray & Tan, 1993; Mowbray et al., 1996; Segal et al., 1995; Sherman & Porter, 1991; Van Tosh & Del Vecchio, 2000). These studies suggest that consumers provide services differently than nonconsumers and are able to perform their jobs competently (Davidson et al., 1999). Schmidt (2005) concluded that the early feasibility studies also suggested that consumer and nonconsumer providers can work well together.

Peer providers bring unique strengths to their work. Among these are life experience, including "street survival" skills, the development of successful coping techniques, and familiarity with successful resource acquisition strategies (Paulson, 1991; Van Tosh et al., 1993). Peer specialists on an intensive case management team developed a distinct advocacy role, representing the client's perspective in discussions with case managers about clients' problems and needs (Felton et al., 1995). Consumer-providers may be especially effective in programs that emphasize mobile outreach and providing services directly to consumers in the community (Lyons et al., 1996). Peer providers are frequently perceived as more credible on medication adherence issues, particularly when they share their own experiences. Along the same lines, they can be particularly effective in helping consumers recognize signs or symptoms that precede acute episodes of mental illness (Paulson, 1991). Also, they are able to provide their peers with important information about their rights and alternative treatment approaches, which allows consumers to choose from a wider array of options than usually offered by nonconsumer providers (Mowbray & Moxley, 1997a).

Van Tosh and her colleagues (1993) observed that peer providers are flexible, patient, dependable, and that the shared experience of having a severe mental illness helps to foster trust and a comfortable rapport, which for some service recipients is difficult to establish with nonconsumer providers. Other reports found the peer providers are more likely to appreciate the strengths of consumers, to understand and respond to consumers' needs, and to promote independence (Davidson et al., 1999; Mowbray & Moxley, 1997a).

A strength of consumer-providers, and perhaps the best reason for promoting consumer involvement in PsyR service provision, is their ability to serve as role models for other consumers. Their presence conveys the important message that people with severe mental illnesses can succeed in a variety of valued social roles. They convey competence and the ability to regain control over their lives to other consumers who may have lost hope of ever moving beyond the role of "mental patient" (Mowbray, 1997; Mowbray et al., 1996; Nikkel, Smith, & Edwards, 1992). Peer providers also deliver a concrete message about empowerment:

> Through the symbol and the reality of consumers who provide services, empowerment is actualized. Power is given (away) to those with a disability label, power to take control over their own outcomes and over systems' operations. (Mowbray, 1997 p. 47)

Are Peer Providers as Effective as Other Providers?

Early studies provided evidence that peer-provided service initiatives are feasible and enhance the provision of supports and services (Davidson et al., 1999; Schmidt, 2005; Solomon & Draine, 2001; Van Tosh & Del Vecchio, 2000). Later studies confirmed that peer-delivered services are probably as effective as services delivered by nonconsumers and may in some cases be more effective (Davidson et al., 1999; Salzer et al., 2002; Schmidt, 2005; Solomon, 2004; Solomon & Draine, 2001).

Several studies found that programs that utilized peer providers were no better or worse in terms of outcomes. Solomon and Draine (1995) compared a peer partnership case management program with a traditional nonpeer case management program. They found that after 2 years both programs were associated with improvements in the lives of the consumers served. There were no significant differences in outcomes of the two types of programs in terms of symptoms, social adjustment, and quality of life. This study was later replicated in a peer-operated agency that operated two assertive community treatment teams, one of which employed peer providers and one that did not. A 2-year comparison also resulted in no significant differences in clinical or social outcomes or in retention rates (Herinckx, Kinney, Clarke, & Paulson, 1997; Paulson et al., 1999; Solomon & Draine, 2001). Chinman, Rosenheck, Lam, and Davidson (2000) compared case management teams serving homeless clients that used peer providers with those that employed nonconsumer staff and found them to be equally effective. Taken as a group, these studies support the assertion that peer providers can be just as helpful to consumers as nonpeer staff.

Are Peer-Delivered Services Better than Other Services?

Another group of studies found that peer-delivered services produced some superior outcomes when compared to services offered solely by nonconsumer providers. Programs that utilized peer providers resulted in a reduction in the use of hospital and crisis services when compared to traditional programs (Clarke et al., 2000; Edmunson, Bedell, Archer & Gordon, 1982; Klein, Cnaan, & Whitecraft 1998). Clarke and colleagues (2000) compared an assertive community treatment (ACT) team that included peer providers with a traditional ACT team without peer providers and found that individuals served by the team with peer providers had both fewer hospitalizations and fewer instances of using crisis services. Klein and colleagues (1998) compared consumers who received both intensive case management and peer-provided social supports with a group who only received case management services. Like the Clarke et al. study (2000), the peer-enhanced group had fewer hospitalizations and used crisis services less frequently than the control group.

Another study compared the outcomes of persons recently discharged from hospitals and referred to traditional community health services to those who received these same services, but also received support from a peer provider (Edmunson et al., 1982). They found fewer hospitalizations among those receiving services enhanced by a peer provider. Dumont and Jones (2002) compared outcomes of consumers utilizing a peer-provided crisis intervention program to those of consumers utilizing traditional crisis intervention services. They found that the group served by peers had fewer days in the hospital and were more satisfied with the services they received than the control group.

In each of these studies (Clarke et al., 2000; Dumont & Jones, 2002; Edmunson et al., 1982), it was unclear whether the peer provider groups did better because they received services from peer providers, or because they received an enhanced form of case management that included additional services (Schmidt, 2005; Solomon & Draine, 2001).

Peer providers were more effective in achieving positive gains in terms of a number of quality-of-life measures including greater satisfaction with housing and financial situation, fewer life problems, and reduced substance abuse among the consumers served (Felton et al., 1995; Klein et al., 1998). Kaufman (1995) examined the outcomes of a peer partnership employment program and found that those assigned to the program achieved superior vocational outcomes when compared to recipients of traditional vocational rehabilitation services. Craig, Doherty, Jamieson-Craig, Boocock, and Attafua (2004) compared two assertive outreach teams that provided case management to a group of high-risk individuals. One of the teams employed peer providers. They found that the consumers who received peer-provided services were better engaged with the team, participated more actively in treatment programs, and had more success in terms of achieving goals identified on their treatment plans.

Between 1998 and 2003 a major, multisite study called the Consumer Operated Service Program Research Initiative (COSP) was funded by SAMHSA's Center for Mental Health Services. The goal of the COSP study was to compare the utilization of peer-operated services as an adjunct to traditional mental health services with the utilization of traditional mental health services alone. Eight peer-operated programs participated in the study and consumers were involved with every aspect of the research project including its design. The service recipient outcomes examined included housing, employment, social inclusion, well-being, and empowerment. As this book was going to press in 2006, the results of this study were still being analyzed. However, initial findings suggest that consumer-operated programs are cost effective and produce positive outcomes beyond traditional services, particularly in the area of well-being (Campbell, 2002; Clay, 2005).

One important benefit of conducting the COSP study was the analysis of common ingredients utilized by various types of consumer-operated programs. The sites in the COSP study included drop-in centers, peer mentoring programs, and education/advocacy programs. Despite the wide variety of program models, six domains of common ingredients were identified:

- *Program structure* emphasizing consumer control, participant responsiveness, and the capacity to link service recipients to other services
- An *environment* that is safe, accessible, informal, and provides reasonable accommodations
- A *belief system* emphasizing the benefits of mutual support, empowerment, choice, recovery, respect for diversity, and spiritual growth
- Formal and informal *peer support strategies* including opportunities to share personal stories and raise consciousness, as well as to provide crisis prevention, peer mentoring, and teaching
- *Education* focusing on self-management/problem solving, skills practice, and job readiness
- *Advocacy* (both self-advocacy and peer advocacy).

The identification of common ingredients led to the development of a fidelity instrument, which was named the *COSP Fidelity Assessment Common Ingredients Tool* or FACIT (Johnsen, Teague & McDonel Herr, 2005).

Benefits to Peer Providers and Mental Health Systems

A number of studies were done to examine the potential benefits of peer-delivered services for the persons providing the services. Most of these studies used qualitative research methods such as interviews with peer providers (Solomon, 2004). Sherman and Porter (1991) found that peer providers had fewer hospitalizations after becoming providers. Peer providers have also reported a number of quality-of-life improvements (Armstrong, Korba, & Emard, 1995; Mowbray, Moxley, & Collins, 1998). Salzer and Shear (2002) conducted in-depth interviews with 14 peer providers and reported improved self-esteem, valuable gains in knowledge and skill development, and help in facilitating their own recovery. Increased independence and enhancement of social support networks are also benefits experienced by peer providers (Mowbray, 1997). To better understand the potential benefits of being a peer provider, consider the following story:

> *Laura, a 38-year-old woman who currently works as a peer advocate on a PACT team, was diagnosed with bipolar disorder when she was 24. A college graduate with a degree in English, Laura hoped for a career in publishing. She had some success as an assistant editor when she was in her early 20s, but her illness interrupted her career and by the time she was 30 she wondered if she could even hold a job. After experiencing success as a cofacilitator of a self-help group, Laura decided to apply for the PACT team position. After 2 years working as a peer provider, she says, "It was one of the best decisions I ever made. For many years my illness got in the way of my career. I felt sorry for myself and thought I was a failure. Now I see that my illness has helped me to become a more compassionate person who can make a difference in other people's lives. My job has done wonders for my self-esteem. I feel like every time I help someone I am taking a step forward in my own recovery."*

Peer-provided services can also have a positive effect on the quality and quantity of mental health services. There is evidence that utilization of peer providers has a positive impact on staff attitudes, helping staff to be more sensitive to the experiences and needs of consumers. Working side by side with consumers forces nonconsumer staff to examine their own prejudices. The experience enables service providers to get to know individuals who have a severe mental illness as colleagues who have strengths, skills, and abilities (Dixon, Krauss, & Lehman, 1994; Doherty, Craig, Attafua, Boocock, & Jamieson-Craig, 2004; Mowbray, 1997; Mowbray et al., 1996; Solomon, 2004). It is hoped that this will allow staff to realize more fully that the consumers they serve are "people first," rather than a manifestation of a psychiatric diagnosis. Mowbray and Moxley (1997a) also suggest that the presence of peer employees helps nonconsumer staff gain a better understanding of the recovery process.

Mental health systems that include peer-delivered services increase their ability to provide an expanded array of services. The inclusion of self-help and peer-provided services within a mental health system expands the number of service and support providers available and increases the capacity of the system (Solomon, 2004). In addition, peer providers can reach a segment of the population that is not easily reached by traditional providers. Individuals who have had negative experiences with professional mental health services are more likely to be engaged by a peer-operated program than traditional services. As mentioned earlier, peer providers are more effective at engaging the high-risk population of individuals who are resistant to accepting services including persons who are homeless, acutely symptomatic, and abusing substances (Craig et al., 2004).

Limitations of the Studies and Ongoing Research Challenges

The studies cited in preceding sections are quite varied in terms of the peer-provided services examined, research design, and results. Many have methodological problems such as small sample sizes. It is unclear whether the results of some of these studies (e.g., Clarke et al., 2000; Edmunson et al., 1982) are due to the receipt of services from peer providers or to the fact that service recipients received an enhanced form of case management (Schmidt, 2005; Solomon & Draine, 2001).

It is difficult to conduct rigorous research on peer support initiatives. Phyllis Solomon, one of the preeminent researchers in this area, stated:

> It's hard to research these kinds of services. It's antithetical in many ways to scientific design . . . and it's hard to get funding for it. It's hard to make as rigorous a study as one would like. (Lundin, 2005, p. 2)

A number of experts, including Solomon, have concluded that while we cannot yet call peer-provided services an evidence-based practice the outcomes research done to date suggests that it is a *promising best practice* (Davidson et al., 1999; Lundin, 2005; Salzer et al., 2002; Schmidt, 2005; Solomon, 2004; Solomon & Draine, 2001). Certainly, more well-designed research studies need to be conducted to increase our understanding of the unique strengths and limitations of peer-delivered services. The COSP study discussed earlier was designed to correct some of the methodological problems inherent in previous studies. The FACIT fidelity tool that came out of the COSP study was also an important step in the study of peer-delivered services and is likely to inspire future research projects.

A participatory action research (PAR) approach, in which the recipients of peer support contribute to the design of the study, may be a promising means of studying self-help and peer-delivered services. This type of research has evolved with the encouragement of the National Institute on Disability and Rehabilitation Research. PAR is a strategy that involves the persons under study fully participating in the research, including formulating research questions and hypotheses, helping to design the study, collecting data, and interpreting findings (Leff, Campbell, Gagne, & Woocher, 1997; Rogers & Palmer-Erbs, 1994).

Challenges for Peer Providers

In their efforts to assist consumers it is important for peer providers to recognize and utilize their unique strengths. At the same time, they need to be aware of some potential limitations and challenges inherent in their dual role as a consumer/provider. One of these limitations is the tendency of some peer providers to generalize their own experiences to the life situations of the individuals they are supporting (Nikkel et al., 1992). They may "fail to fully appreciate the diversity of experiences of persons with major mental illnesses and the individuality of a person's response" (Paulson, 1991, p. 75). For example, a peer provider may make the mistake of thinking that his experience coping with symptoms of depression is typical, whereas it is much more likely that each person he is helping has experienced symptoms somewhat differently. In addition, effective strategies used to relieve symptoms may differ from person to person.

Because mental illnesses are in part stress related, many peer providers and their employers have concerns about coping with the high stress associated with PsyR service provision. Will they be prone to burnout sooner than other providers? Will they need to take a lengthy sick leave if they become acutely ill? If they cannot handle the job stress and become unemployed, will they become eligible or reeligible for disability benefits in a timely manner? Such concerns may plague many peer providers and can even have a negative impact on job performance. Sometimes these concerns may prevent consumers from considering the peer provider role. Nevertheless, research suggests that job retention is longer and career commitment is stronger among peer providers than nonconsumer staff (Basto, Pratt, Gill & Barrett, 2000).

Other challenges involve the potential for dual relationships and role conflict, and the maintenance of confidentiality. Peer providers, particularly those who practice in or near an agency where they are receiving services or have received services in the past, may struggle with boundary issues due to prior relationships they have had with both service providers and service recipients (Carlson, Rapp, & McDiarmid, 2001; Mowbray, 1997; Mowbray et al., 1996). Peer providers may struggle with conflicting roles. In terms of fellow service providers, they should now be relating to them as a colleague, but used to be in the role of service recipient. On the other hand, consumers who used to be acquaintances or friends may now be the individuals for whom they provide services. Complicating problems may include current or past intimate relationships with peers who are potentially future recipients of service. Nonconsumer service providers may also have a hard time relating to a peer or colleague they once served as a consumer.

In terms of confidentiality, access to case records of individuals with whom a peer provider has had a personal relationship raises ethical concerns. While many consumers establish comfortable relationships more easily with peer providers than nonconsumer providers, some are wary of receiving help from a person who may be struggling with his or her own mental illness. These concerns can stem from stigmatizing attitudes since consumers can be both victims and perpetuators of stigma or mistrust of peers once they move into a provider role (Mowbray, 1997). Such reactions can frustrate peer providers in their efforts to provide help, and cause them to question their own capabilities.

Relationships with Nonconsumer Providers

For many peer providers the most formidable challenge is establishing positive relationships with the nonconsumer staff (MaCauley, 1993; Mowbray, 1997). This might come as a surprise for many people entering the field. After all, if PsyR staff internalize PsyR values, goals, and principles, they should be pleased to work side by side with colleagues who are recovering from a mental illness. Unfortunately, this is not always the case. Peer providers frequently report discrimination and the experience of being stigmatized by coworkers. According to Daniel Fisher (1994a), a psychiatrist who is also an activist and self-described "person in recovery from a psychiatric disability":

> *The mental health profession is one of the most discriminating and stigmatizing toward consumer/survivors. Consumer/survivors who work as providers are labeled and objectified in the same fashion as consumers. Their behavior and principles are filtered through their psychiatric disability.* (p. 68)

A common complaint is being eyed suspiciously when expressing anger or simply having a bad day. Nonconsumer colleagues often jump to the conclusion that a peer provider is experiencing symptoms. In such situations peer providers often report being treated in a way that is clearly different than the way other staff are treated when they are in a bad mood or are experiencing the common stresses associated with service delivery. For example, when a peer provider expresses too much emotion, the relationship may suddenly shift from collegial to therapeutic.

Stigmatizing attitudes may be expressed to peer providers in a variety of other ways. Nonconsumer staff may exclude peer providers from social events, eating lunch together, or act in other ways that distance peer providers. Nonconsumer staff may question the professionalism of peer providers, for example, by expressing resentment when reasonable accommodations are made for staff members who have psychiatric disabilities (Mowbray, 1997). Peer providers have also reported hearing comments from colleagues that are mean spirited and hurtful (Roberts, Rotteveel, & Manos, 1995). Stigma may not be the only reason that peer providers are sometimes treated poorly. Staff may fear being displaced by peer providers and thus exhibit resentful behaviors (Mowbray, 1997).

Some agencies employ consumers in order to conform to current trends, but then are not sure how to utilize the individuals that they hire. Such tokenism does little to change skeptical attitudes of professionals and tends to isolate those assuming roles that are not well defined (Griffin-Francell, 1997). Consider the following situation:

> *Tony was initially excited when hired as a part-time consumer case manager for a mobile outreach team. But as he tried to settle into his job he became skeptical. He shared this during a peer provider support group: "They don't seem to know what I should be doing. I volunteer to go out to visit clients, but they always seem to have an excuse why someone else on the team should go instead. The other day when I asked how I could contribute they suggested I should take some clients bowling. I feel I can make more of a contribution, but they don't seem to want to give me a chance."*

Happily, negative treatment of peer providers is not always the case. Many peer providers report very positive, supportive working relationships with nonconsumer colleagues. In fact, many consumers cite a key reason for choosing a career in PsyR is working in an environment that is more supportive and accommodating than other work settings. Peer providers in one study reported higher level of supports from the community mental health organizations that employed them than did their nonconsumer colleagues (Basto et al., 2000).

The Issue of Disclosure

Should a consumer working in a PsyR professional role disclose to other staff or supervisors that he or she is also a recipient of mental health services? While many peer providers are hired, in part, because of their experiences as mental health consumers, others are hired based solely on past work/educational experiences. This latter group may struggle with the issue of whether or not to disclose their experiences as a person living with a psychiatric disability. Past experiences with stigmatizing attitudes of mental health professionals leave some peer providers determined to avoid self-disclosure at all costs. However, many peer providers report that this is a difficult stance to maintain. What if they should come in contact with a consumer who is familiar with their status as a service recipient? Another issue, raised by Patricia Deegan and others, is that one may diminish his or her efficacy by not disclosing relevant personal experiences to consumers (Deegan & Smoyak, 1996). Disclosing one's status as a mental health consumer also provides an important opportunity to act as a positive role model for both consumers and staff (Roberts et al., 1995).

The choice is not only whether or not to disclose. Peer providers must consider a number of related concerns, such as who to disclose to, what to disclose, reasons why it is (or is not) important or useful to disclose, when is an appropriate time to disclose, and how to convey what one chooses to share. Another important consideration is that it is necessary to disclose a disability to at least one staff person in order to access supports and protection via the Americans with Disabilities Act (Fisher, 1994b). Each peer provider must weigh his or her unique circumstances when grappling with the complicated issue of disclosure. However, in all cases, it is essential that the choices be left to the peer provider; disclosure should never be required (Roberts et al., 1995). For more on the issue of disclosure in the workplace, see Chapter 9.

At the 1998 International Association of Psychiatric Rehabilitation Services (IAPSRS, now USPRA) in Minneapolis, workshop participants comprised of self-identified peer providers, nonconsumer providers, and program administrators echoed some of the challenges mentioned here and identified additional issues (Barrett et al., 2000). Their concerns are summarized in Box 12.3.

BOX 12.3
Challenges Identified by Peer Providers

1. Taking on dual roles (e.g., service provider and service recipient), which can be difficult to clarify and can sometimes raise conflict.
2. Role transition can affect relationships with other consumers (changing from consumer to service provider can be similar to changing from colleague to supervisor).
3. Relationship boundary issues with service recipients.
4. Concerns about benefits such as health insurance and the possibility of relapse.
5. Feeling isolated, especially if the person is the sole or "token" consumer-provider.
6. Pressure to be the "standard bearer" for all consumer-providers.
7. Confidentiality issues, such as access to case records for peer providers who received or are still receiving services from the agencies where they work.
8. Dealing with difficult memories and emotions elicited by situations that service recipients' experience that may remind peer providers of their own experiences.
9. Negotiating reasonable accommodations.
10. Stigmatizing job titles (e.g., consumer case manager).
11. Deciding whether to disclose that you have a mental illness, what to disclose, and who to disclose to.
12. Relationships with nonconsumer providers, who may be uncomfortable with the presence of peer providers and/or treat them like service recipients.
13. Job discrimination (e.g., some peer providers receive lower salaries than nonconsumer providers).

Source: Adapted from Barrett et al., 2000, p. 86).

Supports and Professional Development

Considering the many advantages of employing peer providers and the fact that the transition from consumer to provider can be difficult, the ongoing provision of supports both inside and outside of the work environment and the education and training needs of peer providers must be considered. Skilled supervision is essential for peer providers who are dealing with both typical professional growth and development issues and the unique challenges outlined earlier. Supervisors who are working with peer providers may require specialized training (Griffin-Francell, 1997; Mowbray & Moxley, 1997b). Peer provider support groups outside the agency can also be helpful because they allow individuals to openly share feelings and concerns that they may not want to share in the workplace. These groups may also allow peer providers who have not chosen to disclose to obtain support (Fishbein, Manos, & Rotteveel, 1995). Peer providers should also have access to reasonable accommodations in the workplace, as required by the Americans with Disabilities Act. Flexible work schedules, environmental modifications to reduce distractions, and training opportunities that are modified to compensate for cognitive deficits are examples of accommodations that might facilitate the productivity of employees who have a disability. Chapters 9 and 10 provide additional information on reasonable accommodations for employees and students.

It is possible that peer providers who move into professional roles, rather than identified peer provider roles, have a number of advantages. They are less likely to be segregated from other staff and do not have to struggle with role definition issues. They may also encounter less stigma, particularly if their colleagues perceive that they have the requisite qualifications for the position. To move into these roles and become employed as legitimate professionals, rather than being confined to consumer-designated job titles, consumers must have access to appropriate training, as well as opportunities to obtain academic degrees and required credentials. The Certified Psychiatric Rehabilitation Provider (CPRP) credential (discussed in Chapter 1) is an excellent opportunity for peer providers to augment their professional qualifications. Indeed, peer-operated programs in the state of Georgia accord a special status to individuals who have the CPRP. Other peer-operated agencies, such as the Collaborative Support Program of New Jersey (described in Box 12.2) encourage their staff members to obtain the CPRP certification and provide them with resources to do so, such as arranging to have CPRP preparation courses offered on site.

Attending college-level classes or training sessions required for credentialing may not be a viable option for all consumers who choose to provide services and supports to their peers, but these options do provide a distinct advantage, particularly for those seeking an upwardly mobile career path. Many who do not receive additional education face the "glass ceiling" effect (they can see the more desirable positions, but are not allowed to reach them) and remain frustrated in peer-designated positions.

Any discussion of educational opportunities for peer providers must first recognize that many people with psychiatric disabilities who are already practicing in PsyR and related mental health fields have professional degrees and credentials. Some have chosen to disclose their experiences as a consumer and utilize them in providing services. Others have remained silent. Some of these practitioners became ill after receiving their degrees. Others, such as Patricia Deegan, were careful not to disclose their consumer status to college professors and administrators because of expected discrimination (Deegan & Smoyak, 1996). Historically professional degree programs that prepare human service practitioners have shown biases against admitting consumers to their programs (Paulson, 1991). In some universities this trend is changing (Barrett et al., 2000; Gill, Pratt, & Barrett, 1997; Paulson, 1991). Efforts to recruit consumers and integrate them into academic programs with students who are not identified consumers are well known by the authors, who teach in such programs. The University of Medicine and Dentistry of New Jersey offers consumers who want to move into service delivery roles a variety of options including certificate programs and undergraduate and graduate degree programs.

It is important to distinguish between integrated professional training programs and those which are designed solely to prepare consumer providers (Barrett et al., 2000; Housel & Hickey, 1993; Sherman & Porter, 1991). Whereas the latter programs give consumers an opportunity to enter the helping professions and gain knowledge and skills that are essential for practice, they typically prepare consumers for paraprofessional roles. They also ensure that peer providers emerge with a credential that is different than that of their nonconsumer colleagues. Such differences may promote segregation and discriminatory practices.

Supports and education for peer providers are essential, but the field of PsyR also needs to address systemic and work culture changes that will reduce segregation and stigma and provide peer providers with well-defined and meaningful roles. Many mental health professionals have spent years of education and practice creating clear boundaries between what they perceive as the capable helper and the dysfunctional "helpee." Even those who have internalized the PsyR principle of reduced professional boundaries may have difficulty accepting a consumer as a "full-fledged" team member. Programs need to educate and prepare staff before they make a commitment to incorporating peer providers (MaCauley, 1993). In situations where peer employees are already "on board," formal discussions and sensitivity training should be considered to ensure that the culture has adapted in a positive way. The following is an example of a PsyR program that still needs help in this area.

> *Sara works in a clubhouse program as a rehabilitation counselor. She possesses educational and experiential qualifications similar to those of her colleagues, but chose to disclose her status as a consumer when applying for the job. Surface reactions to her have been positive and she has not experienced any direct discrimination. On occasion, some staff members are uncomfortable around her, particularly when clubhouse members are not present. A very unfortunate aspect of the staff culture in this location is that program members are sometimes joked about or imitated during informal staff-only interactions. Sara has noticed people looking at her uncomfortably when this occurs. Sometimes when she enters a room in which staff were talking and laughing she is met with sudden silence.*

CONTROVERSIAL ISSUE

Does the Professionalization of the Peer Provider Role Enhance or Diminish the Potential of the Mental Health System to Become Truly Consumer Directed?

Those peer providers who acquire advanced degrees and professional credentials are in a much better position to move out of designated peer positions and into supervisory and administrative positions that offer them higher status, higher salaries, and more opportunities to make a stronger impact on the mental health service delivery system. These more influential positions allow for opportunities to help transform services and progress to a more consumer-driven and recovery-oriented service system model. Thus, the professionalization of the peer provider workforce offers many potential advantages for both individual peer providers and mental health systems.

Another point of view highlights some possible disadvantages in the professionalization of both peer providers and peer-operated service initiatives. When peer employees are paid by the mainstream mental health system and some obtain degrees and credentials that allow them to move into influential positions in traditional service delivery programs, they may lose the opportunity to bring their unique perspective into the work environment. As a peer provider develops more of a traditional professional identity, he or she may begin to identify less with the consumers served. In addition, service recipients may feel less connected to a peer provider who is viewed as a full-fledged professional, than one who comes across as a true

peer and advocate. The sense of shared experience that helps build rapport and trust may be diminished as a peer provider becomes more comfortable with professional jargon and counseling techniques. Some have used the word *co-opted* to describe a phenomenon in which a peer provider enters the world of professional service providers, perhaps begins to adopt the pretensions associated with the professions, and loses touch with the worldview of consumers who are struggling with both psychiatric symptoms and the experience of being treated by a system that emphasizes their illness rather than their personhood.

Even programs that are fully consumer run may struggle with a similar evolution of identity. Davidson and his colleagues (1999) described the professionalization of consumer-run programs:

> This process involves what have been less formal services, based on such values as flexibility, autonomy and consumer choice, becoming more structured and more driven by their needs to attract and justify funding. To the degree that such a service comes to resemble a more conventional provider agency, it also begins to lose its unique character and role within a system of care. (p. 180)

It may be that systems need to stay focused on the development of two divergent trends: on the one hand, increased opportunities for individuals diagnosed with severe mental illnesses to move into professional roles and influence the evolution of professionally run programs; on the other hand, the ongoing promotion of alternative peer-run programs that stay true to the principles and values of mutual support.

Other Influential Roles for Consumers

In addition to working in a variety of provider roles, consumers make other important contributions to the field of psychiatric rehabilitation. In recent years, more consumers are being asked to participate in governing roles such as membership on agency boards of directors or administrative positions in state mental health departments. Consumers also participate actively in PsyR professional organizations such as USPRA and its state chapters. Increasingly, consumers are also contributing in meaningful ways to program evaluation and research studies. These roles allow consumers to have an impact on practice and policy issues, both on the individual agency level and on the state and national level. However, this can only occur if consumers are allowed to hold real power. As with their provider roles, it is important that the perspective of consumers in these influential positions is used and that they are not simply functioning as tokens to satisfy agency requirements or to help an organization appear progressive.

Activists in the ex-patient/consumer/survivor movement have had a meaningful impact on local, state, and national policy issues that relate to the concerns of people identified as mental health consumers. Typically, they achieve their goals by working outside of the mental health system. But to change a system that many people who have severe mental illnesses are dissatisfied with, the consumer perspective needs to be heard inside of the mental health system as well. In terms of statewide mental health systems, this has been achieved through the establishment of Offices of Consumer Affairs, which now exist within most state mental health authorities (Van Tosh et al., 2000). For example, South Carolina has a director of consumer affairs position. This position is held by an individual who has a mental illness and who reports directly to the state mental health director. Part of this individual's responsibility is to hire consumer affairs coordinators for each of the community mental health centers located throughout the state. The positions are earmarked for self-identified consumers and are funded through the state's mental health plan. The main thrust of this innovative plan is to make consumer satisfaction with mental health services the system's number one goal (Bevilacqua, Gettys, & Cousins, 1997).

Progress has been made on the national level as well. In 1995 SAMHSA's Center for Mental Health Services created the position of consumer affairs specialist. Other examples of consumer involvement on the national level included the appointment of activist Daniel Fisher to the President's New Freedom Commission on Mental Health, which issued its final report, *Achieving the Promise: Transforming Mental Health Care in America,* in 2003.

Consumer involvement on local mental health and PsyR agency boards is essential to the planning and implementation of consumer-centered services. A board of directors that has a substantial percentage of consumers filling meaningful roles is an excellent example of empowerment. It is important to realize that nonprofit agency administrators must answer to their board of directors. The board has the power to hire and fire administrators, develop and refine the agency's mission and goals, and create policies that govern day-to-day service provision. Consumers serving on these boards also have a chance to combat stigma by serving as role models in their communities. For example, residential programs often have to deal with resistant community members when opening new group homes or apartments. Board representatives who are also self-identified consumers can help ease fears and misconceptions by speaking to neighbors and community representatives.

PsyR professional organizations are another place where consumer involvement is essential. Consumer participation on the boards and subcommittees of these organizations provides an excellent opportunity for collaboration between consumers and professionals that can positively influence both local and national service systems. Consumer involvement at local and national professional conferences, as both presenters and attendees, is another way in which consumers can share their perspective with PsyR and mental health professionals. In the 1970s, when PsyR professional associations began to emerge, these conferences were opportunities for professionals to talk with each other about their work with persons with psychiatric disabilities. Now, many of these conferences provide opportunities for professionals, peer providers, consumers, and family members to share concerns and strategies for improving services, with consumers often assuming important roles such as keynote speaker.

Finally, program evaluation and research are areas where consumers are making important contributions. Increased collaboration between providers and consumers in evaluating individual program outcomes is increasingly evident. In terms of more rigorous studies, not only do consumers act as subjects and survey respondents but also as active partners in research projects and even as independent researchers (Campbell, 2002; Van Tosh et al., 2000). Activist Daniel Fisher (1994b) recommends "basing total quality improvement of mental health services on outcome measures designed by survivors and consumers" (p. 915). He cites the formation of the Consumer/Survivor Research and Policy Work Group, an entity that has been supported by SAMHSA's Center for Mental Health Services, as an important example of this goal. Thus, persons who have severe mental illnesses are helping to enhance both our knowledge of best practices and our understanding of recovery through their involvement in planning, designing, conducting, and reporting on important research studies (Van Tosh et al., 2000).

Summary

Peer support is an important component of community support systems. Peer support is offered both through self-help groups and various forms of peer-delivered services. These services include peer-operated programs, and the purposeful inclusion of peer employees in professionally run PsyR programs. While the body of research on the outcomes of self-help and peer-provided services has yet to offer conclusive evidence, it seems clear that people with psychiatric disabilities gain some unique benefits from participation in peer support initiatives. Peer providers themselves, and the nonconsumer staff who they work with, also seem to benefit from these programs. However, there are also a number of challenges faced by peer providers and their colleagues and it is important to address these challenges by providing appropriate supports and training opportunities.

Persons who have severe mental illnesses play other important roles in mental health systems as well. They act as policy makers, advocates, researchers, and board members. Their input into how PsyR services are provided is essential to the development of a truly consumer-driven mental health system. Such input helps to ensure consumer satisfaction and contributes to the protection of the rights and dignity of people with disabilities. It is essential for psychiatric rehabilitation providers who are not diagnosed with a mental illness to learn to work in conjunction with the various types of peer providers, activists, and policy makers and to recognize all of the valuable roles that they can play in transforming mental health systems.

Class Exercises

Exercise 1: Establishing a Self-Help Group

Imagine that you are part of a group of people who have psychiatric disabilities and want to start a self-help group.

1. How would you begin the process?
2. What resources would you need to achieve your goal?
3. Would the group be open to:
   - Anyone with a psychiatric disability?
   - People who had certain issues (e.g. diagnosis) in common?
   - Only your circle?
4. How would you deal with the issue of leadership? Some options are voting on a single leader or co-leaders, shared leadership among all group members, or rotating leadership.
5. Now that you have discussed your hypothetical self-help group in some detail, how would you define the mission and goals of your group?

Exercise 2: Promoting Peer Support

Imagine that you are working in a PsyR program that is primarily operated by nonconsumers in staff roles. From your discussions with some program participants you conclude that many of them would enjoy or profit from participation in peer support self-help activities, such as those offered at a nearby self-help center. You suggest this to a few consumers, but they say that they are not familiar with the self-help center and don't pursue the idea. You don't want to push the idea too strongly because it is contrary to the philosophy of such services, yet you feel many individuals would find self-help to be a beneficial adjunct to the PsyR services they are currently receiving. What other strategies might you pursue to foster their involvement in peer support activities?

References

Ackerman, L. P. (1997). A Recovery, Inc. group leaders story. In C. T. Mowbray, D. P. Moxley, C. A. Jasper, & L. L. Howell (Eds.), *Consumers as providers.* Columbia, MD: International Association of Psychosocial Rehabilitation Services.

Alcoholics Anonymous World Services. (1981). *Twelve steps and twelve traditions.* New York: Author.

Armstrong, M. L., Korba, A. M., & Emard, R. (1995). Mutual benefit: The reciprocal relationship between consumer volunteers and the clients they serve. *Psychiatric Rehabilitation Journal, 19,* 45–49.

Bandura, A. (1977). *Social learning theory.* Englewood Cliffs, NJ: Prentice Hall.

Barrett, N. M., Pratt, C. W., Basto, P. M., & Gill, K. J. (2000). Integrating consumer providers into a service delivery system. *Psychiatric Rehabilitation Skills, 4*(1), 82–104.

Basto, P., Pratt, C., Gill, K., & Barrett, N. (2000). The Organizational Assimilation of Consumer Providers: A Quantitative Examination. *Psychiatric Rehabilitation Skills, 4*(1), 105–119.

Beers, C. W. (1923). *A mind that found itself.* Garden City, NY: Doubleday.

Bevilacqua, J. J., Gettys, D., & Cousins, V. (1997). Mental health systems development: Benefits created by consumer engagement. In C. T. Mowbray, D. P. Moxley, C. A. Jasper, & L. L. Howell (Eds.), *Consumers as providers.* Columbia, MD: International Association of Psychosocial Rehabilitation Services.

Borkman, T. J. (1999). *Understanding self-help/mutual aid: Experiential learning in the commons.* New Brunswick, NJ: Rutgers University Press.

Brown, N. P., & Parrish, J. (1995). CSP champion of self-help. *The Journal of the California Alliance for the Mentally Ill, 6*(3), 6–7.

Caldwell, S., & White, K. K. (1991). Co-creating a self-help recovery movement. *Psychosocial Rehabilitation Journal, 15*(2), 91–95.

Campbell, J. (2002). *Working science: Consumer Operated Service Program. Multi-site research initiative, study overview.* Paper presented at the 12th Annual Conference on State Mental Health Services Agency Research, Program Evaluation and Policy, Baltimore, MD.

Campbell, J. (2005). The historical and philosophical development of peer-run support programs. In S. Clay (Ed.), *On our own together: Peer programs for people with mental illness.* Nashville, TN: Vanderbilt University Press.

Carlson, L. S., Rapp, C. A., & McDiarmid, D. (2001). Hiring consumer-providers: Barriers and alternative solutions. *Community Mental Health Journal, 37*(3), 199–213.

Carpinello, S. E., Knight, E. L., & Janis, L. (1991). A qualitative study of the perception of the meaning of self-help, self-help groups, processes and outcomes by self-help group leaders, members and significant others. Albany, NY: New York State Office of Mental Health.

Chamberlin, J. (1984). Speaking for ourselves: An overview of the ex-psychiatric inmates' movement. *Psychosocial Rehabilitation Journal, 8*(2), 56–64.

Chamberlin, J. (1988). *On Our Own* (2nd ed.). New York: Hawthorne Books, Inc.

Chamberlin, J. (1990). The ex-patients' movement: Where we've been and where we're going. *Journal of Mind & Behavior, Special Issue: Challenging the Therapeutic State: Critical Perspective on Psychiatry and the Mental Health System, 11,* 323–336.

Chamberlin, J., Rogers, E. S., & Ellison, M. L. (1996). Self-help programs: A description of their characteristics and their members. *Psychiatric Rehabilitation Journal, 19*(3), 33–42.

Chinman, M. J., Rosenheck, R., Lam, J. A., & Davidson, L. (2000). Comparing consumer and nonconsumer provided case management services for homeless persons with serious mental illness. *Journal of Nervous and Mental Disease, 188*(7), 446–453.

Clarke, G., Herinckx, H., Kinney, R., Paulson, R., Cutler, D., & Ocman, E. (2000). Psychiatric hospitalizations, arrests, emergency room visits, and homelessness of clients with serious and persistent mental illness: Findings from a randomized trial of two ACT programs vs. usual care. *Mental Health Services Research, 2,* 155–164.

Clay, S. (Ed.). (2005). *On our own together: Peer programs for people with mental illness.* Nashville, TN: Vanderbilt University Press.

Copeland Center for Wellness and Recovery. (n.d.). What Is WRAP? Retrieved January 5, 2006, from *http://www.copelandcenter.com/whatiswrap.html*

Copeland, M. E. (1997). *Wellness recovery action plan.* Brattleboro, VT: Peach Press.

Copeland, M. E., & Mead, S. (2004). *Wellness recovery action plan and peer support.* Brattleboro, VT: Peach Press.

Craig, T., Doherty, I., Jamieson-Craig, R., Boocock, A., & Attafua, G. (2004). The consumer-employee as a member of a mental health assertive outreach team. I. Clinical and social outcomes. *Journal of Mental Health, 13*(1), 59–69.

Davidson, L., Chinman, M., Kloos, B., Weingarten, R., Stayner, D., & Tebes, J. K. (1999). Peer support among individuals with severe mental illness: A review of the evidence. *Clinical Psychology: Science and Practice, 6*(2), 165–187.

Deegan, P. E. (1990). Spirit breaking: When the helping professions hurt. *The Humanistic Psychologist, 18*(3), 301–313.

Deegan, P. E. (1993). Recovering our sense of value after being labeled mentally ill. *Journal of Psychosocial Nursing, 15,* 3–19.

Deegan, P. E. (1996). Using medication as part of the recovery process. Presentation at the New Jersey Psychiatric Rehabilitation Association Annual Conference, December 1996, Eatontown, NJ.

Deegan, P. E., & Smoyak, S. A. (1996). Blending two realities into a unique perspective. *Journal of Psychosocial Nursing, 34*(9), 39–46.

Dixon, L., Krauss, N., & Lehman, A. (1994). Consumers as service providers: The promise and the challenge. *Community Mental Health Journal, 30,* 615–629.

Doherty, I., Craig, T., Attafua, G., Boocock, A., & Jamieson-Craig, R. (2004). The consumer-employee as a member of a mental health assertive outreach team. II. Impressions of consumer-employees and other team members. *Journal of Mental Health, 13*(1), 71–81.

Dumont, J., & Jones, K. (2002, Spring). Findings from a consumer/survivor defined alternative to psychiatric hospitalization. *Outlook, a Joint Publication of the Evaluation Center @ HSRI and NASMHPD Research Institute.* Retrieved November 3, 2003, from http://nri.rdmc.org/Outlook3.pdf

Edmunson, E. D., Bedell, J. R., Archer, R. P., & Gordon, R. E. (1982). Integrating skill building and peer support in mental health treatment: The early intervention and community network development projects. In Jerger M. & Slotnick, R. (Eds.), Community Mental Health and Behavioral Ecology, (pp. 127–139). New York: Plenum Press.

Edmunson, E., Bedell, J., & Gordon, R. (1984). The Community Network Development Project: Bridging the gap between professional aftercare and self-help. In A. Gardner & F. Reissman (Eds.), *The self-help revolution.* New York: Human Services Press.

Felton, C. J., Stastny, P., Shern, D. L., Blanch, A., Donahue, S. A., Knight, E., et al. (1995). Consumers as peer specialists on intensive case management teams: Impact on client outcomes. *Psychiatric Services, 46*(10), 1037–1044.

Festinger, L. A. (1954). A theory of cultural comparison processes. *Human Relations, 7,* 117–140.

Finn, L., & Bishop, B. (2001). Mutual help, an important gateway to well-being and mental health. Retrieved January 4, 2006, from *http://www.communitybuilders.nsw.gov.au/download/mutual.doc*

Fishbein, S. M., Manos, E., & Rotteveel, J. (1995). Helping the helpers: A unique colleague support system for mental health professionals-consumers. *Journal of Psychosocial Nursing, 33*(11), 41–43.

Fisher, D. B. (1994a). A new vision of healing as constructed by people with psychiatric disabilities working as mental health providers. *Psychosocial Rehabilitation Journal, 17*(3), 67–81.

Fisher, D. B. (1994b). Health care reform based on an empowerment model of recovery by people with psychiatric disabilities. *Hospital and community psychiatry, 45*(9), 913–915.

Frese, F. J., & Davis, W. W. (1997). The consumer-survivor movement, recovery and consumer professionals. *Professional Psychiatry, Research and Practice, 28,* 243–245.

Galanter, M. (1988). Zealous self-help groups as adjuncts to psychiatric treatment: A study of Recovery, Inc. *American Journal of Psychiatry, 145,* 1248–1253.

Gill, K. J., Pratt, C. W., & Barrett, N. (1997). Preparing psychiatric rehabilitation specialists through undergraduate education. *Community Mental Health Journal, 33*(4), 323–329.

Griffin-Francell, C. (1997). Consumers as providers of psychiatric rehabilitation: Reflections of a family member. In C. T. Mowbray, D. P. Moxley, C. A. Jasper, & L. L. Howell (Eds.), *Consumers as providers.* Columbia, MD: International Association of Psychosocial Rehabilitation Services.

Herinckx, H. A., Kinney, R. F., Clarke, G. N., & Paulson, R. I. (1997). Assertive community treatment versus usual care in engaging and retaining clients with severe mental illness. *Psychiatric Services, 48,* 1297–1306.

Hix, L. (2005). BRIDGES in Tennessee: Building recovery of individual dreams through education and support. In S. Clay (Ed.), *On our own together: Peer programs for people with mental illness.* Nashville, TN: Vanderbilt University Press.

Housel, D. P., & Hickey, J. S. (1993). Supported education in a community college for students with psychiatric disabilities: The Houston Community College model. *Psychosocial Rehabilitation Journal, 17*(1), 41–50.

Jacobs, E., Masson, R., & Harvill, R. (2005). *Group counseling: Strategies and skills* (5th ed.). Belmont, CA: Brooks/Cole.

Johnsen, M., Teague, G., & McDonel Herr, E. (2005). Common ingredients as a fidelity measure for peer-run programs. In S. Clay (Ed.), *On our own together: Peer programs for people with mental illness.* Nashville, TN: Vanderbilt University Press.

Kaufman, C. (1995). The self-help employment center: Social outcomes form the first year. *Psychosocial Rehabilitation Journal, 18*(4), 145–162.

Kaufman, C. L., Freund, P. D., & Wilson, J. (1989). Self-help in the mental health system: A model for consumer-provider collaboration. *Psychosocial Rehabilitation Journal, 13*(1), 5–21.

Kaufman, C. L., Ward-Colasante, C., & Farmer, J. (1993). Development and evaluation of drop-in centers operated by mental health consumers. *Hospital and Community Psychiatry, 44*, 675–678.

Kennedy, M. (1989). Psychiatric hospitalizations of GROWers. Paper presented at the 2nd biennial conference of Community Research and Action, East Lansing, MI.

Klein, A. R., Cnaan, R. A., & Whitecraft, J. (1998). Significance of peer social support with dually diagnosed clients: Findings from a pilot study. *Research on Social Work Practice, 8*(5), 529–551.

Lee, D. T. (1995). Professional underutilization of Recovery Inc. *Psychiatric Rehabilitation Journal, 19*(1), 63–70.

Leff, H. S., Campbell, J., Gagne, C., & Woocher, L. S. (1997). Evaluating peer providers. In C. T. Mowbray, D. P. Moxley, C. A. Jasper, & L. L. Howell (Eds.), *Consumers as providers.* Columbia, MD: International Association of Psychosocial Rehabilitation Services.

Low, A. A. (1950). *Mental health through will training* (15th ed.) Boston, MA: Christopher.

Luke, D. A. (1989), The measurement of change in a self-help context. Unpublished doctoral dissertation, University of Illinois, Urbana–Champaign.

Lundin, R. (2005). Phyllis Solomon speaks on consumer operated services and jail diversion. *American Journal of Psychiatric Rehabilitation, 8*(1), 1–7.

Lyons, J. S., Cook, J. A., Ruth, A. R., Karver, M., & Slagg, N. B. (1996). Service delivery using consumer staff in a mobile crisis assessment program. *Community Mental Health Journal, 32*(1), 33–40.

MacAuley, R. (1993). Professionals need training to accept ex-patients as colleagues. *Resources, 5*(1), 18.

Magura, S., Laudet, A., Mahmood, D., Rosenblum, A., Vogel, H., and Knight, E. (2003). The role of self-help processes on achieving abstinence in dual recovery. *Addictive Behaviors, 28*(3), 399–413.

Manos, E. (1993). Prosumers. *Psychosocial Rehabilitation Journal, 16*(4), 117–120.

Mead, S., Hilton, D., & Curtis, L. (2001). Peer support: A theoretical perspective. *Psychiatric Rehabilitation Journal, 25*(2), 134–141.

Mowbray, C. T. (1997). Benefits and issues created by consumer role innovation in psychiatric rehabilitation. In C. T. Mowbray, D. P. Moxley, C. A. Jasper, & L. L. Howell (Eds.), *Consumers as providers.* Columbia, MD: International Association of Psychosocial Rehabilitation Services.

Mowbray, C. T., Chamberlain, P., Jennings, M., & Reed, C. (1988). Consumer-run mental health services: Results from five demonstration projects. *Community Mental Health Journal, 24*, 151–156.

Mowbray, C. T., & Moxley, D. P. (1997a). Consumers as providers: Themes and success factors. In C. T. Mowbray, D. P. Moxley, C. A. Jasper, & L. L. Howell (Eds.), *Consumers as providers.* Columbia, MD: International Association of Psychosocial Rehabilitation Services.

Mowbray, C. T., & Moxley, D. P. (1997b). Futures for empowerment of consumer role innovation. In C. T. Mowbray, D. P. Moxley, C. A. Jasper, & L. L. Howell (Eds.), *Consumers as providers.* Columbia, MD: International Association of Psychosocial Rehabilitation Services.

Mowbray, C. T., Moxley, D. P., & Collins, M. (1998). Consumers as mental health providers: First person accounts of benefits and limitations. *The Journal of Behavioral Health Services & Research, 25*, 397–411.

Mowbray, C. T., Moxley, D. P., Thrasher, S., Bybee, D., McCrohan, N., Harris, S., & Clover, G. (1996). Consumers as community support providers: Issues created by role innovation. *Community Mental Health Journal, 32*(1), 47–67.

Mowbray, C. T., & Tan, C. (1993). Consumer-operated drop-in centers: Evaluation of operations and impact. *The Journal of Mental Health Administration, 20*, 8–19.

Moxley, D. P., & Mowbray, C. T. (1997). Consumers as providers: Forces and factors legitimizing role innovation in psychiatric rehabilitation. In C. T. Mowbray, D. P. Moxley, C. A. Jasper, & L. L. Howell (Eds.),

Consumers as providers. Columbia, MD: International Association of Psychosocial Rehabilitation Services.

Murray, P. (1996). Recovery, Inc., as an adjunct to treatment in an era of managed care. *Psychiatric Services, 47*(12), 1378–1381.

New Jersey Self-Help Clearinghouse. (2005). *The self-help group directory* (20th ed.). Cedar Knolls, NJ: Saint Clare's Health System.

Nikkel, R. E., Smith, G., & Edwards, D. (1992). A consumer operated case management project. *Hospital and Community Psychiatry, 43*(6), 577–579.

Noordsy, D. L., Schwab, B., Fox, L., & Drake, R. E. (1996). The role of self-help programs in the rehabilitation of persons with severe mental illness and substance use disorders. *Community Mental Health Journal, 32*(1), 71–81.

Paulson, R. I. (1991). Professional training for consumers and family members: One road to empowerment. *Psychosocial Rehabilitation Journal, 14*(3), 69–80.

Paulson, R., Herinckx, H., Demmler, J., Clarke, G., Cutler, D., & Birecree, E. (1999). Comparing practice patterns of consumer and non-consumer mental health service providers. *Community Mental Health Journal, 35*, 251–269.

Perron, B. (2002). Online support for caregivers of people with a mental illness. *Psychiatric Rehabilitation Journal, 26*(1), 70–77.

Petr, C., Holtquist, S. & Martin, J. (2000). Consumer-run organizations for youth. *Psychiatric Rehabilitation Journal,24,* 142–148.

Powell, T., Yeaton, W., Hill, E., & Silk, K. (2001). Predictors of psychosocial outcomes for patients with mood disorders: The effects of self-help group participation. *Psychiatric Rehabilitation Journal, 25*(1), 3–11.

Presidents New Freedom Commission on Mental Health. (2003). *Achieving the promise: Transforming mental health care in America, Final Report.* Retrieved June 3, 2005, from *http://www.mentalhealthcommission.gov*

Raiff, N. (1984). Some health related outcomes of self-help participation: Recovery, Inc. as a case example of a self-help organization in mental health. In A. Gardner & F. Reissman (Eds.), *The self-help revolution.* New York: Human Services Press.

Rappaport, J. (1993). Narrative studies, personal stories and identity transformation in the mutual help context. *The Journal of Applied Behavioral Science, 29*, 239–256.

Rappaport, J., Seidman, E., Toro, P. A., McFadden, L. S., Reischl, T. M., et al. (1985). Collaborative research with a mutual help organization. *Social Policy, 15*, 12–24.

Reissman, F. (1965). The "helper-therapy" principle. *Social Work, 10*, 27–32.

Roberts, M., Rotteveel, J., & Manos, E. (1995, Spring). Mental health consumers as professionals: Disclosure in the workplace. *American Rehabilitation*, pp. 20–23.

Robertson, N. (1988). *Getting better: Inside Alcoholics Anonymous.* New York: William Morrow.

Rogers, E. S., & Palmer-Erbs, V. (1994). Participatory action research: Implications for research and evaluation in psychiatric rehabilitation. *Psychosocial Rehabilitation Journal, 18*(2), 3–12.

Rogers, S. (1996). National clearinghouse serves mental health consumer movement. *Journal of Psychosocial Nursing, 34*(9), 22–25.

Salzer, M. S., & Shear, S. L. (2002). Identifying consumer provider benefits in evaluations of consumer-delivered services. *Psychiatric Rehabilitation Journal, 25*(3), 281–288.

Salzer, M. S., & The Mental Health Association of Southeastern Pennsylvania Best Practices Team. (2002). Consumer-delivered services as a best practice in mental health care delivery and the development of best practice guidelines. *Psychiatric Rehabilitation Skills, 6*(3), 355–382.

Sarason, I., Levine, H., Basham, R., & Sarason, B. (1983). Assessing social support: The social support questionnaire. *Journal of Personality and Social Psychology, 44,* 127–139.

Schmidt, L. T. (2005). *Comparison of service outcomes of case management teams with and without a consumer provider.* Unpublished dissertation.

Segal, S. P., Silverman, C., & Temkin, T. (1993). Empowerment and self-help agency practice for people with mental disabilities. *Social Work, 38*(6), 705–712.

Sherman, P. S., & Porter, R. (1991). Mental health consumers as case management aides. *Hospital and Community Psychiatry, 42*(5), 494–498.

Skovholt, T. M. (1974). The client as a helper: A means to promote psychological growth. *Counseling Psychologist, 43,* 58–64.

Solomon, P. (2004). Peer support/peer provided services: Underlying processes, benefits and critical ingredients. *Psychiatric Rehabilitation Journal, 27*(4), 392–401.

Solomon, P., & Draine, J. (1995). The efficacy of a consumer case management team: Two-year outcomes of a randomized trial. *Journal of Mental Health Administration, 22*(2), 135–146.

Solomon, P., & Draine, J. (1996). Perspectives concerning consumers as case managers. *Community Mental Health Journal, 32*(1), 41–46.

Solomon P., & Draine, J. (2001). The state of knowledge of the effectiveness of consumer provided services. *Psychiatric Rehabilitation Journal, 25*(1), 20–27.

Stroul, B. A. (1989). Community support systems for persons with long-term mental illness: A conceptual framework. *Psychosocial Rehabilitation Journal, 12*(3), 9–26.

Stroul, B. (1993). Rehabilitation in community support systems. In R. Flexer & P. Solomon (Eds.), *Psychiatric rehabilitation in practice.* Boston, MA: Andover Medical Publishers.

Swarbrick, M. (2005). *Consumer-operated self-help centers: The relationship between the social environment and its association with empowerment and satisfaction.* Unpublished dissertation.

Swarbrick, M., & Brice, G., Jr. (2006). Sharing the message of hope, wellness and recovery with consumers and staff at state psychiatric hospitals. *American Journal of Psychiatric Rehabilitation.*

Turner, J. C. (1977). Comprehensive community support systems for mentally disabled adults: Definitions, components, guiding principles. *Psychosocial Rehabilitation Journal, 1*(3), 39–47.

U.S. Department of Health and Human Services. (1999). *Mental health: A report of the surgeon general.* Rockville, MD: U.S. Department of Health and Human Services, Substance Abuse and Mental Health Services Administration, Center for Mental Health Services, National Institutes of Health, National Institute of Mental Health.

Van Tosh, L., & Del Vecchio, P. (2000). *Consumer-operated self-help programs: A technical report* (DHHS Publication No. SMA 01–3510). Rockville, MD: Center for Mental Health Services. Retrieved November 3, 2003, from *http://www.mentalhealth.org/publications/ allpubs/SMA01–3510/SMA01–3510.pdf*

Van Tosh, L., Finkle, M., Hartman, B., Lewis, C., Plumlee, L. A., & Susko, M. A. (1993). Working for a change: Employment of consumer/survivors in the design and provision of services for persons who are homeless and mentally disabled. Rockville, MD: Center for Mental Health Services.

Van Tosh, L., Ralph, R. O., & Campbell, J. (2000). The rise of consumerism. *Psychiatric Rehabilitation Skills, 4*(3), 383–409.

Vogel, H. S., Knight, E., Laudet, A. B., & Magura, S. (1998) Double Trouble in recovery: Self-help for the dually-diagnosed. *Psychiatric Rehabilitation Journal, 21*(4), 356–364.

Whitecraft, J., Scott, J., Rogers, J., Burns-Lynch, B., Means, T., & Salzer, M.S. (2005). The Friends Connection, Philadelphia, Pennsylvania. In S. Clay (Ed.), *On our own together: Peer programs for people with mental illness.* Nashville, TN: Vanderbilt University Press.

Zinman, S., Harp, H. T., & Budd, S. (1987.) *Reaching across.* Sacramento, CA: California Network of Mental Health Clients.

Chapter 13

The Role of the Family in Psychiatric Rehabilitation

Introduction   *374*

Working with Families and Psychiatric Rehabilitation Principles   *375*

The Family as a "Caring Agent"   376

Dual Diagnosis and the Family   376

Independence/Dependence   377

Burden and Stigma   377

Troublesome Actions that Contribute to Burden   378

Family Dissatisfaction   379

Three Levels of Family Involvement   380

Kevin's Story: A Confidentiality Issue   *381*

The Unique Burdens of Spouses   382

Siblings and Children   382

People with Mental Illness as Parents   383

The Anguish of the Individual   386

The Burdens of Family Living for the Person with Mental Illness   *386*

The Dilemma of Functional Expectancy and Independence/Dependence Revisited   386

Loneliness   387

Goals for Helping Families   387

Family Interventions   *387*

Summary of the Empirical Evidence   389

The Effectiveness of Family Education and Support   391

Main Benefits of Family Intervention   392

Family Psychoeducation: An Evidence-Based Practice   *392*

Critical Ingredients of Family Psychoeducation   392

Outcomes of Family Psychoeducation   393

Other Family Psychoeducation Approaches   *394*

Professional and Consumer Collaboration   394

The Concept of Family Recovery   *395*

Stage 1: Discovery/Denial   396

Stage 2: Recognition/Acceptance   396

Stage 3: Coping/Competence   396

Stage 4: Personal/Political Advocacy   396

The Story of NAMI   *396*

History of NAMI   397

Families Helping Each Other   398

Familial Strengths and Resilience   *399*

Summary   *399*

Class Exercise   *400*

References   *401*

The role of the family in psychiatric rehabilitation and treatment has gone through many changes. Formerly, family influences were viewed as a contributing cause of mental illnesses; today, the family is seen as an important partner in the rehabilitation process. Family interventions focusing on psychoeducation and coping strategies have been proven to be effective and are now considered an established evidence-based practice. This chapter will describe the effects on the family of having a member with mental illness and how families can contribute to the recovery of a person with mental illness. Finally, we will review the development of family advocacy movements such as the National Alliance on Mental Illness (NAMI), which help to keep the needs of people with mental illness prominent in state legislatures, administrative offices, and public policy forums. In addition, NAMI and its affiliates have disseminated their own mutual self-help family intervention, "Family to Family," and have made special efforts to educate professionals through the NAMI Provider Education Program.

This chapter will answer the following questions:

1. *What is the effect on the family of having a member with severe and persistent mental illness?*
2. *How does living with the family affect the adjustment and recovery of a person with major mental illness?*
3. *What kinds of family interventions have been shown to be effective for family members with mental illness?*
4. *How does the family fit into the concept of recovery?*
5. *What is the role of NAMI in supporting people with mental illness?*

Introduction

In many ways, the catastrophe of mental illness strikes not only the individual but also his or her entire family, placing an undue burden on them (Hatfield, 1987a). The role of the family in recovery from severe and persistent mental illness has become increasingly important as community integration has become more of a reality. Many of the first community-based psychiatric rehabilitation services were designed for single, deinstitutionalized adults, many of whom were completely estranged from their families. Today, when long-term hospitalization is the exception rather than the rule, families have once again become primary agents of care (Hatfield, 1987a). At the same time, the opportunity for the individual to maintain a family life is greater than ever before. Today, people with mental illness are likely to stay involved with their family of origin including parents and siblings. They are more likely to marry or stay in other long-term relationships, and to have children.

At the same time, community-based care has also increased the burden that family members must bear, both subjectively and objectively. Shorter hospital stays often mean that many acutely ill individuals return home for continuing care in the community with their family.

In the past, families were incorrectly identified as etiological agents, literally causing serious mental illness. Mothers, in particular, have borne the brunt of these assertions. In fact, familial psychosocial factors, such as an environment high in criticism, hostility, and levels of emotional overinvolvement may contribute to relapses in some cases (Anderson, Reiss, & Hogarty, 1986). This type of environment has been termed high in *expressed emotion* (EE). Nevertheless, most family households with members who have mental illness do not have high EE environments (Lefley, 1989). In addition, high EE environments can also be found outside family settings such as other residential settings and some clinics (Hogarty, 1993).

A paradigm shift has taken place. Families were assumed to be dysfunctional, illness-causing systems. Now, many families are recognized as surprisingly resilient and resourceful with a potentially important role to play in treatment and rehabilitation. Despite the burden that a family member's illness often presents, some individuals have reported discovering strengthened familial bonds, stronger commitments, and a clearer identification of familial strengths and resources. Family members are finding they can make important contributions to the recovery process (Mannion, 1996).

Family interventions, based on the strengths of families are among the most successful categories of psychosocial treatment and rehabilitation, actually reducing the frequency and length of psychotic relapse (Dixon & Lehman, 1993; Dixon et al., 2001; Hogarty, 1993; McFarlane, Dixon, Lukens, & Lucksted, 2003). These family interventions are typically designed around illness education, support, problem solving, and crisis intervention. Indeed, a body of data shows that the decompensation and/or hospital recidivism of persons with mental illness who reside with their families can be significantly reduced by this type of intervention in combination with psychotropic medication (Lehman & Steinwachs, 1998; Pharoah, Mari, & Streiner, 2004). This reduction in relapse is significantly greater than when medication alone is employed.

Working with Families and Psychiatric Rehabilitation Principles

Like the rest of society, mental health professionals have traditionally let fear and blame dominate their interactions with the families of persons who have a mental illness (Lundwall, 1996). All professionals, including psychiatric rehabilitation (PsyR) practitioners, need to be willing to create better options and resources for families and their members. One of the guiding principles of psychiatric rehabilitation is that the involvement and partnership of persons receiving services, as well as their family members, is essential to effective operation, evaluation, and governance of PsyR services (IAPSRS, 1996). Thus, family involvement in treatment, rehabilitation, and support are recognized as important elements in a person's rehabilitation (Cook & Hoffschmidt, 1993). In particular, the *psychoeducation* of families and consumers helps ensure that they have reasonable expectations regarding the disease, its treatment, and rehabilitation (Hatfield, 1990).

Because psychiatric rehabilitation is about community-based services, integrated settings, and natural supports, the involvement of family members (parents, spouses, children, and others) is essential in order to provide maximally normalized services. Clearly, many consumers may need treatment and a great deal of support for their entire lives. Thus, it is probably best if family members, when willing, are engaged as partners in the long-term rehabilitation process (Cook & Hoffschmidt, 1993).

The Family as a "Caring Agent"

Today with very short hospital stays, and deinstitutionalization a reality, many families have become primary care providers. Since the early 1980s, more than half of all persons leaving state hospitals are sent to live with their family members. Among short-stay patients, as many as four out of five individuals return to their families for care (Hatfield, 1987b).

Lefley (1989) notes that families must cope with both the positive and negative symptoms of severe mental illness (as discussed in Chapter 2). But it is often the negative symptoms that have the most devastating effect on both the individual and the family. Impaired levels of functioning are related to loss of old skills and the failure to acquire new ones. This affects the person's productivity, self-concept, and potential for positive change. This, in turn, increases the family burden, both perpetuating and increasing the individual's dependence, socially and economically.

Dual Diagnosis and the Family

The impact on the family unit of a member with a dual diagnosis of psychiatric disability and either a substance abuse disorder or a developmental disability can be complex. (The topic of dual diagnosis, mental illness and substance abuse, is given more thorough treatment in chapter 8.) Depending on the severity and duration of the person's disabilities, the family may have expended considerable emotional and financial resources in coping with the situation. All areas of family functioning may be affected by the presence of a dual diagnosis in a family member, including the general atmosphere, the ways family members communicate with each other, and the relationships, roles, and responsibilities that family members assume or are assigned (Daley, Moss, & Campbell, 1993). Likewise, families affect the family member with a disability. In their attempts to "control the uncontrollable," some family members may become overinvolved or enmeshed. Others become completely shut off or "disengaged" from their family member with a disability (Evans & Sullivan, 1990). In the case of a substance abuse disorder, sometimes well-intentioned behavior on the part of caring family members has the unintended effect of enabling the person to continue to abuse substances. For example, money given to the individual for living expenses or rent may actually be spent on alcohol or drugs (Evans & Sullivan, 1990).

Nevertheless, families have often developed skills and strategies for coping with a very difficult situation and services to families should build on those strengths. Evans and Sullivan (1990) address the need for families dealing with substance abuse and mental illness to enter a recovery process of their own. Education about chemical dependence and psychiatric disability, support groups such as Al-Anon, the 12-step program for families, and skill development in problem solving, negotiation, and communication are all services that are helpful to families in recovery (Evans & Sullivan, 1990). The concept of family recovery is addressed in more detail later in this chapter.

Independence/Dependence

Hatfield (1992) defines the central dilemma facing adults with serious and persistent mental illness and their families as being centered on the issue of independence/dependence. In Western culture, the independence of young adults or even adolescents is seen as an important developmental goal. For many adults with severe and persistent mental illness, continued dependence on others is a virtual necessity. This requirement of continuing dependence often leads to great tension among family members. This is particularly true for parents who see fostering independence in their adult offspring as an important goal of parenting.

Burden and Stigma

Lefley (1989) discussed both the *family burden* and the *family stigma* associated with major mental illness. She noted that the emphasis on the family in terms of experience of mental illness has shifted from causing the disorders to being viewed as "potential precipitants of relapse" (Lefley, 1989, p. 556). Both the earlier and more recent views cast the family in a very negative light and contribute to the stigma experienced.

Lefley (1989) also reports that families fear, sometimes with good reason, that the behavior of a relative with mental illness diminishes their reputation as individuals and as a family, jeopardizing their relationships with friends and neighbors. Because of this stigma, family members wish to distance themselves from their ill relative, but often feel guilt if they do so.

In one study, half of the parents and spouses of persons hospitalized for a mental disorder reported concealing the hospitalization to some degree (Phelan, Bromet, & Link, 1998). Indeed, a significant portion of family members (16%) reported that they believed other people were avoiding them, suggesting a strong awareness of stigma by family members (Phelan et al., 1998).

Marsh and colleagues (1996) collected many comments regarding familial burden. The burden the family bears has been described as suffering, very sad, draining, and lonely. Family members speak of the care of their loved one as being a full-time job. Some report the abandonment of their own jobs and careers. Often, they feel as if they have not done enough. Some report permanent distraction. Others report anger toward their spouses or other family members. For example, parents of adults may be angry with the siblings of the person who is ill for their lack of support, involvement, and sometimes their lack of acknowledgment of the existence of the sick family member to other people.

Families coping with any chronic medical condition, mental illness or otherwise, attempt to adjust. Under conditions of constant strain regardless of the diagnostic category, family members see the illness as cycles or patterns of exacerbation with contrasting periods of remission. Thus, they experience many cycles of hope and disappointment.

Families experience a variety of stresses. These stresses can be very tangible, such as the economic burden of high health care costs or the loss of insurance. They can also be less tangible, but no less real, such as fear, anxiety, and fatigue. Thus, the stress on the family has been categorized into two broad areas: objective burden and subjective burden. Both types of burden will be discussed next.

The Objective Burden

Objective burden deals with specifically identifiable, observable problems associated with the person's mental illness. The objective burdens of families in which a member has a chronic developmental, mental, or physical disability have a degree of commonality. Objective burden includes financial hardships due to medical bills, the cost of the consumer's economic dependence, disruptions in household functioning, restriction of social activities, and altered relationships because of the demands of caregiving. There is often a significant time commitment to the mental health consumer's needs at the expense of other family activities. Individual members of the family, particularly the primary caregiver, may often need to change their role in the family, often at the expense of their own careers.

The Subjective Burden

Subjective burden refers to the psychological distress borne by family members, which is engendered by the illness. Subjective burden is related to objective burden, but not always directly. A caregiver may carry the highest objective burden in the family, yet because she has accommodated herself to it, may feel a relatively lower subjective burden than other family members. Other family members who are caregivers often bear a smaller objective burden, but feel they have a greater burden because of the apparently abrupt disruptions in their routine, which they experience as a significant burden.

Besides some of the chronic burdens families face, there are certain acute ones that are no less troublesome. Families may have periodic crises involving interactions with emergency services and the police. In addition, in most states, involuntary commitment procedures can pit family members against one another in an adversarial manner that is often poorly understood and causes resentment.

> Gina, a 28-year-old woman with four children had become very distressed. Her husband, Mike, had stopped seeing his psychiatrist. He had not bathed in months and had literally stopped speaking. He was not working and remained in the house. For weeks, she had begged him to get help. When he became completely mute, she finally called crisis services and later filed the complaint to commit him. He was hospitalized, received medication, improved markedly, and went back to work. But, he was very resentful. Gina's father-in-law, Ralph, who was normally supportive and mild mannered, said years later, "Do you realize she had Mike COMMITTED! I will never forgive her for that!" When other relatives pointed out it was the only option she had left to get Mike help, Ralph refused to listen.

Troublesome Actions that Contribute to Burden

In describing family life with a person with severe and persistent mental illness, Lefley (1987a, 1987b, 1989) noted a variety of behaviors of some persons with serious mental illness that contribute to the burden borne by their family members:

- Hostile, abusive, or assaultive behaviors (even if rare)
- Mood swings, other unpredictable behavior
- Socially offensive or embarrassing behavior
- Poor motivation, apparent malingering (often due to negative symptoms)
- Apparently self-destructive actions such as poor handling of money, deteriorated personal hygiene, and neglect or damage of property.

The burden that family members must bear occasionally includes abusive and assaultive behaviors in acute phases of the illness, especially in the earlier years. While infrequent or even based on a single instance, these incidents within a family are very memorable and may be dwelled on for years to come. There are a variety of other troublesome behaviors that are particularly upsetting, including symptoms such as paranoid ideation about family members and negative symptoms that lead to poor self-care.

As if these problems were not enough, parents also worry about what will happen to their adult child "when I am gone." That is, they worry about who will provide care after their own deaths, although there are efforts to help parents with estate planning that will help care for their children, a practice begun for parents of persons with developmental disabilities. Lefley (1987a) also stated that many families experience a "dilemma of functional expectancy" (p. 114). This dilemma refers to the idea that having normal expectations for the role of a family member with mental illness sometimes leads to frustration because the person has difficulty meeting these expectations. For example, parents may attempt to promote the independence of their son or daughter, that is, expect that as an adult he or she should be able to maintain his or her own apartment. Yet, when the person fails, the parents may think it is too much to expect. At the same time, if expectations are inordinately lowered, the individual may tend to live up to these low expectations, rarely reaching a level of functioning that would be considered normal.

The situation of adult children living with parents is often very stressful regardless of the presence or absence of mental illness. Indeed, the variance in burden experienced by the parents is directly related to the degree of dependence of the adult on their parents, whether or not a psychiatric illness was present. Nevertheless, the situation is not hopeless. Today's family psychoeducation and support interventions, while they involve the family very extensively, actually succeed in promoting independence (Pharaoh et al., 2004) and reducing family burden (McFarlane et al., 2003). This evidence is discussed in more detail later in this chapter.

Family Dissatisfaction

Given the numerous burdens families must deal with, one would hope that the mental health system would be responsive to their concerns. Unfortunately, families are often unhappy with the way their relatives are served. They express general dissatisfaction with the service delivery system and often with mental health professionals themselves. They have frequently been subjected to irrelevant treatment models that do not meet their expressed needs. Traditional approaches often leave them with inappropriate expectations about their family member. The expectations offered by professionals are often too low, too high, or absent altogether. For a number of reasons professionals frequently withhold relevant information and do not help in managing difficult behaviors.

Consider the lot of the mother of a person with serious mental illness, living at home after hospital discharge:

> She is suffering the pain of her child's illness, the stigmatization of having caused it, the burden of overseeing a treatment plan that may be unrealistic . . . at the same time, she is trying to balance conflicting advice. . . . (Lefley, 1989, p. 557)

Seemingly logical instructions from professionals can be clearly contradictory. Family members can be accused of being overprotective at the same time they are being told to discourage their family member from taking unnecessary risks. For example, a mother may be told that she has been neglectful or rejecting in the past, but that now she must encourage independence. If she does not take the advice of the professional, she may be accused of sabotaging treatment (Lefley, 1989).

Too often professionals have been basically disapproving in the messages they give family members. Their overt or covert disapproval evokes defensive reactions on the part of the family members, thus fulfilling the bias of clinicians that the family is "too defensive."

Given these communication problems, family members may become alienated and resentful. Other families may become overly submissive, inordinately deferring to the professionals. Some families, following instructions, have disengaged from or abandoned their family member with mental illness.

Three Levels of Family Involvement

The burden experienced by family members varies based on their level of involvement with the member who is ill. Terkelson (1987a) proposed that there are three tiers of family involvement. In the immediate family, most often one individual, usually (but not always) a woman who is the mother, wife, sister, or daughter of the person with mental illness, assumes the role of principal caregiver. Much of her daily life becomes a series of illness-related occupations and preoccupations. She acknowledges the illness more than others and also suffers its impact more than others in this family. This individual, especially if she is the mother of the ill relative, may also feel responsible for the illness itself, an idea sometimes foisted on her by professionals. Terkelson (1987a) notes:

> She witnesses the impatient naiveté of overworked, well meaning professionals. She takes in their suggestions for modifying family life and suffers from the implications. . . . (p. 131)

Often these implications are significant, asking a family to change its entire lifestyle, resulting in understandable resistance. Terkelson describes this sort of caregiver as living a life that is a stream of nursing activities. Other activities include attempting to keep the illness from disrupting the rest of the family members' lives. Relief is found only when the consumer shows some progress. Time away from caring for the consumer is often filled with worrying or at least thinking about the person.

Second-tier relatives may live with or near the person with mental illness, but they are less intimately exposed to the "ups" and "downs" of the person's life. Thanks to the primary caregiver or first-tier relatives, as well as their own efforts, these second-tier relatives experience less frequent intrusions on their lives. However, occasionally they experience a more noticeable disruption when some troublesome aspect of the illness inserts itself into their lives. For example, while their daily routine is not burdened by the care of a relative with a disability, their lives may be more abruptly disrupted in the midst of an exacerbation of that person's symptoms. More than the primary caregiver or first-tier relatives, they may come to dread both the illness and interaction with the consumer, avoiding involvement whenever possible. In addition, to avoid indirect involvement with the mental health consumer, they often avoid involvement with the primary caregiver. Thus, a husband may become estranged from a wife, siblings from each other, a child from a parent, and so forth.

By contrast, there are also some second-tier relatives who, although they detach themselves from daily involvement with the consumer, involve themselves actively only during times of crises.

Third-tier relatives are not in the immediate household, but still share a common interest in the well-being of the consumer. At times, these individuals may play down or deny the presence of the illness and associated disability. Sometimes they regard the person with the illness as faking or lazy. Others may feel helpless in the face of the problem and wonder what they can do to help. They may also wonder if they have contributed to the adverse situation. Some may also have fantasies about rescuing the ill person. Occasionally, they may blame the primary caregiver or underinvolved second-tier relatives for the person's mental illness. As you can see by Terkelson's very insightful description of the situation, the objective and subjective burdens of each group vary markedly.

Kevin's Story: A Confidentiality Issue

Maintaining the confidentiality of a person receiving services is considered a person's right as well as a good thing. Even with something as obvious as confidentiality, however, problems can arise. Consider the following situation.

Kevin is a semi-retired man in his early 60s. Almost everyday, he drives his son, Brian, who is about 30, to the local psychosocial rehabilitation day program. He drops him off at about 9 a.m. and picks him up about 3 p.m. One day, Kevin thinks he ought to talk things over with the staff at the center because Brian is sleeping poorly and often paces all night. He decides to call the center after he arrives at his part-time job. He asks for Brian's case manager, who gets on the phone. Brian's case manager makes the following response to Kevin's queries, ostensibly to protect confidentiality, "I cannot even say whether your son is served here or not." In fact, the case manager is upholding the agency's policy of not revealing information about the people they serve to anyone, unless the client expressly consents to the disclosure. Enraged at this "snippy" attitude and the rejection of his attempts to share information for his son's benefit, Kevin responds: "I know damn well he is there. I drive him there everyday and pick him up, so don't give me that nonsense. Besides you call my wife and I when it suits you, we have spoken before!"

Mental health professionals who are also members of families experiencing mental illness make up an interesting group of individuals in this regard. In many ways they are not different from other family members, except they may bear an additional stigma. Lefley (1987a, 1987b) found that mental health clinicians did not differ from lay family members in some important ways. Their assessment of the psychological burden or subjective burden of a having a family member with mental illness was very similar to that of all family members. Like other family members, they assigned a high priority to the need for education on symptoms and medications, techniques for managing difficult behavior, and involvement in support groups. Yet, they were very uncomfortable in discussing their family's experience with mental illness with their colleagues. The great majority had frequently heard colleagues make negative or otherwise disparaging remarks about family members of people with mental illness.

The Unique Burdens of Spouses

Spouses of persons with severe mental illness bear a unique burden. Mannion (1996) estimated that 35% to 40% of people hospitalized for psychiatric disabilities are discharged to live with their spouses. Mannion reported that the great majority of spouses surveyed reported a process of adaptation and recovery. Nevertheless, the burden of spouses includes these problems:

- Marital dissatisfaction and disruption
- Financial problems
- Socialization difficulties
- Personal experience of emotional and mood symptoms
- Separations and divorce.

Clearly, when one's spouse has a major mental illness it puts a great deal of stress on the marriage. Despite this, it is often difficult for the well spouse to receive help to keep the marriage together. A reciprocal flow of information between spouses and professional caregivers would improve the quality of care and effectively reduce relapse, but unfortunately, this is all too rare.

Siblings and Children

Siblings of people with mental illness also experience significant stresses (Kinsella, Anderson, & Anderson, 1996). Young family members, both siblings and children of people with the disorders, share a special vulnerability to the familial experience of mental illness (Marsh et al., 1993). For example, one grown child of a mother with mental illness reported "The mental illness shaped my life . . . it revolved around her problems."

Adults who dealt with the mental illness of a relative during their own childhood reported a variety of difficulties, including subjective burden in the form of feelings of grief and loss, empathy for the suffering of other family members, stigma on the individual and family, and objective burden in needing to deal with symptomatic behavior and illness related crises. Specific problems include the following:

- Absence of a model of normal development
- Difficulty determining which experiences were "normal" and which were not normal
- Altered roles, for example, "parentification," a child having to care for the sick parent
- Their own mental health problems
- Strain in relationships outside family, for example, at school
- Fear of developing mental illness themselves.

In adulthood, these individuals attribute impaired self-esteem and self-concept and fear of rejection to their childhood experience (Marsh et al., 1993).

People with Mental Illness as Parents

Parents with a serious mental illness face the challenges that every other parent faces, often have the additional burden of being a single parent, and, in addition, they have specific, unique challenges associated with having a severe and persistent mental illness. Some of the universal challenges of parenthood include the economic burdens of caring for children, the need to develop and apply new skills to provide effective childrearing, and the need for social support from the extended family, their own parents, or friends who can provide advice, encouragement, and emotional support for their efforts. Parents with mental illness face these same challenges, often exacerbated by their mental illness, poverty, and social isolation. For example, people with mental illness face particularly serious economic challenges, particularly if they are dependent on public benefits, which are barely adequate for their own support, let alone those of dependent children. Many individuals, because of the nature of the course of their illness, have had the development of parenting skills and household management skills disrupted. In addition, they often have small social networks and do have others available to support them in their role as parents.

Single mothers with a mental illness report experiencing more financial strain and health problems even when compared to other low-income, single mothers (Mowbray et al., 2000). They also experience a disproportionate number of losses, crises, assaults, negative life events, and chronic hassles. Like other parents, they find religion, interpersonal support, and help from mental health professionals to be useful (Mowbray et al., 2000).

Most of the research on this topic is about mothers with mental illness because they are more likely to be the custodial parent, the one who has responsibility for daily care of the child in her household, than a father. Yet, the number of single fathers rearing a child is increasing (Styron, Pruett, McMahon, & Davidson, 2002) and in many ways they are very similar to single mothers with a mental illness (Nicholson, Nason, Calabresi, & Yando, 1999). As single parents, these parents are very likely to be impoverished, fairly isolated, and often unskilled as a parent. A fairly large number of men with serious mental illness are fathers (20% to 33%), and among these fathers a majority wish to be involved with their children even if they do not have custody (Styron et al., 2002).

The timing of the onset of mental illness is associated with the adaptation to motherhood. Those whose illness began well after the birth of a child had the best adaptation to the role of mother. Those who had the second best adaptation were individuals whose onset of the illness was before the birth of their children. Those who had the worst adaptation to motherhood were women whose onset of the illness coincided with the birth of one of her children (Mowbray, Bybee, Oyserman, & MacFarlane, 2005). These women tended to be younger at the birth of their first child and have more children. This is an alarming finding considering the relatively high incidence of postpartum mental illnesses.

Parents and their children can engage in a number of strategies to successfully cope with a mental illness. These have been summarized by the University of Pennsylvania's Rehabilitation Research and Training Center on Community Integration in their publications, which are available through their website. Applicable publications include *Parenting with a Mental Illness: Positive Parenting & Child Resilience* (2005a) and *Parenting with a Mental Illness: Child Welfare & Custody Issues* (2005b).

Some of the most important strategies include the following:

1. *Development of natural supports for both parent and child:* There is a folk expression that it takes a village to raise a child. Along the same line of thinking, it takes at least a parent with his or her own support network to more effectively raise a child. Those persons with mental illness who become parents and/or are considering becoming parents need to have a social support network to help with daily coping and emotional support, but also to assist during periods of stress and crisis situations. Similarly children need and benefit from the supports of family, friends, classmates, participation in school, and community activities. Parents need to make the effort to integrate their children in supports outside the home.

2. *Parenting skills:* Parenting is a complicated role and includes complex cognitive and emotional tasks. In most communities, little attention is paid to this very unique form of skill development, and it is virtually nonexistent in psychiatric rehabilitation services. Like other new or inexperienced parents, or parents facing challenges of disciplining children, parents who have a mental illness could benefit greatly from a parenting skills training program. A number of models are available for parents of children with attention deficit disorder that are based on behavioral principles that would be helpful to all parents, even those who have children who do not have these difficulties.

3. *The necessity of a relapse plan:* Every person with a severe and persistent mental illness should have a plan for relapse both for the management of their own illness and the maintenance of their jobs, homes, and other aspects of their lives. For persons with these mental illnesses who are parents, a plan to manage relapse is particularly critical for many reasons, particularly the safety and well-being of their children for time periods when they may not be able to care for them. This is essential for the child's health and emotional well-being, but also to establish that the parent should retain legal custody

because the children were never endangered. Thus, it is most essential that preplanning for child care in case of relapse and/or rehospitalization be done.

4. *Normal interests outside the home:* It is important that both child and parent have normal interests outside the home. These interests are a source of natural supports as alluded to earlier, but also provide relief from each other. While parents and children are capable of providing mutual support, it is also important that each have interests and supports other than their all-important first-tier relative. When a parent or child is the only support available to the other, a great deal of pressure on each can result. Indeed, if mothers have too high an expectation of support from their child/children, it is a predictor of maternal behavior that puts a child at risk for abuse, neglect, or other maltreatment (Mullick, Miller, & Jacobsen, 2001).

5. Awareness *of legal rights:* Parents need to be aware of their legal rights and responsibilities in terms of maintaining custody and legal recourse for regaining child custody. There is often a great deal of pressure to relinquish custody. In contrast, understanding about alternatives such as adoption, including open adoption, is important, as is understanding the limitations and problems with foster care.

6. *Professional supports:* Maintaining regular contact with mental health professionals to continue to receive appropriate medication and psychosocial interventions is essential. Sometimes, children are also in need of these professional supports.

7. *Age-appropriate education of children regarding mental illness:* Parents, in collaboration with professionals, should educate their children regarding mental illness with accurate information the child can assimilate, with its complexity increasing as the child becomes older. In this way, unnecessary stigma is avoided and as an adolescent and adult, the child can later support his or her parent in managing the illness

How well adjusted are the children of persons who have a mental illness? Contrary to popular belief, all the children of persons with severe and persistent mental illness do not have severe emotional problems or mental illnesses themselves. As reported in Chapter 2's discussion of etiology, only 10% to 20% will have a similar diagnosis. In fact, there is a broad range of outcomes. Mowbray and colleagues (2000) found that about 15% of the children of mothers with serious mental illness exhibited psychiatric symptoms, 27% had possible behavior problems, and about 4% had social isolation problems. Slightly more than half were socially and academically competent. Fifty-two percent had average or above-average academic functioning, although among this group a number of children were very adult oriented, as opposed to oriented toward age-appropriate peer activity.

Being a parent is a normal adult role that many people with severe and persistent mental illness must fulfill or wish to pursue. Like other roles, it often requires skills and resources to pursue and often the assistance of professionals, but also natural supports such as family, neighbors, and friends. Of course, there are the unique challenges that are added by parenthood and children. There is evidence that the better the parent's understanding of his or her own illness, the better the adjustment of his or her child (Mullick et al., 2001). In addition, as discussed earlier, it is *critical* for parents to have a relapse plan that includes the uninterrupted care of their children.

The Anguish of the Individual

Lefley (1987a, 1987b) suggests that the most devastating stressor for family members may be that of learning to cope with the person's own anguish over an impoverished life; that is, his or her acute awareness of what he or she has missed out on or will miss out on. Not only does the individual with mental illness experience this extended grieving, so do the relatives who mourn the loss of the personality, skills, and strengths of the person due to the illness.

The Burdens of Family Living for the Person with Mental Illness

Up to this point this chapter has dealt with the burden of care associated with living with a relative with mental illness. But does family life present any unique stresses or burdens to the person with mental illness? As already stated, in the past, it was inaccurately assumed that family living was not only stressful, but also a possible cause of mental illness. Today we understand that this is not the case, but there is some evidence that a particular emotional environment of high expressed emotion may contribute to the relapses of some people with mental illness (Anderson et al., 1986).

British researchers observed an association between living arrangements and relapses among persons with schizophrenia (Anderson et al., 1986). Independent groups of investigators found that the emotional level within family groups with close ties presented a specific stress. Specifically, consumers whose families manifested high EE as demonstrated by criticism, hostility, and levels of emotional overinvolvement were at higher risk for relapse (sometimes 50% or more over a 9-month period), compared to consumers returning to low EE families (13% to 15% relapse rate). If a consumer had frequent contact (more than 35 hours per week) with a high EE relative, the increased relapse rate occurred even if they were compliant with their regimen of antipsychotics. A high EE environment apparently serves as a trigger for relapse. This negative high EE effect seems to be most relevant for unmarried men living in their parental homes (Harding & Zahniser, 1994).

A climate of high EE in one's family or other social unit apparently contributes to the onset of psychotic symptoms among people genetically at risk for schizophrenia (Anderson et al., 1986). However, it has also been found that most families with members who have schizophrenia do not have this high EE pattern; only those with high EE environments are more likely to relapse. Therefore, high EE does not appear to be either necessary or sufficient to cause schizophrenia (Harding & Zahniser, 1994).

The Dilemma of Functional Expectancy and Independence/Dependence Revisited

The dilemma of "functional expectancy" and the independence/dependence dilemma were discussed earlier in terms of their burden to family members. These two factors also present a potential burden to the person with mental illness. Living with one's family, especially one's family of origin, presents constant reminders of disabilities and unfulfilled plans and aspirations that may not be helpful at all. For example, there may be the daily stress of being presented with the fact that one is not making a normal, expected contribution to family life. On the other hand, the lack of this expectation on the part of others may harm self-esteem. In addition, failing to achieve independence is also constantly thrown in one's face by having to depend on one's family for basic needs. These clearly are significant stresses that are more acutely felt in a family environment as opposed to solitary living.

Loneliness

One of the major complaints of persons with serious mental illness is their persistent loneliness. Are persons who live with family members less lonely than those who do not? The answer appears to be "not necessarily" (Brown, 1996). Both men and women with serious mental illness are significantly more lonely than the general population, as measured by the UCLA loneliness scale. In one study (Brown, 1996), consumers with mental illness were grouped according to different living situations, that is, alone, with a roommate, with family, or in a group home. Those living with their families were no less lonely than those living in other situations.

Goals for Helping Families

Because families are the primary care agent, an enormous source of social support, and a strong contributing factor to recovery, the family–professional relationship should be one of collaboration, avoiding blaming and pathologizing family members. Given the objective and subjective burden of family members and the needs of their relative with mental illness, Anderson and colleagues (1986) specified the following goals in trying to help families:

- Establish a relationship with the family in which there is a genuine working alliance that is a partnership in order to help the consumer.
- Attempt to comprehend familial problems that may be contributing to both the stress level of the consumer and the family members.
- Gain an understanding of the family's resources and what successful and unsuccessful attempts have been made to cope with the illness they have faced.
- Build rehabilitative and educational endeavors around the family's strengths.
- Develop appropriate expectations for the rehabilitation and treatment process through a contract that includes specific goals that are both mutual and attainable.

Family Interventions

Given the importance of the family in the rehabilitation process, a great deal of work has gone into studying how families can be assisted. During the last two decades, sophisticated psychosocial interventions involving family members have been developed to assist in the rehabilitation of persons with severe and persistent mental illness (Dixon et al., 2001; McFarlane et al., 2003). These methods have been studied empirically and rigorously evaluated, and have been found to be effective (Dixon et al., 2001). As it turns out, family interventions are one of the leading PsyR strategies whose effectiveness has been confirmed by research. In other words they are evidence-based practices. (See the discussion of family psychoeducation as an evidence-based practice later in this chapter.) Some common assumptions are shared in all of these approaches:

- Schizophrenia and other major mental illnesses are regarded as medical, biological conditions.
- The family environment is not seen as an etiological factor.
- Social and emotional support is provided, often including support from other families.
- Routine psychotropic medication management is included as an essential component.

These approaches are emphatically in contrast to traditional family therapies based on etiological theories that assert the family and/or its communication patterns are a major causative factor of the illness.

These rehabilitation-oriented interventions also tend to have common components that only differ in emphasis or in the specific technique employed. These components include the following:

- *Psychoeducation:* Information about mental illness and its treatment, similar to the content of Chapters 1, 2, and 3 of this book
- *Behavioral problem solving:* Structured problem solving about daily issues, crises, and so forth, often beginning with brainstorming and moving to evaluation of specific alternatives (Hatfield, 1990)
- *Family support:* Empathy from other families and professionals regarding the plight of the family
- *Crisis management:* Concrete information on de-escalation of crises, coping with symptom exacerbation, and so forth.

These interventions are delivered in a variety of formats that vary along a number of dimensions (Hatfield, 1990; McFarlane 1994). For example, sometimes interventions are aimed at a single family or at groups of families. Interventions are provided in different settings such as clinics, hospitals, homes, or church halls. The length of these interventions may range from a one-day workshop to several years of monthly meetings. Also, the intervention may be designed to take place during different phases of the illness or to be carried out without regard for the phase of the illness. Some family interventions are conducted without the relative who has mental illness present, while others are only implemented with the relative present. In addition, professionals, family members, or a team consisting of both family members and professionals can conduct these interventions. Thus, in many family psychoeducational efforts, family members have leadership roles.

Similar to other psychiatric rehabilitation techniques, family psychoeducation involves connecting with family members by focusing on the "here and now" (Cnaan, Blankertz,

Messinger, & Gardner, 1993). Anderson and colleagues (1986) advise mental health practitioners to make themselves available to families immediately and not just at scheduled times. The initial focus must be on the present crisis that has brought them to seek assistance: a recent hospitalization, an impending hospital discharge, or a recent escalation in symptoms. In this collaborative approach it is important not to treat the family as a patient, but instead to treat it as a partner (Anderson et al., 1986). Some older family intervention models saw the family as "a system" that maintained pathology. Newer family interventions see families as having both strengths and weaknesses that, like many other psychosocial factors, impact the course and adjustment of a person with serious mental illness. Working with families is a joint project with the staff, individual family members, and the consumer collaborating in the rehabilitation process.

Sometimes, family members lack basic information regarding schizophrenia or other major mental illnesses. To address this deficit, Hogarty and his colleagues (Anderson et al., 1986) devised a single-day "Survival Skills Workshop." This approach has been adopted in various formats and is often spread out over a series of sessions (Hatfield, 1990). This type of training provides family members with important knowledge about mental illness and its treatment, working on the premise that knowledge is power in itself. Typically, a survival skills workshop includes discussions on the following topics:

- Definitions of diagnoses such as schizophrenia
- History and prevalence of the disorder
- Personal and public experience
- The role of biology in the illness
- The role of antipsychotic medications, how they work, impact on outcome, therapeutic and side effects
- Psychosocial treatments
- Course of the illness and impact of treatment on course
- Impact on family
- Familial responses
- Common problems families face
- Strategies for family coping including revising expectations, avoiding overstimulation, selectively ignoring certain behavior, setting expectations, identifying signals of impending trouble, effectively using professionals.

Other groups (e.g., Hatfield, 1990) have expanded on this approach and spend a good deal of time teaching families to create supportive environments. In addition, there is explicit training around problem-solving skills and dealing with crises (Hatfield, 1990). Hatfield also recommends that besides addressing immediate family needs, realistic long-range planning should also take place to balance the needs of the family as well as the individual.

Summary of the Empirical Evidence

As mentioned earlier family interventions, particularly psychoeducational and problem-solving approaches, are among the best methods of promoting better outcomes among people with severe and persistent mental illness (Dixon et al., 2001; Lehman & Steinwachs, 1998). If family members can be engaged, certainly these interventions are among the most effective social techniques that can be employed to improve the course and outcome of illnesses such as schizophrenia (Hogarty, 1993). Family interventions that are primarily psychoeducational are particularly effective (Dixon & Lehman, 1995). Secondly, those that include the patient in the family intervention also appear to be superior. Multiple family groups working together are particularly effective, perhaps because of the mutual emotional support and practical advice they can share (McFarlane et al., 2003).

Many of these studies of family interventions began as part of an aftercare program following discharge from a psychiatric hospital. Some others began as families simply providing support to other families in distress. Goldstein, Rodnick, Evans, May, and Steinberg (1978) found that even as few as six weekly sessions focusing on education and building acceptance and planning for the future resulted in significantly lower relapses. Some family interventions were developed as explicit efforts to change high EE family environments, although as discussed earlier, most families who have persons with mental illness do not exhibit this high EE style. Nevertheless, Falloon and his colleagues (1982, 1985) studied this minority of families with a high EE environment. All of the families had members diagnosed with schizophrenia who were predicted to be at high risk for relapse because they were living with high EE relatives. His treatment group included behavioral family therapy, problem solving, and communication skills designed to promote a low EE style. Training lasted for 3 months at the family's home with a 6-month follow-up period to provide familial support. This family intervention approach was compared to supportive individual psychotherapy and brief family counseling. Measured at 9 months and 2 years, the comprehensive family intervention produced significantly fewer relapses, increased patient functioning, reduced family burden, and lowered overall treatment costs.

Similarly, Leff and colleagues (1982, 1985) worked with the families of people with schizophrenia who were also classified as high EE. Psychoeducation of family members, a relatives' group, and individualized problem-solving–oriented family therapy in the home were compared to minimal family contact and regular hospital follow-up. Measured at 9 months, it was found that the comprehensive family intervention reduced relapses.

As mentioned earlier, Hogarty and colleagues (1986, 1991) developed an approach that was very family centered and sought to empower families by promoting useful skills, knowledge and attitudes. The family treatment focused on (1) building an alliance with the family, (2) providing concrete information and management suggestions, (3) building a support network at a 1-day survival skills workshop, and (4) providing workshop skills in individual family therapy with the patient included.

There is empirical support for the efficacy of Hogarty's approach. One of the most compelling findings from his studies, which employed random assignment, was that after 2 years, 25% to 29% of the individuals who received the family treatment relapsed, compared to relapse rates as high as 62% for individuals who received social skills training or day treatment alone.

McFarlane expanded Hogarty's approach to multiple family groups, which were later found to be superior. McFarlane (1994) and McFarlane and colleagues (1995, 2003) conducted studies of a psychoeducational family intervention delivered in a multiple-family group format. Using content similar to that developed by Hogarty and colleagues (1991) to serve one family at a time, McFarlane and his colleagues began serving multiple families simultaneously.

The first study they conducted compared three groups: (1) psychoeducation and multiple-family group, (2) psychoeducation and single-family therapy, and (3) multiple-family groups without psychoeducation, known as *family dynamic group*. Both psychoeducational conditions were similar in content. The psychoeducational interventions included initial family engagement and educational sessions followed by 2 years of biweekly sessions on illness management with clinicians using formal problem-solving techniques. This was followed by an additional 2 years of monthly sessions. Consumers did not attend initial family engagement and educational sessions, but did attend the later monthly sessions. In the single-family condition, clinicians met with one family at a time, but covered the same areas over the same period of time at the same intensity of service as the multiple-family groups. In the multiple-family group without psychoeducation (dynamic multiple group), no education was provided. The methods used by clinicians in this approach included opening intrafamilial communication, sharing emotional responses, and attempting to resolve familial conflicts. These groups met weekly for the first 2 years and twice monthly in the second 2 years.

After 1 year, the dynamic multiple-family group condition was discontinued for ethical reasons, due to the inordinately high relapse rate. In the other treatments, after both 2 and 4 years, the relapse rates were significantly lower in the multiple-family condition compared to the single-family group. After 4 years, 78% of the single-family condition patients had relapsed, compared to only 45% of the multiple-family condition sample. McFarlane replicated this study using 172 families at six sites throughout New York state (McFarlane et al., 1995). The multiple-family group condition again proved superior to the single-family condition. A number of studies with related findings support the efficacy of educational interventions with families and consumers (McFarlane, 1994).

The Effectiveness of Family Education and Support

In the report on the Schizophrenia Patient Outcomes Research Team (PORT), Lehman and Steinwachs (1998) summarized the research regarding family interventions and offered the following two recommendations about people with schizophrenia who have continuing contact with their families:

1. They should be offered a family psychosocial intervention that lasts at least 9 months.
2. This intervention should include education about mental illness, support for family members, formal behavioral problem solving, and crisis intervention skills.

These recommendations were based on the fact that these packages of interventions have been found to reduce typical 1-year relapse rates of 40% to 53% to as low as 2% to 23%. They are excellent examples of how a psychosocial intervention can help the course of a biological disorder.

Initially, it had been thought that these interventions should be limited to families classified as having high EE (criticism, hostility, and overinvolvement). Although there is substantial benefit to these families, these interventions have been found to be helpful regardless of the level of EE (Lehman & Steinwachs, 1998). Lehman and Steinwachs also added that family therapies based on the premise that family dysfunction is the etiology of a person's schizophrenic disorder should definitely not be used:

> The presumption that family interaction causes schizophrenia . . . has led to serious disruption in clinician/family trust without evidence of therapeutic effectiveness. (p. 3)

Main Benefits of Family Intervention

In the most rigorous studies, randomized controlled trials of family psychoeducation that includes mental illness education, problem solving, and social support have been found to have numerous benefits for consumers:

- Decreased risk of relapse and decreased number of days spent hospitalized (Leff et al., 1989; McFarlane et al., 1995; Xiong et al., 1994)
- Reduction in the tension of family life (Tarrier et al., 1988) and better relations with specific relatives (Falloon et al., 1982)
- Significant reductions in the number and length of hospital admissions (Pharoah et al., 2004), including time in the hospital reduced by up to 67% (Xiong et al., 1994)
- Improved social functioning and overall level of functioning (Barrowclough et al., 2001; Xiong et al., 1994)
- Improved employment outcomes in terms of length of time employed (Xiong et al., 1994)
- More independent living by people allocated to individual family intervention.

In addition, positive outcomes for family members that translate into positive influences on the recovery of consumers include the following:

- Improved families' ability to understand the patients' needs (Bloch, Szmukler, Herrman, Benson, & Colussa, 1995)
- Reduced burden felt by family caregivers (Xiong et al., 1994)
- Quality of life for family significantly improved (Shi, Zhao, Zu, & Sen, 2000)
- Decreased levels of overinvolvement, criticism, and hostility toward the person with mental illness among high EE families (Leff et al., 1989).

Family Psychoeducation: An Evidence-Based Practice

Family psychoeducation is one of the six evidence-based practices (EBPs).

Critical Ingredients of Family Psychoeducation

1. Mental illness education
2. Problem solving

3. Stress reduction
4. Long-term duration
5. Family and consumer involvement.

Outcomes of Family Psychoeducation

1. Reduces relapse.
2. Reduces hospitalizations.
3. Improves family knowledge of mental illness, symptoms, medications, therapeutic effects, and side effects.
4. May improve family problem solving.
5. May reduce family stress.
6. May assist family "recovery."

As this chapter has pointed out, families are often the principal support providers for people with severe mental illness. Effectively educating and supporting these families has been shown to have very positive effects for the family member with mental illness as well as the entire family. For many years, under the influence of psychodynamic thinking, parents were blamed for contributing to their child's illness (e.g., the "schizophrenogenic" mother). Later professionals reawakened to the fact that families were important caregivers with the ability to affect the course of the illness. A number of different family psychoeducation and support strategies have been employed (e.g., Anderson, Reiss, & Hogarty, 1986; Falloon, Boyd, & McGill, 1984). This has produced a sufficient body of research to be considered an EBP.

The elements considered critical to effective family psychoeducation include the following:

- *Mental illness education:* This consists of providing the family with information about the probable etiology, course, and treatment of the mental illness in question. Additional information about medications, medication side effects, treatment options, and psychiatric rehabilitation services is also provided.
- *Problem solving:* Families are taught problem-solving strategies that they role-play and practice on a regular basis. Besides improving the family's response to crisis, this training helps to improve family morale and confidence. An important aspect of family psychoeducation is that it provides support to the caregivers as well as the consumer.
- *Stress reduction:* Family members and the consumer are taught stress reduction techniques. In combination with problem solving, this helps to improve morale, reinforce caregiving, and sometimes forestall crisis.
- *Long-term duration:* Supports are provided as long as they are needed. This is similar to other EBPs. Families are different, they exist in different circumstances and their ill members are different. The family psychoeducation services are tailored to the needs of the individual family.

- *Family and consumer involvement:* Family psychoeducation training is conducted with the consumer present as an integrated member of the family.

Psychoeducation with high fidelity to these approaches results in reductions in the number of relapses, fewer and shorter hospitalizations, and increased knowledge of mental illness, medications, and their side effects and the services available. Additionally, family psychoeducation may improve family problem solving, may reduce family stress, and is theorized to assist with family "recovery."

Studies of the effectiveness of family psychoeducation raise some important issues about how the effectiveness of EBP is assessed. In fact, family interventions of this type actually reduce the number of relapses and rehospitalizations in the long run.

McFarlane et al. (2003) summarized the state of the empirical evidence on family interventions:

> Family psychoeducation has emerged as a treatment of choice for schizophrenia, bipolar disorder, major depression, and other disorders. More than 30 randomized clinical trials have demonstrated reduced relapse rates, improved recovery of patients, and improved family well-being among participants. Interventions common to effective family psychoeducation programs have been developed, including empathic engagement, education, ongoing support, and clinical resources during periods of crisis, social network enhancement, and problem-solving and communication skills. (p. 223)

Unfortunately, this evidence has not been broadly incorporated into general practice:

> Application of family psychoeducation in routine settings where patients having these disorders are usually treated has been limited, reflecting attitudinal, knowledge, practical, and systemic implementation obstacles.

McFarlane et al. (2003) continue to say that in order for it to be implemented, there needs to be: "Consensus among patient and family advocacy organizations, clinician training, and ongoing technical consultation and supervision (p. 223)."

Other Family Psychoeducation Approaches

The family self-help movement has also been active in designing interventions including programming sponsored by NAMI (formerly the National Alliance for the Mentally Ill, which in 2005 was renamed the National Alliance on Mental Illness), is discussed in a later section. In this framework, family education is targeted not only to help the consumer, but to help the family as well. These family education models reject the medical model concept that treatment is something done to the individual and families must just comply. At the same time, they incorporate the reality that major mental illnesses are biological disorders. Like other rehabilitative approaches, these interventions concentrate on the competencies and strengths of family members.

Professional and Consumer Collaboration

Lundwall (1996) reported on an innovative approach that combines psychoeducation, support, and familial empowerment. The psychoeducational group is initially led by professionals and later is turned over to family members with the staff remaining in a case management or supportive role. Initially, the professional leads the rehabilitation process by providing psychoeducation, concrete guidelines, and coordination of service. Later, the leadership of the group is turned over to family members who have been empowered to lead their own group. The professional(s) continues in an advocacy, liaison, and service coordination role. The combination of education and support, followed by the assumption of leadership by family members, serves to increase the confidence of family members and, it is hoped, improve their ability to care for familial needs. In addition, the coordination of services helps meet the many needs of consumers and families. Families are supported in the experience of "grief" and "loss" of the ill family member. Also, the group empowers family members to help create positive changes in the service systems.

The Concept of Family Recovery

In our efforts to help consumers and their families, it might be helpful to recognize that, like the individual with mental illness, families may also go through a process of recovery. Spaniol and Zipple (1994) described *family recovery* as an essential goal for helping people with mental illness and their families. Their conception of family recovery parallels the concept of recovery for individuals discussed throughout this text. Spaniol and

---

CONTROVERSIAL ISSUE
Supervision versus Self-Determination

In a new bill a state legislator proposes that all state-licensed residences serving people with mental illness provide 24-hour supervision for their residents. This bill would even cover those programs that intentionally have minimal staff intervention because they are designed to promote independence. Not surprisingly, this bill receives a very mixed review from different groups. Some of the family advocates groups in the state praise the legislator for her vision, while other family advocates are uncomfortable with such a sweeping proposal. Some particularly vocal consumer advocates vigorously oppose the measure, while some other consumers prefer staff in the homes at all times.

What psychosocial rehabilitation principles are at stake here? Why are some of the family member advocates and consumer advocates on opposing sides here? Basically, they share the same concerns: the well-being of mental health consumers. One family advocate says he is for promoting quality of life and the 24-hour supervision will ensure good medication compliance and prompt crisis intervention. A consumer advocate says he is seeking a better quality of life by opposing the measure for his constituents, which he says will only hinder community integration, consumer choice, and self-determination. One wise observer comments, "I guess where you stand on this issue depends on where you sit." That is, some of the family advocates simply want their family member cared for, while some consumer advocates want to promote independence.

Zipple identified four stages in a family's recovery from serious and persistent mental illness: (1) discovery/denial, (2) recognition/acceptance, (3) coping/competence, and (4) personal/political advocacy. These four stages are discussed next.

Stage 1: Discovery/Denial

Family members' initial response to severe and persistent mental illness may range from minimizing the importance of the condition ("it's not so serious") to active denial ("it's just a phase" or "he is experimenting with drugs"). A lack of information and poor communication with professionals about what is happening can aggravate this situation. Sometimes, the best way to describe this stage is one characterized by a state of disbelief.

Stage 2: Recognition/Acceptance

As they become aware of the seriousness of the illness, family members may experience feelings of guilt, embarrassment, and self-blame. As they accept the reality of the illness, they experience a deep sense of loss. This sense of loss is often made more difficult by the cyclical nature of the illness, especially the periods of improvement that can cause a roller coaster of repeated hope followed by disappointment.

Stage 3: Coping/Competence

After acceptance, most families marshal their resources as they try to cope with the illness. Coping strategies may be effective or ineffective, informed by so-called expert opinion, or devised on their own. As outlined earlier in this chapter, a variety of effective approaches are available to help families cope better and become competent in their crisis intervention, problem solving, and understanding of mental illness.

Stage 4: Personal/Political Advocacy

Finally, many families reach the stage of personal/political advocacy. This stage is characterized by efforts to influence how the mental health system responds to the needs of the family member with mental illness and other individuals in the same predicament. These advocacy efforts often involve attempts to influence public policy through groups such as the National Alliance on Mental Illness and its local affiliates, which are discussed next.

The Story of NAMI

Family members are, and always have been, the caregivers for the majority of people with severe and persistent mental illness. Now, in many U.S. states and in other countries they have assumed an organized advocacy role. The largest and most successful American group is the National Alliance for the Mentally Ill (NAMI), renamed the National Alliance on Mental Illness in 2005. NAMI's major activities include families providing mutual support, sharing information, educating the public, and advocating for improved public policy and legislation.

Thanks in part to the efforts of NAMI, new and productive alliances between professionals and families are developing. These alliances are manifest with family representation on the advisory and governance boards of mental health services, as well as through family and consumer input in treatment, rehabilitation, and research. Family groups, in particular NAMI, have been very active in advocating, sponsoring, and raising funds for mental illness research.

History of NAMI

NAMI was founded in 1979, in Madison, Wisconsin, by people who wanted to help their relatives with mental illness and themselves. The first meeting included about 250 people who spent an emotional and memorable weekend together. Although professionals were in attendance, family members who founded this organization were determined to have it governed by and for families and consumers (NAMI, 1996, 1998).

Within 1 year, NAMI was incorporated, achieved nonprofit status, and elected a board of directors. Early efforts centered on making connections with small family support groups that had already been initiated throughout the United States. An annual conference was begun and a newsletter was published. By 1982, NAMI opened its first national office in Washington, D.C., and began the work of trying to influence legislation and policy with Congress, the administration, and other key lawmakers. NAMI describes itself as "A grass roots, self-help, support, and advocacy organization of families and friends of people with serious mental illness, and those persons themselves" (NAMI, 1996, 1998).

NAMI has focused on the unfulfilled needs of persons with the most serious forms of mental illness including those served in PsyR programs. Many of the members of NAMI are parents who were blamed for their child's mental illness. As such, they have firsthand understanding of the social stigma their son or daughter has experienced.

NAMI families join together to advocate for both needed changes in public attitudes and public policy. They have been supportive of current research that has been demonstrating the biochemical basis of what they now call brain diseases. Unlike most other advocacy or professional organizations, NAMI's exclusive focus is on serious mental illnesses or brain disorders. It now has more than 140,000 members and approximately 1,100 state, county, and local affiliates throughout the United States. The stated mission is as follows: "NAMI is dedicated to the eradication of mental illnesses and to the improvement of the quality of life of all whose lives are affected by these diseases" (NAMI, 2005).

NAMI's advocacy efforts have focused on many public policy issues facing mental illness, including achieving parity for mental disorders in all insurance plans. At both the federal and state levels, NAMI is working with legislators to introduce and pass laws that would end the discriminatory treatment of serious mental illness by insurance plans and companies. In short, they want mental illness to be treated like any other serious medical disorder. According to Dausey (2004), there is empirical evidence that the likelihood and speed of passing an insurance parity bill is directly correlated with the extent of NAMI advocacy in a state.

As of 2006, NAMI and its state chapters were playing an important role in a number of important public mental health system issues, such as the promotion and dissemination of the assertive community treatment (ACT) model throughout the United States (see Chapter 7 of this text and http://www.nami.org). NAMI and its chapters are very supportive of ACT, sometimes known as PACT (programs of assertive community treatment).

Another treatment approach promoted by some NAMI chapters and members is assisted outpatient treatment, also known as involuntary outpatient commitment. This involves court-ordered, community-based treatment for persons who are likely to become a risk to themselves or others by dropping out of treatment or as a result of medication nonadherence. Although NAMI and most of its affiliates support the extension and enforcement of commitment laws in many states, some chapters such as Connecticut NAMI do not favor this form of commitment (Dausey, 2004). Advocates who oppose outpatient commitment are concerned about the civil rights of persons with severe mental illnesses and also question the efficacy of forced treatment.

Families Helping Each Other

One of NAMI's education and support endeavors include the "Family to Family" education course. This is, in fact, a family-to-family program that is usually provided free of charge. In an intensive weekend training, family members are trained as teachers and facilitators to provide both education and support to other families. The educational component consists of a 12-week course. Teams of two members cover the following areas regarding serious mental illness:

- Learning about feelings, learning about facts
- Introduction to schizophrenia (e.g., diagnosis, crucial periods, etc.)
- Introduction to depression
- Basics about the brain
- Problem-solving skills workshop
- Medication review
- "What Is It Like to Be Mentally Ill?" empathy workshop
- Relative groups and self-care
- Communication skills
- Rehabilitation
- Advocacy (fighting stigma)
- Certification and celebration.

NAMI has also implemented a provider education program with family members and consumers educating helping professionals about the family perspective and experience. In addition, they offer "In Our Own Voice," a presentation by consumers that creates awareness about what is involved in recovery from mental illness. Thus, NAMI offers a broad array of education programs including Family-to-Family, a provider education program, as well as a peer-to-peer education program. Other state and local educational programs are also offered by trained family and consumer teachers to help inform and support other families, consumers, and professionals.

Familial Strengths and Resilience

As discussed in Chapter 2, the available evidence suggests that schizophrenia and other major mental illnesses, like many other biologically caused disorders such as asthma or hypertension, have a large genetic component. Persons with this genetic component are often vulnerable to environmental stresses or triggers that promote specific biological events, such as changes in neurotransmitter functioning. Some aspects of family life may cause stress, which in turn may trigger relapse or the recurrence of symptoms. In any case, families are neither a necessary nor sufficient cause of serious mental illness.

This discussion of the role of stress in the etiology of schizophrenia and other disorders is not to deny the fact that some people with serious and persistent mental illness have had traumatic or difficult childhood experiences involving their families (as have many people who do not have serious mental illnesses). Nor is it to deny that many individuals with serious mental illness live under adverse familial circumstances as adults.

Equally undeniable, however, is evidence of the resilience and strength of some families despite the objective and subjective burdens they face. Mannion (1996) reports:

> There have been few attempts to go beyond the concept of family burden and examine family resilience . . . a process of constructive change and growth in response to a serious psychiatric disorder in a loved one. (p. 4)

This positive outlook may strike some family members as looking at the world through rose-colored glasses, prompting some to note: "We are all surviving schizophrenia." (excerpted from Marsh et al., 1996, p. 11).

At the same time, it has also been demonstrated that family members can do effective problem solving, intervene in crises, and promote recovery for their relative with mental illness (Lehman & Steinwachs, 1998).

Summary

The influence of family life on the lives of persons with mental illness can be both positive and negative. The effect of the person's illness on the family can be burdensome, although many families prove very resourceful and resilient. At the same time, characteristics of some families, those with high expressed emotion for example, may present specific stresses to the relative who has a mental illness and produce negative outcomes.

The disorder in the lives of these families does not cause serious mental illness. Although such influences as hostile remarks, critical comments, and other high EE behavior have been found to be harmful to the course of serious mental illness, these same families have also been found to be capable of changing this style of interaction to promote coping, competence, and recovery.

Families go through their own process of recovering, adapting, and incorporating severe and persistent mental illness into their self-image as a family. They can be a great source of support not only to their own members, but also other families. In the face of serious mental illness, many families are found to be ultimately resilient and quite capable. Many family members, after struggling with their own member's illness, become advocates for improved psychiatric rehabilitation policies and increased mental illness research. The PsyR practitioner must take the stance of partnership with family members. There is no other position that could be considered responsible or ethical.

If mental health consumers desire family involvement and if family members can be successfully engaged, they are among the most important partners in the processes of rehabilitation and recovery. Most families can become competent in their knowledge of mental illness and its treatment. These families can effectively solve problems presented by their member's illness and disability. Most importantly, these families can be effective agents for promoting the attainment of their loved one's rehabilitation goals.

Class Exercise

Designing a Family Intervention and Support Program

Question 1

It is clear that family interventions that are primarily psychoeducational have been found to be very effective, especially if started when the ill relative is in the acute phase of his or her illness. In this exercise the task is to generate the variety of possible reasons that family psychoeducation can lead to a reduction in both the number and frequency of relapses. For example: How do knowledge and skills translate into a lower likelihood of relapse? Remember, this effect can take place in both high EE and low EE families. Also, consider the following questions about what these interventions actually accomplish for the family. Do they help families to (1) be better observers, (2) intervene sooner when relapse is coming, or (3) be better symptom management agents?

Based on the information in this chapter, generate a list of possible reasons why these psychoeducational family interventions have positive effects for a person with mental illness. Provide the rationale for each reason on your list.

Question 2

Those family interventions that include people with mental illness directly in the training or group result in better outcomes. Is this fact consistent with PsyR principles? If so, which principles does it relate to and why?

Question 3

Mowbray, Bybee, Harris, and McCrohan (1995) found that high family contact was associated with poorer vocational outcomes, while less contact was associated with better outcomes. Alternatively, McFarlane's group (1995) found that families can help to promote vocational outcomes. Are these two sets of findings inconsistent? If they are reconcilable, what do they imply about the role of families in the vocational rehabilitation of people with severe and persistent mental illness?

References

Anderson, C. M., Reiss, D. J., & Hogarty, G. E. (1986). *Schizophrenia and the Family*. New York: The Guilford Press.

Barrowclough, C., Haddock, G., Tarrier, N., Lewis, S. W., Moring, J., & O'Brien, N. (2001). Randomized controlled trial of motivational interviewing, cognitive behavior therapy, and family intervention for patients with co-morbid schizophrenia and substance use disorders. *American Journal of Psychiatry*, *158*(10), 1706–1713.

Bloch, S., Szmukler, G. I., Herrman, H., Benson, A., & Colussa, S. (1995). Counseling caregivers of relatives with schizophrenia: themes, interventions, and caveats. *Family Process, 34*, 413–425.

Brown, C. (1996). A comparison of living situation and loneliness for people with mental illness. *Psychiatric Rehabilitation Journal, 20*(2), 59–63.

Cnaan, R. A., Blankertz, L., Messinger, K. W., & Gardner, J. R. (1990). Experts assessment of psychosocial rehabilitation principles. *Psychosocial Rehabilitation Journal, 13*(3), 59–73.

Cook, J. A., & Hoffschmidt, S. J. (1993). Comprehensive models of psychosocial rehabilitation. In R. W. Flexer & P. A. Solomon (Eds.), *Psychiatric rehabilitation in practice* (pp. 81–97). Boston, MA: Andover Medical Publishers.

Daley, D. C., Moss, H. B., & Campbell, F. (1993). *Dual disorders: Counseling clients with chemical dependency and mental illness* (2nd ed.). Center City, MN: Hazelden Foundation.

Dausey, D. J. (2004). Mental health policy innovation in the American states. Yale University. *Dissertation Abstracts International: Section B: The Sciences and Engineering, 64*(10-B), p. 4859.

Dixon, L. B., & Lehman, A. F. (1995). Family interventions for schizophrenia. *Schizophrenia Bulletin, 21*(4), 631–644.

Dixon, L., McFarlane, W. R., Lefley, H., Lucksted, A., Cohen, M., Falloon, I., et al. (2001). Evidence-based practices for services to families of people with psychiatric disabilities. *Psychiatric Services, 52*(7), 903–910.

Evans, K., & Sullivan, J. M. (1990). *Dual diagnosis: Counseling the mentally ill substance abuser*. New York: The Guilford Press.

Falloon, I. R. H., Boyd, J. L., & McGill, C. W. (1984). *Family care of schizophrenia: A problem solving approach to the treatment of mental illness*. New York: The Guilford Press.

Falloon, I. R., Boyd, J. L., McGill, C. W., Ranzani, J., Moss, H. B., & Gilderman, A. M. (1982). Family management in the prevention of exacerbation of schizophrenia. *New England Journal of Medicine, 306*, 1437–1440.

Falloon, I. R., & Pedersen, J. (1985). Family management in the prevention of morbidity of schizophrenia: The adjustment family unit. *British Journal of Psychiatry, 147*, 156–163.

Goldstein, M. J., Rodnick, E. H., Evans, J. R., May, P. R., & Steinberg, M. R. (1978). Drug and family therapy in the aftercare of adult schizophrenics. *Archives of General Psychiatry, 35*, 1169–1177.

Harding, C. M., & Zahniser, J. H. (1994). Empirical correction of seven myths about schizophrenia with implications for treatment. *Acta Psychiatrica Scandanavica, 90*, 140–146.

Hatfield, A. B. (1987a). Families as caregivers: A historical perspective. In A. B. Hatfield & H. P. Lefley (Eds.), *Families of the mentally ill: Coping and adaptation* (pp. 3–29). New York: The Guilford Press.

Hatfield, A. B. (1987b). Coping and adaptation: A conceptual framework for understanding families. In A. B. Hatfield & H. P. Lefley (Eds.), *Families of the mentally ill: Coping and adaptation* (pp. 60–84). New York: The Guilford Press.

Hatfield, A. (1990). *Family education in mental illness*. New York: The Guilford Press.

Hatfield, A. B. (1992). Leaving home: Separation issues in psychiatric illness. *Psychosocial Rehabilitation Journal, 15*(4), 37–47.

Hogarty, G. E. (1993). The prevention of relapse in chronic schizophrenic patients. *Journal of Clinical Psychiatry, 54,* 18–23.

Hogarty, G. E., Anderson C. M., Konrblith, S. J., Greenwald, D. P., Javana, C. D., & Moadonia, M. J. (1986). Personal indicators in the course of schizophrenia research group. Family psychoeducation, social skills training, and maintenance chemotherapy in the aftercare treatment of schizophrenia: I. One-year effects of a controlled study on relapsed and expressed emotion. *Archives of General Psychiatry, 43,* 633–642.

Hogarty, G. E., Anderson C. M., Konrblith, S. J., Greenwald, D. P., Ulrich, R. F., & Carster, M. (1991). Family psychoeducation, social skills training, and maintenance chemotherapy in the aftercare treatment of schizophrenia: II. Two-year effects of a controlled study on relapse and adjustment. *Archives of General Psychiatry, 48,* 340–347.

IAPSRS (1996). *Core principles of psychiatric rehabilitation.* IAPSRS, Columbia, Maryland.

Kinsella, C. B., Anderson, R. R., & Anderson, W. T. (1996). Coping skills, strengths, and needs as perceived by adult offspring and siblings of people with mental illness: A retrospective study. *Psychiatric Rehabilitation Journal, 20*(2), 24–32.

Leff, J. P., Berkowitz, R., Shavit, N., Strachan, A., Glass, I., & Vaughn, C. (1989). A trial of family therapy versus a relatives' group for schizophrenia: Two year follow-up. *British Journal of Psychiatry, 154,* 58–66.

Leff, J. P., Kuipers, L., Berkowitz, R., Eberlein-Fries, R., & Sturgeon, D.A., (1982). A controlled trial of social intervention in schizophrenia families. *British Journal of Psychiatry, 146,* 594–600.

Leff, J. P., Kuipers, L., Berkowitz, R., & Sturgeon, D.A. (1985) A controlled trial of social intervention in schizophrenia families: Two year follow-up. *British Journal of Psychiatry, 146,* 594–600.

Lefley, H. P. (1987a). Culture and mental illness: The family role. In A. B. Hatfield & H. P. Lefley (Eds.), *Families of the mentally ill: Coping and adaptation* (pp. 30–64). New York: The Guilford Press.

Lefley, H. P. (1987b). Behavioral manifestations of mental illness. In A. B. Hatfield & H. P. Lefley (Eds.), *Families of the mentally ill: Coping and adaptation* (pp. 107–127). New York: The Guilford Press.

Lefley, H. P. (1989). Family burden and stigma in major mental illness. *American Psychologist, 44*(3), 556–560.

Lehman, A. F., & Steinwachs, D. M. (1998). At issue: Translating research into practice: The Schizophrenia patient outcomes research team (PORT) treatment recommendations. *Schizophrenia Bulletin, 24*(1), 1–10.

Lundwall, R. R. (1996). How psychoeducational support groups can provide multi-disciplinary services to families of people with mental illness. *Psychiatric Rehabilitation Journal, 20*(2), 64–72.

Mannion, E. (1996). Resilience and burden in spouses of people with mental illness. *Psychiatric Rehabilitation Journal, 20*(2), 13–23.

Marsh, D. T., Dickens, R. M., Koeske, R. D., Yackovich, N. S., Wilson, J. M., et al. (1993). Troubled journey: Siblings and children of people with mental illness. *Innovations and Research, 2*(2), 13–23.

Marsh, D. T., Lefley, H. P., Evans-Rhodes, D., Ansell, V. I., Doerzbacher, B. M., et al. (1996). The family experience of mental illness: Evidence for resilience. *Psychiatric Rehabilitation Journal, 20*(2), 3–12.

McFarlane, W. R. (1994). Multiple family groups and psychoeducation in the treatment of schizophrenia. *New Directions in Mental Health Services, 62,* 13–22.

McFarlane, W. R., Dixon, L., Lukens, E., & Lucksted, A. (2003). Family psychoeducation and schizophrenia: A review of the literature. *Journal of Marital & Family Therapy, 29*(2), 223–245.

McFarlane, W. R., Lukens, E., Link, B., Dushay, R., Deakins, S. A., et al. (1995). Multiple family group and psychoeducation in the treatment of schizophrenia. *Archives of General Psychiatry, 52,* 679–687.

Mowbray, C. T., Bybee, D., Harris, S. N., & McCrohan, N. (1995). Predictors of work status and future work orientation in people with a psychiatric disability. *Psychiatric Rehabilitation Journal, 19*(2), 17–28.

Mowbray, C. T., Bybee, D., Oyserman, D., MacFarlane, P. (2005). Timing of mental illness onset and motherhood. *Journal of Nervous & Mental Disease, 193*(6), 369–378.

Mowbray, C., Schwartz, S., Bybee, D., Spang, J., Rueda-Riedle, A. & Oyserman, D. (2000). Mothers with a mental illness: Stressors and resources for parenting and living. *Families in Society, 81*(2), 118–129.

Mullick, M., Miller, L. J., & Jacobsen, T. (2001). Insight into mental illness and child maltreatment risk among mothers with major psychiatric disorders. *Psychiatric Services, 52*(4), 488–492.

National Alliance of the Mentally Ill. (1996, 1998). *History of NAMI.* Washington, DC: Author. (Courtesy of NAMI-New Jersey.)

National Alliance on Mental Illness. (2005). Retrieved October 19, 2005, from http://www.nami/org.

Nicholson, J., Nason, M. W., Calabresi, A. O., & Yando, R. (1999). Fathers with severe mental illness: Characteristics and comparisons. *American Journal of Orthopsychiatry, 69*(1), 134–141.

Pharoah, F. M., Mari, J. J., Streiner, D. (2004). *Family intervention for schizophrenia. The Cochrane Database of Systematic Reviews.* The Cochrane Collaboration.

Phelan, J., Bromet, E. J. & Link, B. J. (1998). "Psychiatric illness and family stigma." *Schizophrenia Bulletin, 24,* 115–126.

Shi, Y., Zhao, B., Xu, D., & Sen, J. (2000). A comparative study of life quality in schizophrenic patients after family intervention. *Chinese Mental Health Journal, 14*(2), 135–137.

Spaniol, L., & Zipple, A. M. (1994). The family recovery process. *Journal of the California Alliance of the Mentally Ill, 5*(2), 57–59.

Styron, T. H., Pruett, M. K., McMahon, Y. J., & Davidson, L. (2002). Fathers with mental illness: A neglected group. *Psychiatric Rehabilitation Journal, 25*(3), 215–222.

Tarrier, N., Barrowclough, C., Vaughn C., Bamrah, J. S., Porceddu, K., Watts, S., & Freeman H. (1988) The community management of schizophrenia: a controlled trial of a behavioural intervention with families to reduce relapse. *British Journal of Psychiatry, 153,* 532–542.

Terkelson, K. G. (1987a). The meaning of mental illness to the family. In A. B. Hatfield & H. P. Lefley (Eds.), *Families of the mentally ill: Coping and adaptation.* New York: The Guilford Press, pp. 128–150.

Terkelson, K. G. (1987b). The evolution of family responses to mental illness over time. In A. B. Hatfield & H. P. Lefley (Eds.), *Families of the mentally ill: Coping and adaptation.* New York: The Guilford Press, pp. 151–166.

University of Pennsylvania RRTC Collaborative on Community Integration. (2005a). *Parenting with a Mental Illness: Positive Parenting & Child Resilience.* Retrieved October 18, 2005, from http://www.upennrrtc.org/issues/Resilience.pdf

University of Pennsylvania RRTC Collaborative on Community Integration. (2005b). *Parenting with a Mental Illness: Child Welfare & Custody Issues.* Retrieved October 18, 2005, from http://www.upennrrtc.org/issues/ChildWelfareCustodyFS.pdf.

Xiong, W., Phillips, M. R., Hu, X., Wang, R., Dai, Q., et al. (1994). Family-based intervention for schizophrenic patients in China: A randomised controlled trial. *British Journal of Psychiatry, 165,* 239–247.

Chapter 14

Psychiatric Rehabilitation in Hospital Settings

Introduction 406

A 19th-Century Institution in the 21st Century 407

Comparison and Contrast with Today's Hospitals 408

Many Meanings of "The Shame of the States" 409

Functions of State Psychiatric Hospitals 410

Length of Hospital Stay and Rehabilitation Outcome 412

Population Served by State Psychiatric Hospitals 412

Stan's Story 412

Julie's Story 414

Challenges in the Hospital Environment 416

Seclusion and Restraint: Definitely Not Psychiatric Rehabilitation 416

Beyond Eliminating Restraints: Is Psychiatric Rehabilitation Possible in the Hospital Setting? 417

Psychiatric Rehabilitation Goals 417

Values of Psychiatric Rehabilitation 417

Guiding Principles of Psychiatric Rehabilitation 418

Psychiatric Rehabilitation Models within Hospitals 420

Social and Independent Living Skills (SILS) Model 420

Psychiatric Rehabilitation Integrated Service Model 421

Treatment Mall 421

Case Study of a Hospital Implementing Individualized Psychiatric Rehabilitation 422

Implementing Psychiatric Rehabilitation at Eastern State Hospital 422

Is Hospitalization Always Necessary? 423

Addressing Acute Care Needs without Large Hospitals 423

Intermediate and Long-Term Care Needs without Large Institutions 424

Summary 425

Class Exercise 426

References 426

Most of the chapters of this book are devoted to the implementation of the guiding principles of psychiatric rehabilitation (PsyR) in community settings in the pursuit of recovery, community integration, and improved quality of life. Can these goals be pursued in hospitals as well? Are the principles of PsyR applicable to hospital settings? As this chapter will explain, the barriers to the pursuit of these goals in hospital settings are often formidable. The treatment values and assumptions of hospital settings are literally different from those of community settings. Traditionally, there have been significant restrictions on the freedom of choice of persons in psychiatric hospitals. An individual's stay in these hospitals often begins involuntarily. By design and definition, they are rarely integrated with the community. Yet, in many places psychiatric hospitals remain a critical part of the mental health service system. The people served in state psychiatric hospitals are very often the same individuals who are served by community psychiatric rehabilitation.

This chapter will answer the following questions:

1. *Can the principles of psychiatric rehabilitation be applied in hospitals?*
2. *Are psychiatric hospitals an impediment or can they help foster community integration?*
3. *Can recovery and quality of life be fostered by hospitalization experiences?*
4. *What are the common barriers to both the application of PsyR principles and the pursuit of PsyR goals in hospitals?*

Introduction

Large psychiatric hospitals around the world have been plagued by well-documented reports of patient neglect or abuse (e.g., Geller, 2000). In addition, there are many reports of deteriorating, unhealthy, and unsanitary living conditions. There is also strong evidence that the psychiatric care in some of these institutions is quite inadequate, with even basic guidelines for the prescription of medications not being followed.

Many of the so-called reform movements aimed at these hospitals have focused primarily on improving the physical plant, reducing the size of institutions, building smaller wards with private or semiprivate bedrooms, and generally reducing the buildings' resemblance to prisons. Given the reports of neglect and abuse and the iatrogenic effects of institutional treatment, can these hospitals where involuntary care is the norm rather than the exception, possibly promote recovery, enhance quality of life, and promote community integration?

Experts disagree. Two of these experts, E. Fuller Torrey (2003) and Patrick Corrigan (2003) give the qualified answer of "yes." Other experts assert that psychiatric patients would be better off without these institutions. While neither Corrigan nor Torrey report being pleased with the overall quality of care offered, each sheds light on how hospitalization can play a positive role. Torrey suggests that the relative lack of availability of hospitalization, the difficulties of getting into a hospital, and the short, inadequate lengths of stay all inhibit the recovery of persons with mental illness, detracting from their integration in the community and harming their quality of life. Corrigan indicates that hospitals can, in fact, be one of the settings, like other types of residential programs (described in Chapter 11), where successful rehabilitation interventions can be implemented. Strategies such as goal setting, skills training, and cognitive rehabilitation can all be initiated in the hospital. Reduced symptoms, improved skills, and increased supports can also be achieved in hospital settings. Nevertheless, many barriers must be overcome. Hospital policies and rules rarely promote key values of PsyR such as empowerment and choice. There is little emphasis on skills training in the hospital environment. Finally, community and family coordination is typically postponed until the individual is close to being discharged.

If hospital administrators and staff members adhere to PsyR values, is it possible to promote recovery, improve quality of life, and foster community reintegration? In short, can hospitals be organized to deliver psychiatric rehabilitation?

A 19th-Century Institution in the 21st Century

To understand both the barriers to implementing psychiatric rehabilitation in hospitals, as well as the potential for its success, it may be instructive to briefly review the history of such institutions. Large public, psychiatric hospitals include those run by most state governments of the United States, the Veterans Administration in the United States, other units of government (such as county or city governments), and occasionally charities. They exist in some other countries, often state run. They are, in large part, 19th-century institutions struggling to adapt to the demands and conditions of the 21st century. Most of these institutions grew out of faith in the potential for large, orderly institutions, to promote the safety of society and provide peaceful sanctuary for those disturbed by troubling mental disorders. In the United States, the large institution-asylum concept also grew out of a concern for the inhumane treatment and the neglect of persons with mental illness who often were jailed in poorhouses as debtors, were homeless, or living under extremely restrictive and inadequate conditions (Rothman, 2002).

The movement to develop these institutions peaked in the mid-19th century. Many are still in existence today. These institutions were clearly meant to be a reform to provide an orderly environment that helped individuals manage the chaos of their illness through participation in a self-sustaining community that kept individuals occupied by useful activity (Rothman, 2002). This movement coincided with the development of a variety of other large institutions with a significant moral or ethical purpose, such as state penitentiaries directed toward moral reform of criminals and large state schools that taught practical skills to people who were blind (Rothman, 2002).

Before the development of state institutions, private charities rather than governments were the primary helpers of persons with mental illness. There were some rare exceptions such as Eastern State Hospital operated in the city of Williamsburg, Virginia, and founded in 1773. Eastern State actually sought out psychiatric patients by making an appeal to their friends and loved ones.

National reform took place in the United States in the mid-19th century, led by the social activist Dorothea Dix. Dix established psychiatric hospitals for the first time. This movement was part of a paradigm shift with larger units of government accepting greater responsibility for societal problems. In the United States, the states themselves, as opposed to cities or towns, began to take on the burden of operating these institutions. The other issue addressed by the development of this type of facility was the thinking that such institutions could have some curative impact, indeed a *rehabilitative* impact (Rothman, 2002). Dorothea Dix's mark remains today. She lived for a long time at Trenton (New Jersey) Psychiatric Hospital and died there. At least one hospital in North Carolina bears her name.

Comparison and Contrast with Today's Hospitals

In some ways, the 19th-century state hospital bears little resemblance to today's hospitals. Although the locations are often literally the same, these were usually remote settings at the time and were often self-sustaining communities. Many had large working farms, produced crops, and raised livestock. Most of the support services needed: hardware, blacksmiths, and later central heating plants or power plants were on the grounds. Some hospitals their own factories. Until the 1950s, everyone associated with such a hospital—staff, nurses, and doctors—lived on the grounds near the patients. These institutions literally maintained themselves with the goods, services, and products they required to have a functioning community (Rothman, 2002). They were their own worlds or at least their own separate communities.

At the peak of what was known as the "moral" treatment era, the precursors of two intervention strategies, which later became more prominent in the PsyR field, were initiated in these hospitals. *Milieu therapy* and the *work-ordered day* (discussed in Chapter 6) were attempted to a large extent in the new institutions, although neither of these phrases was employed. There was a strong belief, for example, that the environment was in fact the treatment, as is asserted in milieu therapy. In addition, when feasible for persons who had uncontrolled psychotic symptoms, the idea of the work-ordered day actually prevailed in psychiatric hospitals. Later it was adopted and popularized by the clubhouse model.

To give an idea of the size and complexity of these state institutions, consider the example of one state hospital in New Jersey, Greystone Park, which was founded in 1876 by Dr. Thomas Story Kirkbride. The Greystone campus covers a square mile. Its 43 buildings once included housing for more than 6,000 patients as well as about the same number of staff. The buildings themselves offer a remarkable record of 19th- and 20th-century institutional and residential architecture. From 1876 to 1943, the main administration building, the Kirkbride Building, was the largest structure on a single foundation in the United States. According to the Morris County Preservation Society (Preservation New Jersey, 2003):

> *Dr. Kirkbride believed that patients should recuperate in a calm setting. Their light, airy rooms afforded views of a soothing landscape punctuated by elaborate flowerbeds and fountains. Greystone was once a self-contained community that included staff housing, a post office, fire and police stations, a working farm, vocational and recreational facilities, and its own gas and water utilities.*

In its history, the hospital saw the introduction of a number of positive developments including occupational therapy, antipsychotic medication, and the use of small cottage residences organized around psychiatric rehabilitation principles. However, other treatment approaches actually proved to be harmful to many patients such as psychosurgery, the outmoded severing of nerve fibers in the brain's frontal lobes (sometimes referred to as a lobotomy).

In 2006, Greystone still had more than 600 patients at any given time, half of whom were awaiting placement in the community. The hospital is scheduled for a downsizing by 250 beds, accompanied by a significant expansion in community services. Greystone Park still has its own post office and police. While the farms are gone, Greystone Park has a working greenhouse and horticultural program. Its fallow farmland has only recently been sold. Its administration building still has some offices and a chapel decorated from the Victorian era (Preservation New Jersey, 2003). Although it contracts for many outside services, there is still an in-hospital work program for patients.

State hospitals have other continuing legacies, besides their architecture and physical plant. In some places, large dormitory-style housing without privacy for the patients still exists. Other elements of the legacy include separation from the rest of the world, including a psychological distance from communities. In many hospital settings, there is another vestige from an earlier time: the belief that recovery of any sort from a serious mental illness is not a likely outcome (Birkman, Sperduto, Smith, & Gill, 2006; Dhillon & Dollieslager, 2000).

Dhillon and Dollieslager (2000), as well as Birkmann and his colleagues (2006), report that one of the greatest barriers to implementing PsyR in hospitals may be an attitudinal one, embedded in the culture and practices of the institutions. Many staff members in these institutions simply do not believe that persons with severe and persistent mental illness can actually recover to any meaningful extent. In part, this may be due to the fact that hospital staff, due to the nature and locale of their jobs, rarely get to see persons with severe and persistent mental illness who are not symptomatic coping well in the community and living independently. This is a version of what Harding & Zahniser (1994) refers to as the *clinician's mistake based on experience*. Staff in hospitals literally get to see people at their worst, never or rarely at their best. As a result, they infer that everyone with these disorders always looks like the patients they believe they know so well (Harding & Zahniser, 1994).

Many Meanings of "The Shame of the States"

As mentioned earlier, Dorothea Dix devoted her life to developing psychiatric hospitals and advocating for their establishment in various states in the mid-19th century. About 100 years later, Deutsch (1948) referred to the "shame of the states," because they did little or nothing for persons with mental illnesses except house them in facilities that were beginning to deteriorate. This phrase continued to be relevant in the years that followed. In the 1960s and 1970s, the shame of the states remained the hospitals themselves, rocked with scandals about inhumane conditions and the lack of treatment (Geller, 2000).

The scandalous conditions that preceded deinstitutionalization continue today. Some state psychiatric hospitals in the United States have been under federal supervision by the U.S. Department of Justice because of evidence of violations of civil rights. Concerns about treatment and conditions have led other states to eliminate or very significantly curtail the number, size, and census of their state hospitals. Several state mental health departments have instituted major projects in collaboration with universities and community providers to improve the conditions at their institutions.

At the same time, the insufficient availability of hospital beds or alternate forms of providing acute and intermediate psychiatric care are equally shameful. E. Fuller Torrey (2003) points out that we may have turned the clock back further than the mid-19th century. In many places there are more persons with mental illness in state prisons and county jails than in hospitals operated by states and counties. In fact, in the United States, the most populous institutions housing the most persons with mental illness are the following county or city jails: Los Angeles, California; Cook County, Illinois; and Rikers Island, New York (Torrey, 2003).

Functions of State Psychiatric Hospitals

State psychiatric hospitals formerly served one primary function, the maintenance (providing for the physical needs) and care (often lifelong) of persons with psychotic disorders. A number of important developments since the 1950s (Geller, 2000) have changed this situation:

1. *The advent of psychotropic medications, first introduced in the late 1950s,* did a great deal to provide symptom relief and promote some level of recovery. For many individuals these medications eliminated the necessity of lifelong confinement.
2. *Changes in the U.S. Social Security laws in 1965 and 1966* provided income support and medical coverage that permitted persons with disabilities in all states to be maintained outside institutions.
3. A *series of U.S. Supreme Court cases in the 1960s and 1970s* affirmed the civil rights of patients. For the first time, discharge planning and linkage to the community became an important state hospital role. A series of U.S. Supreme Court cases including *Wyatt v. Stickney* and *Donaldson v. O'Connor* found that state psychiatric hospitals often deprived individuals of basic civil rights.

These U.S. Supreme Court rulings resulted in changes in the involuntary commitment laws, raising the bar of who could be confined against their will (i.e., only those who pose an imminent risk to themselves, other people, and sometimes property due to a mental illness). In addition, one could no longer be committed without being offered active treatment. *Active treatment* refers to the requirement that individuals who are committed to state institutions cannot be deprived of liberty for public safety purposes alone. Rather, during their confinement, individuals who are committed must also receive an active program of care to address the symptoms and deficits associated with their psychiatric illness. Thirty-five years later many hospitals are still trying to achieve these standards (Dhillon & Dollieslager, 2000; Geller, 2000).

According to Leona Bachrach (1999), today's state psychiatric hospitals serve a number of functions including care of persons who require one of the following:

- *Short stays* (less than 1 month) are used for the management of acute symptoms and quick symptom reduction.
- An *extended stay* provides time to stabilize symptoms. For some individuals, longer stays (several weeks to months) are required for stabilization as compared to the very short stays that are typically provided in the psychiatric units of general hospitals.
- *Long stays* (several months to many years) are experienced by individuals for whom the hospital provides both residential and case management services (care coordination) in addition to their psychiatric services.

In addition, many state hospitals also serve the following functions:

- *Forensic care:* Hospitals serve a heterogeneous population of persons with legal involvement including those who are not guilty by reason of insanity, are on other types of court retainers for criminal charges, or are sexual offenders who have been civilly committed under special *sexual predator laws*. After serving a jail sentence for sexual offenses, in many states, these individuals are committed to a hospital stay based on the premise that they are a danger to others.
- *Geriatric care:* This type of care is provided for elderly psychiatric patients who have numerous medical concerns, but nowhere to go in the community to have their multiple health care needs served.

Most state psychiatric hospitals provide care primarily to individuals under court-ordered involuntary commitment. Because of this, they are likely to admit: (1) individuals in the acute phase of their illness, (2) individuals who are not responding to treatment for one reason or another, and (3) persons who are potentially harmful to themselves or others. Thus, these hospitals face great challenges.

A variety of factors have contributed to this multiplicity of demands on state psychiatric hospitals. However, the primary problem is that these hospitals are often the "last stop" or a state's only alternative to providing care when other parts of the system are uninterested, unwilling, or incapable.

In some places state psychiatric hospitals provide acute care services because local community hospitals have no psychiatric units. Due to changes in insurance practices and managed care policies, many hospitals have very short lengths of stay of 7 to 10 days or less. This persists despite the fact that it takes 4 to 6 weeks for antipsychotic medication to develop its full therapeutic effect. A lack of hospitals to provide intermediate or long stays often necessitates the transfer of individuals to state hospitals.

Length of Hospital Stay and Rehabilitation Outcome

Evidence has accumulated that neither very short nor very long hospital stays are helpful for recovery. Very long stays are associated with iatrogenic effects, referred to in Chapter 1 as "institutionalization syndrome." These include extreme dependence and passivity. Very short stays allow insufficient time to manage and reduce symptoms. Is there an optimal length of hospital stay for recovery from severe and persistent mental illnesses?

The lengths of hospital stays have been drastically reduced during the last 30 years, although not in all U.S. locations, nor all other countries, notably Japan (Tsuchiya & Takei, 2004). Some argue that this reduction has led to a pattern of revolving door admissions and worsening mental health outcomes despite apparent cost savings (Talbott, 2004). In contrast, others suggest longer stays may be more harmful in the long term by fostering dependence on institutions.

Johnstone and Zolese (2001) completed a review of the studies examining lengths of hospital stays for people with serious mental illness. Short stays varied from 1 week (Herz, Endicott, & Spitzer, 1975) to 3 to 4 weeks (Glick, Hargreaves & Raskin, 1975, Glick, Hargreaves, Drues, & Showstack, 1976) and, in all the studies reviewed, ranged from an average of 11 to 25 days. In these studies, those randomly assigned to short stays received treatments such as medication, crisis resolution, and discharge planning (Glick, Hargreaves, & Raskin, 1975; Glick, Hargreaves, Drues, & Showstack, 1976). These short-stay studies focused on short length of stay by state hospital standards, but not by today's community hospital standards. Antipsychotic drugs were the main treatment for participants and most studies reported similar use of these medications in both long- and short-stay participants. Persons assigned to planned short stays experienced no more readmissions, were not harder to follow up, and were more successfully discharged compared to those who received longer stays, an average of 28 to 94 days (Johnston & Zolese, 2001). The short-stay patients had a greater chance of becoming employed. These findings suggest that a planned short-stay policy does not, in itself, encourage a "revolving door" pattern of admission or a lack of continuity of care and may foster community integration (Johnstone & Zolese, 2001).

Population Served by State Psychiatric Hospitals

In large part, the persons served in state psychiatric hospitals are the same individuals described throughout this text who receive PsyR services. The two stories that follow illustrate common profiles of persons currently residing in state hospitals. When reading their stories, consider the following questions: In addition to a psychiatric disorder, what other challenges are they facing? Are other factors contributing to the lengthening of their hospitalization? Does the hospital environment foster their recovery?

Stan's Story

Consider Stan's story, which describes the lifestyle of a wanderer not fully aware of his illness, a pattern of revolving door admissions, and some unnecessarily long lengths of stay in hospitals.

Stan is now in his late 40s. He remembers an incident from his early 20s that resulted in his having a psychiatric evaluation performed in an emergency room (ER). "My girl-friend kicked me out of her house and called the police. I was calm and cool with the cops but they didn't know what to do with me." He remembers talking to a counselor and a psychiatrist in the ER and being informed that he had "delusions" and that they were going to prescribe medication that would help alleviate this problem. "They gave me the prescription which I filled and the number of some sort of clinic to follow up with . . . but I was ready to move on even though I had a pretty good job." For a period of a few years he traveled around the East Coast looking for work and living in various unsafe situations, including on the street. During this period he is sure that he had no treatment and took no medication.

"Looking back, I can't quite believe that I stayed alive. I was extremely confused. I believed at one point that I was a famous Hollywood actor starring in a movie that was my life. It led to one really bad decision." After conferring with some acquaintances from his boarding home, Stan attempted to rob a gas station and was immediately apprehended. The court-appointed attorney recommended that he plead "not guilty by reason of insanity" with the promise that he would be out of the hospital in 6 months. He accepted this advice and was admitted to a state psychiatric hospital. The 6-month stay according to Stan was "good news and bad news."

"It was good that I was in the hospital and realized that I've got this illness, that it's real, it is probably not going away, and that I need to take medicine. The bad news is that six months became three years." At the end of 6 months he was recommitted because of "erratic behavior." He also continued to be on the state list of those patients that had criminal charges pending a disposition from the justice system. Somewhere in the second year of his hospitalization his social worker began to emphasize plans for discharge.

"This was very good news for me. I felt ready to leave and that I had done my time, so to speak. The problem was that my plans and the social worker's were not the same." Stan was looking forward to living on his own, and his social worker felt that he needed to live in a group home for people with psychiatric diagnoses. Stan went to a series of interviews and visits with residential providers.

"They seemed more interested in whether my beard was trimmed than anything else and whether I was ever going to rob a gas station again. I finally ended up on a waiting list. I was at the point where I would go anywhere to get out, but no one would take me." After 3.5 years in a state hospital he was discharged to a group home in a nearby suburb. He lived in the group home and attended a day program for 9 months but says:

"I never really felt at home, I wanted to work, maybe get off disability and find a place on my own. The staff always told me to wait for the right time. I sort of went along with it and finally just left."

For the next 3 years he repeated the earlier pattern of intermittent work, marginal housing, and no psychiatric or support services. While traveling through a small city he was questioned by police and evaluated once again in an ER. He had an untreated wound on his leg from a construction work accident and also recounted his history of hospi-talization and psychiatric services. He was readmitted to the same state hospital. He was stabilized on medication and within 6 months was determined to be ready for discharge. Once again he cited his preference for independent living, but he had to repeat the process of interviewing for group homes. The main concern now was his "elopement" from the previous group home. A series of failed interviews resulted in his transfer from a unit that had high expectations for discharge to a unit that had minimal expectations. He then found himself on a list of patients who do not meet criteria for commitment but for whom no residential program is available.

"I have tried to get my social worker and the team to work with me on this. I know I need help when I get out there. I've brought up going to the city where I have family and I know there are programs. They won't go for it."

After 4 years he remains in the hospital.

Stan's story resembles that of many people served by state hospitals. His struggle with mental illness is long term. When it began he was not even aware it was an illness. His poor judgment, poorly thought-out plans, and indeed his symptoms led to encounters with law enforcement. Currently, like many hospital patients, he remains in the hospital not for a medical or psychiatric reason, but simply because no community placement is available to him.

Julie's Story

Now consider Julie's story. Like Stan, she faces multiple challenges in addition to her mental illness, but there are also a number of differences.

Julie is a 43-year-old, single woman who was admitted to the state hospital in 1996 at age 35 and has been hospitalized there on and off through 2005. Her IQ is 55, putting her in the range for mental retardation. Before being hospitalized, she was living with her sister. On the day of her admission, she felt depressed when her sister left the house. She called the police threatening to harm herself. Previously, she had been hospitalized twice at the Elm Foundation Hospital. She was exhibiting self-mutilating behaviors, depression, and suicidal ideation. She was diagnosed as suffering from impulse control disorder and returned to live with her sister. Julie has numerous medical problems including diabetes, obesity, anemia, and ovarian cysts. She lived with her parents until her father died in 1995. Then she went to live with her sister. Julie has several close relatives who are mentally ill and/or mentally retarded and has a daughter who is around 17 years old, who lives with her sister. She has exhibited so-called "behavioral" problems without much improvement since the time she was admitted. These problems have included banging walls and doors, verbal and physical threats and assaults, blocking doorways, swallowing inedible objects, and attempting to escape. She has difficulty trusting others and hears voices. She has been depressed occasionally.

Julie also has a good sense of humor, can be playful, and teases other people. She has earned the highest level of hospital privileges in the past and was conditionally released to her sister's care in May 1997 but remained in the community for only 2 months and was returned because she refused to take her medications and became self-destructive.

At a special case conference Julie complained of hearing her father's voice often (he had died 6 years previously). She also stated that he was coming to get her. The treatment team requested she be transferred to another ward where she would be with other "higher functioning" patients who could be good role models for her. Unfortunately, she continued her disruptive behaviors and was transferred to the state's forensic hospital.

She improved significantly at the forensic hospital and was returned to the previous ward. She has remained on the same ward since her transfer. She has been prescribed many different medications including antipsychotics, mood stabilizers, antidepressants, and benzodiazepines. Team members report no significant improvement except when Clozaril was prescribed. Unfortunately, she refused to comply with required blood tests and the medication was withdrawn. Julie has a "behavioral plan" but the team members report that it has been difficult to implement throughout the three work shifts of the day because of staff changes.

She has maintained contact with her sister and her daughter only by phone. Julie had a boyfriend, Bob, at the hospital and liked to talk about the relationship. She was proud of the bracelet he had given her. They broke up on a day she was not feeling well. She didn't go out for the "smoke break" and she did not want to talk with Bob when he called the unit later that day. When informed of the latter, Bob told another patient who answered the phone to "tell Julie we're through." When Julie was informed of this, she initially was sad, but later would smile when staff kidded her that "men do dumb things sometimes."

After several days, Julie's mood became increasingly depressed and she was constantly crying. She would sit on the floor with tears streaming down her face. She described feeling depressed and frightened that she was "losing her mind." When asked why, she said she was hearing the voices of "some men" who were telling her to "scratch and cut" herself. She said the "voices" woke her up at 2 o'clock in the morning. She also said the voices made it difficult for her to focus.

After a time, she was no longer crying and she looked less depressed, but she was relatively nonverbal and extremely self-abusive. As a result, she was repeatedly placed in restraints. She would scream that she wanted her restraints loosened only to use this little bit of freedom to scratch her face or arms. On one occasion, she rubbed the side of her hand on the metal bedside. She was rubbing so hard that she was removing her skin. When a staff person said it was better to talk about her feelings than to hurt herself, she stared at him, as if infuriated, and rubbed her hand harder and more rapidly.

Several weeks later, Julie was talking about her medication and she said she needed something to make her feel better, but she didn't want the medicine that made her "so sleepy." She noted that she even fell asleep while going to the bathroom. Later she discussed with her doctor how Haldol had helped her in the past. Although initially dismissed by some staff, her doctor decided to try it and her symptoms significantly subsided.

Like many people in state hospitals, Julie has at least two diagnoses, in her case a developmental disability and a mental illness. She also has many other health problems. Her psychiatric diagnosis is in question as well. Which severe and persistent mental illness does she have? After all these years, there is no consensus among the professionals. It is not an academic question, because if an accurate diagnosis were known it would imply a specific treatment. The hospital setting does not seem to be conducive to her recovery, yet no community option is available for her.

Also implied in Julie's story is how "abnormal" or "un-normalized" Julie's life is in the hospital. Indeed she must bear additional stresses that most people do not experience. She only knows about her teenage daughter's life through the phone or by mail. She does not get to experience the normal rewards and challenges that being the mother of a young girl involves. Also, note that Julie's boyfriend lived in another hospital unit. To carry on that relationship, other patients had to pass personal messages through a ward telephone shared by all who live there. How does one carry on a relationship with such indirect and nonprivate circumstances? The circumstances of Julie's life in the hospital are very different than the lives of other women her age who are living in the community.

Challenges in the Hospital Environment

Many large psychiatric institutions have been plagued by well-documented reports of patient neglect or abuse and reports of deteriorating, unhealthy, and unsanitary living conditions. Also, there is growing evidence that the psychiatric care in these institutions is inadequate, with even basic guidelines for the prescription of medications not being followed.

Seclusion and Restraint: Definitely Not Psychiatric Rehabilitation

One traditional feature of many psychiatric hospitals has been seclusion and restraints. *Seclusion* is being segregated from others in a supposedly quiet and low-stimulation environment. *Restraint* is restricting the physical movement of the individual, including binding individuals to beds by the arms and legs for hours, days, and even longer periods of time. These techniques have been traditionally used to restrict the movement of individuals acutely distressed and displaying aggressive behavior. However, there was never any evidence that it succeeded in doing anything to the individual other than humiliating and exhausting the person. Often restraint took place when other approaches had failed and sometimes when staff had contributed to the escalation of the person's distress. In any case, restraints have been primarily used for staff safety, as opposed to care of persons with mental illness. In many countries and some states of the United States, seclusion and restraints have been completely eliminated; in other places, their use has been severely reduced. Busch (2005) wrote:

> Seclusion and restraint are increasingly controversial, and with good reason. Seclusion and restraint can be deadly. However, no medical literature guides as to which methods are safer and under which circumstances. Patients have described these experiences as negative at best, and as traumatic at worst. Of further concern, seclusion and restraint are not applied uniformly—numerous studies have shown considerable variation in their frequency and duration. Non-clinical factors, such as patients' ethnicity and level of staff experience, are known to be associated with the use of seclusion and restraint (p. 1104).

Medication used for solely sedative purposes and not for symptom management is another form of physical restraint, sometimes called *chemical restraint* (Donat, 2005). A number of treatment improvement programs aimed at reducing seclusion and restraint have proved successful, without increased risk to patients or staff (Busch, 2005; Curie, 2005; Donat,

2005; Smith et al., 2005). These techniques generally involved improved communication, with staff becoming more sensitive to cues of escalating aggression; engaging in speech and making comments that are de-escalating, as opposed to antagonistic; reducing unnecessary stimulation in quiet but nonsecluded areas; and rewarding the individual for nonaggressive acts, as well as other behavioral techniques.

Beyond Eliminating Restraints: Is Psychiatric Rehabilitation Possible in the Hospital Setting?

Given the context and history of psychiatric hospitalization, can hospitals be organized to deliver psychiatric rehabilitation? Consider the following analysis of how the goals, values, and guiding principles of psychiatric rehabilitation introduced in Chapter 4 may relate to psychiatric hospitalization.

Psychiatric Rehabilitation Goals

The goals of psychiatric rehabilitation include the following:

- *Recovery:* Potentially, hospitals can provide the best setting for the resolution of acute symptomatology through the use of psychotropic medication. There is ample opportunity to titrate or "adjust" dosages and observe the individual's responsiveness to medication. Thus, the portion of recovery that involves symptom amelioration can be very well managed if quality psychiatric care is provided. Unfortunately, there is evidence that the medication management services of many hospitals are very poor. In any case, symptom reduction is only one component of recovery. Recovery is further enhanced through community integration.
- *Community integration:* To promote community integration, close coordination with community providers is necessary, if community agency staff have access to hospital treatment team meetings, participate in hospital treatment teams, work on discharge planning, and meet with the consumer before they leave, community reintegration can be promoted. Visits by the consumer to the community, before discharge, are often helpful.
- *Quality of life:* A reasonable quality of life is more likely to be ensured if the concerns of symptom amelioration and reintegration in the community are addressed. Yet, as illustrated earlier in Julie's story, normal privacy, an important component of quality of life, can be impossible to achieve in a state hospital setting.

Values of Psychiatric Rehabilitation

A great challenge to the implementation of PsyR in hospital settings is the fact that the values of PsyR clash directly with those of the medically oriented asylum:

- *Self-determination* is in some ways not possible, certainly under conditions of involuntary commitment for psychiatric care. Yet, subsequent treatment planning and interventions can be used to engage the consumer and promote self-determination. Stan's story illustrates the importance of this value. Stan was dismayed when he was not included in his treatment and discharge planning; if he had been, a successful life in the community would have been more likely. In Julie's story, she finally got some relief from her symptoms when hospital staff listened to her input and responded to her description of which medicines helped her in the past. Giving each individual input on their goals and interventions is an example of what can be done within the hospital to promote self-determination (Starkey & Leadholm, 1997). Being able to choose activities, such as in the treatment mall approach described later in this chapter, is another example (Bopp, Ribble, Cassidy, & Markoff, 1996).

- Hospitals that are overcrowded and focused primarily on custodial maintenance care have little chance of creating an environment where people are *treated with dignity*. Indeed, decades of scandal suggest that many hospitals definitely do not treat individuals with dignity. However, it is certainly possible for hospital staff to communicate respect. Communication skills training has been found to be effective in this regard (Smith, 1998). More respectful communication is also associated with less violence and a reduced need for restraints in hospitals (Smith, 1998).

- *Promoting optimism and hopefulness* is also needed, but not typically emphasized in psychiatric hospitals. Learning about the findings of longitudinal studies (as discussed in Chapters 1, 2, and 3 of this text) and meeting with consumers who have left the hospital and are doing well are among strategies that help staff become more optimistic and promote this optimism.

- The *capacity of every individual to learn and grow* should be nourished. Although some hospitals do little more than provide custodial care, they can develop a wide range of programming, services, and activities that appeal to people of different abilities and interests (Bopp et al., 1996; Tsang, Liberman, Hilty, & Drake, 2002). This can include skills training activities, career exploration and opportunities to pursue hobbies and other interests.

- Many hospitals struggle with the issue of *cultural sensitivity*. Too often, cultural activities within the hospital actually reflect cultural preferences of the dominant staff culture. Staff should attend to the cultural interests of the patient population and plan activities consistent with the interests and backgrounds of the people they serve.

Guiding Principles of PsyR

Equally challenging is the implementation of the guiding principles of PsyR:

- *Individualization:* Hospitals are geared toward serving groups, sometimes very large groups in a similar, apparently efficient manner. This works against the individualization of all services. Mall programs, discussed later, are an example of how programming can be individualized.

* *Maximum client involvement, preference, and choice:* In the acute phase of the illnesses, maximum involvement by the patient is difficult, because symptoms often interfere. Nevertheless, as symptoms subside, more opportunities for participation arise if staff members are open to patient involvement. Participation in treatment planning, choosing of activities, and contributing to discharge preferences can allow for the partial implementation of this principle. An example is the use of recovery-oriented action plans or advanced directives by which consumers can express their treatment preferences prior to the onset of an acute episode.

* *Normalized, community services:* On the face of it, normalized community-based service seems impossible. Yet some hospitals do pursue this principle: (1) They provide living quarters that resemble community residences more than hospital wards. This principle is partially addressed in some hospitals that are organized around small homes or cottages, similar to group homes, rather than large wards. (2) They begin participation in normalized community service activities prior to discharge. This is probably best addressed by continued communication with community service providers and supports that can maintain the person's job and housing while still hospitalized.

* *Strengths' focus:* By their nature, hospitals and their staff focus on patient deficits and weaknesses. However, hospital staff could focus on patients' skills (i.e., strengths) in recovering from acute episodes in the past. Their attention can also be focused on different services that can potentially engage and interest these individuals by having a variety of activities available that permit the individual to demonstrate his or her potential. This thinking can extend to discharge planning by choosing placements and services that capitalize on individuals' prior successes in the community.

* *Situational assessments:* These types of assessments are important and are not typically carried out in hospital settings. Even when hospital settings are appropriate for such an assessment, they are often biased. Different hospital wards and programs lead to different responses and better or worse coping. The sometimes hostile or overwhelming environments of a hospital can negatively affect an individual's coping skills. Staff can be trained to assess the impact of the ward environment on each individual, rather than assume that symptoms and challenging behaviors are caused by internal factors.

* *Holistic approach:* This refers to integration of a treatment/rehabilitation plan and services. A holistic approach should be the goal of every psychiatric hospital. Unfortunately, many hospitals focus only on symptom management, sometimes at the expense of the whole individual. This is unfortunate since most hospitals have a variety of professionals and resources available. If the treatment/rehabilitation team offers services collaboratively, an integrated, holistic program of care can be provided.

* *Ongoing, accessible, coordinated services:* These types of services are possible in hospital settings, but large bureaucracies characterized by overlapping multiple reporting lines among the staff and narrow divisions of responsibilities create many barriers to the coordination of services. Ongoing coordination with community providers to make services accessible is equally challenging. Hospitals need to explore simplified reporting lines, work on team functioning by including all relevant staff in discussions, and

coordinate with community providers whenever possible. Community providers should respond in kind.

• *Skills training:* Skills training is a favorite intervention in certain hospital settings. However, to promote ongoing recovery, provision must be made for the transferability or generalization of skills to the community. This is a difficult task, especially since behaviors tend to be situation specific and difficult to generalize to other settings.

• *Environmental modifications and supports:* Hospital staff and administration typically resist modifying the environments of their institutions to accommodate individual patient preferences. But care should be taken to make ward environments less noisy or overstimulating. Environments may also need to be modified to accommodate the cultural preferences of the patients.

• *Partnership with the family:* When family is involved, their full participation with the treatment team and on discharge planning is critical. Involvement in the treatment team, support groups on hospital grounds, and a family advisory group are all possible steps to encourage this.

• *Vocational focus*: A vocational focus has been a part of hospitals but success in a hospital work program does not readily translate to the community (see Chapter 9). Any vocational work should focus on clarification of the individual's employment preferences and the pursuit of opportunities in the individual's home community.

Psychiatric Rehabilitation Models within Hospitals

There are, in fact, some examples of PsyR program models within psychiatric hospitals. These include (1) the social and independent living skills (SILS) model, a skills training approach that focuses on social learning principles and was promoted initially by Liberman and his colleagues (Wallace, Liberman, MacKain, Blackwell, & Eckman, 1992); (2) the psychiatric rehabilitation integrated service model (PRISM) (Starkey & Leadholm, 1997), a comprehensive PsyR approach; and (3) the treatment mall model, which incorporates changes in the physical plant with programming changes (Bopp et al., 1996). These three models are discussed in more detail in the following subsections.

Social and Independent Living Skills (SILS) Model

With the SILS approach (Wallace et al., 1992), staff teach specific skills and skill training modules relevant to social and independent living. The modules provide step-by-step training activities for patients to learn the skills they will need outside the hospital. SILS has been used effectively in both community-based and hospital settings. Modules focus on these broad areas:

• Social skills
• Symptom management skills
• Medication management skills
• Community reentry skills.

The modules consist of an overview and explanation of the relevant skill, demonstration of the skill by staff, group member participation in practicing the skill, and "homework" assignments to practice skills between sessions. In addition, the groups include suggestions on how to apply the skills outside the groups. A number of hospitals have been very successful implementing these skills training modules (e.g., Smith, 1998).

Psychiatric Rehabilitation Integrated Service Model (PRISM)

The PRISM approach, described by Starkey and Leadholm (1997), is far more comprehensive than the SILS approach. The goal of PRISM is to increase patients' participation in their own treatment through these means:

- Patient participation in treatment planning meetings
- Treatment plans with a rehabilitation focus that emphasizes goals, skill development, and development of external supports
- Problem reconceptualization as obstacles that need to be overcome to reach independent living goals
- True patient participation in treatment team meetings, with the patient identified as a *member* of the team
- Involvement of family members (with consent of the patient) and community providers directly in the treatment team

PRISM also focuses on improving the ward atmosphere and promoting patient involvement there. These improvements require significant restructuring of ward activities, including the following:

- Community meetings co-led by patients and staff
- The development of patient committees on each unit to advise unit staff leaders regarding patient concerns
- Meetings of patient representatives or advisors from each ward with hospital staff and administrators

The PRISM approach requires extensive staff training, particularly emphasizing interaction with the patients and promotion of patient choice (Starkey & Leadholm, 1997).

Treatment Mall

The treatment "mall" is another PsyR approach. With this approach, most daily programming is conducted off the ward in a central location, where a variety of programming options are available to people attending the activities. Wards are solely dormitories or living space. The mall, located in a separate building, offers a variety of activities both occupational and recreational. The patients choose to attend the activities they prefer. It differs from some traditional hospitals where only one activity at a time is offered in the same location as one's main living space. The mall model is a strategy to increase normalization (leaving one's sleeping space) that offers some degree of consumer choice by offering an array of activity options.

Case Study of a Hospital Implementing Individualized Psychiatric Rehabilitation

Dhillon and Dollieslager (2000) described turning around a troubled state psychiatric hospital by adopting a PsyR treatment philosophy. The story of Eastern State Hospital in Virginia and the problems it has faced are similar to the situations faced by many state psychiatric hospitals. This hospital, like many others, has been under the supervision of both the U.S. Department of Justice and the Health Care Financing Administration (HCFA, now the Center for Medicare and Medicaid Services, CMS). The deteriorating physical plant of the hospital, insufficient staffing, and inadequately credentialed staff all contributed to the inability to provide active treatment of severe and persistent mental illness. They obtained external consultation and a hospital-wide mandate for psychosocial (psychiatric) rehabilitation services to be developed.

Recognizing and overcoming obstacles to incorporating the principles and practices of psychiatric rehabilitation were essential to their success. Here are some of the barriers they had to overcome:

- Many staff members believed that television watching and naps were acceptable for most patients most of the time.
- Team members often expressed the belief that acutely ill patients were generally unable to participate in activities. This prevailing attitude is a barrier in many hospitals.
- Staff members viewed psychosocial treatment as being solely in the realm of occupational, recreational, and activity therapists, not doctors, nurses, and social workers.

Like most hospitals, Eastern State also had:

- A history of emphasizing biological treatment, primarily medication
- A necessary emphasis on maintaining a safe environment for staff and patients
- A lack of treatment team ownership of responsibility for individual patients
- Numerous patients with chemical or substance dependency
- Programming that was not individualized to the patient's unique needs.

These sorts of barriers, attitudinal and otherwise, seem prevalent in state hospital settings. For example, Birkmann and colleagues (2006) reported similar attitudes among staff.

Implementing Psychiatric Rehabilitation at Eastern State Hospital

An essential component of the intervention at Eastern State Hospital was the use of *peer coaches,* who were assigned to each team to encourage an interdisciplinary focus that included an emphasis on psychiatric rehabilitation. Corrigan and McCracken (1995) suggested a similar strategy, proposing that "champions" of the cause of PsyR be identified to help design and initiate the implementation of PsyR principles.

For Eastern state, adopting PsyR meant the following:

- Clarifying each person's goals, promoting their freedom of choice, enhancing their privacy and dignity, and increasing their time with friends and family when they were still in the hospital setting.
- Educating each individual about the nature of his or her illness and how medications work to restore self-control (illness management).
- Teaching about medication and its side effects, self-monitoring, and communicating with the psychiatrist and other members of the treatment team
- Connecting with the family or other natural supports in the community
- Enabling the patient to make appropriate aftercare plans for residential and continuing treatment needs postdischarge.

Dhillon and Dollieslager (2000) viewed treatment and rehabilitation as complementary; that is, as components of the same holistic approach. They integrated psychiatric rehabilitation into more traditional methods of treatment that blended rehabilitation programming with medication interventions, efforts to improve the supervision of staff, and efforts to promote safety.

Is Hospitalization Always Necessary?

Any large-scale changes or reconfigurations of mental health delivery systems focused on deinstitutionalization should include the consideration and exploration of alternatives to hospitalization. The goal should be to make the use of a state psychiatric institution unnecessary—or minimally necessary. At present, the best evidence is that nonhospital alternatives are available for most of the services and functions provided within the institutions such as crisis residences and early intervention teams. The alternatives, which are described next, are generally more consistent with PsyR principles than hospitalization in large psychiatric institutions.

Addressing Acute Care Needs without Large Hospitals

There are numerous alternatives to the provision of acute inpatient psychiatric care in large institutions. Some of the alternatives described here rely on the availability of hospital beds in local community hospitals, sometimes subsidized by the state mental health authority.

• *Acute partial hospitalization:* There is a very large body of evidence that acute partial hospitalization is an excellent alternative to inpatient care with equal or better efficacy than inpatient care, yet without some of its deleterious side effects (Horvitz-Lennon, Normand, Gaccione, & Frank, 2001). Generally programming is available 7 days per week for 6 to 12 hours per day, with a maximum length of stay of 4 to 8 weeks. More than 30 years of research supports the efficacy of these programs.

• *Crisis residential care:* Crisis residences which offer 24-hour, 7-days-a-week acute care are another alternative to inpatient hospitalization (Rakfeldt et al., 1997). These well-staffed programs provide residential and psychiatric care around the clock in a setting with a very small census. In many ways, they look more like a group home than a hospital and are usually located in a regular house in the community. Some geographic areas in the United States, including parts of California and other states, have turned over all acute care to this type of setting, reserving inpatient care solely to those requiring the very severe restriction of locked wards.

• *Early intervention teams:* Another alternative is comprehensive multidisciplinary treatment and rehabilitation teams that resemble ACT, but may be employed even before a person's diagnosis as severely and persistently mentally ill is confirmed. Comprehensive integrated early intervention teams intervene at the time of the first psychotic episode and continue to follow the person as long as needed. This strategy has been found to help reduce persistent symptomatology, the revolving door effect (cycling in and out of the system), and the (unnecessary) deterioration in functioning that often takes place before the person receives effective care. Where used, these teams have significantly reduced the need for public psychiatric hospital care (Abas et al., 2003; Thornicraft & Tansella, 2004).

• *In-home crisis intervention and psychosis management:* A number of strategies are used to manage psychotic disorders in the home through crisis intervention approaches, personal assistants, and intensive familial support where appropriate.

• *Combination of one or more of these approaches:* Using the approaches outlined above in combination is another viable alternative. For example, there is strong empirical evidence that partial hospitalization and crisis residence programs can work effectively in tandem to provide 24-hour acute care (Budson, 1994).

Intermediate and Long-Term Care Needs without Large Institutions

In some places, the mental health authority subsidizes—in part or fully—*subacute* psychiatric wards in general hospitals for longer term care than is typically provided in acute units. These units allow for longer hospitalization than is permitted in most short-term acute units.

For individuals who might require and/or prefer 24-hour care, long-term residences in the community have been developed. Typically, these long-term residences consist of several individuals living in a group setting with on-site staff present 24 hours per day. These facilities usually have indefinite lengths of stay.

An enhanced community mental health service system will reduce the need for state hospital care. For example, in Pennsylvania it was found that 300% to 400% more residential placements were needed than the number the state hospital beds eliminated (Kamis-Gould, Snyder, Hadley, & Casey, 1999; Rothbard, Kuno, Schinnar, Hadley, & Turk, 1999; Rothbard, Schinnar, Hadley, Foley, & Kuno, 1998). That is, to reduce a hospital census by 300 beds, for example, required additional enhanced services for 900 to 1,200 adults residing in the community. This increase in the number of residential place-

CONTROVERSIAL ISSUE
Large Public Psychiatric Hospitals:
Should They All Be Closed?

Are large psychiatric hospitals necessary or useful? To many consumer advocates and PsyR practitioners, large public psychiatric hospitals are a waste of money and, perhaps worse than that, a potentially harmful form of care. In many U.S. states and in some other countries, state hospitals account for more than 50% of the state's mental health budget. Often, much of this expense goes to maintaining an outdated physical plant that provides for very unpleasant congregate (group) living.

Others argue that these hospitals are a necessary evil and some say they are clearly beneficial, preventing even more negative outcomes. On the whole, deinstitutionalization is judged to have been good for those individuals actually deinstitutionalized. But that may not be the whole story. What about those individuals who formerly would have entered these institutions but now must stay in the community? There is evidence that some of these individuals are served poorly and are at risk for many difficulties (Shepherd, 1998).

The necessary evil argument proceeds as follows. There are individuals who are so symptomatic (either on a long- or short-term basis) that local community hospitals and outpatient programs cannot serve them. Community living is not an option for them, and community providers are either not equipped or are unwilling to help them. Therefore, large psychiatric hospitals are needed as the last stop or last resort. Following this line of thinking, hospitalization actually prevents homelessness, unnecessary victimization, and incarceration in jail or prison (Lamb, Weinberger, & Gross, 2004; Perez, Leifman, & Estrada, 2003; Talbott, 2004).

There are numerous alternatives to the provision of inpatient psychiatric care in large institutions, although many places do not have these alternatives in place. Some of the alternatives rely on the availability of hospital beds in local community hospitals, sometimes subsidized by the state mental health authority. Others do not. As discussed in this chapter, these alternatives include acute partial hospitalization, crisis residential care, in-home illness management, and a combination of these approaches. Indeed with very comprehensive crisis services and long-term community services, large public psychiatric hospitals have been eliminated without negative outcomes, for example, in parts of Italy (Ruggieri et al., 2004).

What is the best way to view these large psychiatric hospitals? It depends on a number of factors, primarily the quality of the hospitals involved and their level of integration with the community system. To what extent does a particular hospital provide best practices that foster recovery? Are the staff members there unprepared to offer these? Does the living environment provide for some dignity or privacy or is it a setting without any of the comforts of home where individuals are ignored and sometimes abused (Miller, 2005)? Does the hospital foster community reintegration by working closely with community providers?

ments seems to be the rule. In the Netherlands, for instance, a fivefold increase in community-based services was needed. Why is this? In the hospital, in the course of a year, three or four different individuals fill each bed. Therefore, to eliminate the need for one bed, at least three hospitalizations must be prevented.

Summary

Public psychiatric hospitals remain a part of the mental health system in many places, despite the fact that a body of evidence has emerged indicating that their closure and planned deinstitutionalization result in better outcomes for persons formerly hospitalized and that comprehensive community services can fill the needs met by state hospitals. Their closure does present challenges in serving persons who community providers may be reluctant to serve when seriously ill. Given that in many areas hospitals remain a large part of the system of care, inpatient stays, if needed, must provide for continuity with community life and not be disruptive to rehabilitation efforts and the person's individual recovery.

Psychiatric hospital stays that are long enough to provide for stabilization of symptoms, usually a period of several weeks, can be conducive to recovery. At the same time, very long stays work against recovery by promoting passivity and contributing to a deterioration of community living skills. Treatment programming in the hospital should be offered according to psychiatric rehabilitation principles and be based on known evidence-based practices. In addition, during the course of a hospital stay, a sustained effort should be made to coordinate the hospital and community-based services on the part of both hospital and community staff in order to facilitate reintegration.

Class Exercise

Question 1

Given the constraints inherent in public psychiatric hospitals, give two specific examples of how the guiding principles of psychiatric rehabilitation described in Chapter 4 could be implemented. When developing these examples consider the following:

- The types of activities that can be offered
- The rules or policies the hospital would need to use to implement these activities.

Question 2

What can hospital and community staff do to ensure continuity of care for the individual across treatment settings in different phases of the illness? What are some specific steps they can take to ensure they are working together to enhance recovery and promote community reintegration?

References

Abas, M., Vanderpyl, J., Prou, T. L., Kydd, R., Emery, B., & Foliaki, S. A. (2003). Psychiatric hospitalization: Reasons for admission and alternatives to admission in South Auckland, New Zealand. *Australian & New Zealand Journal of Psychiatry, 37*(5), 620–625.

Bachrach, L. L. (1999). The state of the state mental hospital at the turn of the century. In W. D. Spaulding (Ed.), *The role of the state hospital in the twenty-first century* (Vol. 84, New Directions for Mental Health Services, pp. 7–24). San Francisco, CA: Jossey-Bass.

Birkmann, J. C., Sperduto, J., Smith, R. C., & Gill, K. J. (2006). A collaborative rehabilitation approach to inpatient treatment. *Psychiatric Rehabilitation Journal*, 29157–29165.

Bopp, J., Ribble, D., Cassidy, J., & Markoff, R. (1996). Re-engineering the state hospital to promote rehabilitation and recovery. *Psychiatric Services*, 47(7), 697–698.

Budson, R. D. (1994). Community residential and partial hospital care: Low-cost alternative systems in the spectrum of care. *Psychiatric Quarterly*, 65(3), 209–220.

Busch, A. B. (2005). Introduction to the special section. *Psychiatric Services*, 56(9), 1104.

Corrigan, P. W. (2003). Towards an integrated, structural model of psychiatric rehabilitation. *Psychiatric Rehabilitation Journal*, 26(4), 346–358.

Corrigan, P. W., & McCracken, S. G. (1995). Psychiatric rehabilitation and staff development: Educational and organizational models. *Clinical Psychology Review*, 15(8), 699–719.

Curie, C. G. (2005). SAMHSA's commitment to eliminating the use of seclusion and restraint. *Psychiatric Services*, 56(9), 1139–1140.

Deutsch, A. (1948). *The shame of the states*. Oxford, England: Harcourt, Brace.

Dhillon, A. S., & Dollieslager, L. P. (2000). Overcoming barriers to individualized psychosocial rehabilitation in an acute treatment unit of a state hospital. *Psychiatric Services*, 51(3), 313–317.

Donat, D. C. (2005). Encouraging alternatives to seclusion, restraint, and reliance on PRN drugs in a public psychiatric hospital. *Psychiatric Services*, 56(9), 1105–1108.

Geller, J. L. (2000). The last half-century of psychiatric services as reflected in *Psychiatric Services*. *Psychiatric Services*, 51, 41–67.

Glick, I. D., Hargreaves, W. A., & Raskin, M. (1975). Short versus long hospitalization. II. Results for schizophrenia in-patients. *American Journal of Psychiatry*, 123, 385–390.

Glick, I. D., Hargreaves, W.A., Drues, J. M. A., & Showstack, J. A. (1976). Short versus long hospitalization: a controlled study. III. Inpatient results for nonschizophrenics. *Archives of General Psychiatry*, 33, 78–83.

Harding, C. M., & Zahniser, J. H. (1994). Empirical correction of seven myths about schizophrenia with implications for treatment. *Acta Psychiatrica, Scandanavica*, 90, 140–146.

Herz, M. I., Endicott, J., & Spitzer, R. L. (1975). Brief hospitalization of patients with families: initial results. *American Journal of Psychiatry* 132, 413–418.

Horvitz-Lennon, M., Normand, S.-L. T., Gaccione, P., & Frank, R. G. (2001). Partial versus full hospitalization for adults in psychiatric distress: A systematic review of published literature (1957–1997). *American Journal of Psychiatry*, 158(5), 676–685.

Johnstone, P. & Zolese, G. (2001). Length of hospitalization for people with severe mental illness. *The Cochrane Database of Systemic Reviews* accessed at http://www.umdnj.edu/librweb.

Kamis-Gould, E., Synder, F., Hadley, T. R., & Casey, T. (1999). The impact of closing a state psychiatric hospital on the county mental health system and its clients. *Psychiatric Services*, 50, 1297–1302.

Lamb, H. R., Weinberger, L. E., & Gross, B. H. (2004). Mentally ill persons in the criminal justice system: Some perspectives. *Psychiatric Quarterly*, 75, 107–126.

Miller, R. (2005). Publicity re: past abuses of patients in mental hospitals. *Australian & New Zealand Journal of Psychiatry*, 39(5), 425–426.

Perez, A., Leifman, S., & Estrada, A. (2003). Reversing the criminalization of mental illness. *Crime & Delinquency*, 49(1), 62–78.

Preservation New Jersey. (2003). Retrieved from http://www.preservationnj.org/ten_most/ten_most_property_detail.asp?COUNTY=Morris%20County&PropID=98

Rakfeldt, J., Tebes, J. K., Steiner, J., Walker, P. L., et al. (1997). Normalizing acute care: A day hospital/crisis residence alternative to inpatient hospitalization. *Journal of Nervous & Mental Disease*, 185(1), 46–52.

Rothbard, A. B., Kuno, E., Schinnar, A. P., Hadley, T. R., & Turk, R. (1999). Service utilization and cost of community care for discharged state hospital patients: A 3-year follow-up study. *American Journal of Psychiatry*, 156(6), 920–927.

Rothbard, A. B., Schinnar, A. P., Hadley, T. P., Foley, K. A., & Kuno, E. (1998). Cost comparison of state hospital and community-based care for seriously mentally ill adults. *American Journal of Psychiatry*, 155(4), 523–529.

Rothman, D. J. (2002). *The discovery of the asylum: Social order and disorder in the New Republic.* New York: Walter de Gruyter.

Ruggeri, M., Leese, M., Slade, M., Bonizzato, P., Fontecedro, L., & Tansella, M. (2004). Demographic, clinical, social and service variables associated with higher needs for care in community psychiatric service patients: The South Verona outcome project 8. *Social Psychiatry & Psychiatric Epidemiology, 39*(1), 60–68.

Shepherd, G. (1998). System failure? The problems of reductions in long-stay beds in the UK. *Epidemiologia e Psichiatria Sociale, 7*(2), 127–134.

Smith, G. M., Davis, R. H., Bixler, E. O., Lin, H.-M., Altenor, A., et al. (2005). Pennsylvania State Hospital System's seclusion and restraint reduction program. *Psychiatric Services, 56*(9), 1115–1122.

Starkey D., & Leadholm B. A. (1997). PRISM: the Psychiatric Rehabilitation Integrated Service Model—A public psychiatric hospital model for the 1990s. *Administration and Policy in Mental Health, 24,* 497–508.

Smith, R. C. (1998). Rehab rounds: Implementing psychosocial rehabilitation with long-term patients in a public psychiatric hospital. *Psychiatric Service, 49,* 593–595.

Talbott, J. A. (2004). Deinstitutionalization: Avoiding the disasters of the past. *Psychiatric Services, 55*(10), 1112–1115.

Thornicroft, G., & Tansella, M. (2004). Components of a modern mental health service: A pragmatic balance of community and hospital care: Overview of systematic evidence. *British Journal of Psychiatry, 185*(4), 283–290.

Torrey, E. F. (2003). Keynote address at the World Association of Psychosocial Rehabilitation Congress, New York, August 4, 2003.

Tsang, H. W. H., Liberman, R. P., Hilty, D. M., & Drake, R. E. (2002). "Requirements for multidisciplinary teamwork in psychiatric rehabilitation": Reply. *Psychiatric Services, 53*(6), 768–769.

Tsuchiya, K. J., & Takei, N. (2004). Focus on psychiatry in Japan. *British Journal of Psychiatry, 184*(1), 88–92.

Wallace, C. J., Liberman, R. P., MacKain, S. J., Blackwell, G., & Eckman, T. A. (1992). Effectiveness and replicability of modules for teaching social and independent skills to the severely mentally ill. *American Journal of Psychiatry, 149,* 654–658.

Glossary

action stage—At this stage of change the individual is actively changing his or her behavior.

acute (active) phase—The phase of an illness in which the most severe symptoms are experienced.

acute care—In the context of psychiatric hospital stays, a service intended to manage the acute phase of a psychiatric illness, lasting from a few days to several weeks in length.

addiction—The persistent voluntary and/or involuntary use of chemicals, including alcohol and other drugs, to the detriment of one's physical and mental health.

algorithm—A process or set of rules for problem solving; for example, the rules being developed for the titration (adjustment) of psychotropic medications based on symptoms, responsiveness, side effects, and other factors.

amygdala—A subcortical (below the cortex) brain structure.

anosognosia—Literally, not knowing what you do not know; the lack of awareness that a psychotic symptom is actually present.

antidepressant—A medication that reduces or eliminates one or more symptoms of depression.

antimanic—A medication that reduces or eliminates one or more of the symptoms of mania.

antipsychotic—A medication that reduces or eliminates one or more of the symptoms of psychosis.

assertive community treatment (ACT)—A full support approach to the provision of case management, rehabilitative, and treatment services. ACT programs utilize assertive outreach and *in vivo* service provision techniques.

benzodiazepines—A form of minor tranquilizer, used to relieve anxiety or induce sleep; chemically similar to alcohol and cross-tolerant with alcohol.

biological treatment—Also known as *somatic treatment;* the biological treatment of choice for severe mental illness is medication (e.g., antipsychotic medications, antidepressant medications, or mood stabilizers).

burnout—Reaction by some psychiatric rehabilitation practitioners who have experienced frustration and a sense of failure in their work with people who have severe mental illness.

career development—Persons diagnosed with psychiatric disabilities need assistance in building a career that matches their interests and abilities, rather than being steered toward entry-level, low-paying jobs. Psychiatric rehabilitation programs that integrate supported education and supported employment strategies emphasize this concept.

chronic—Meaning "over time," from the Greek *Kronos,* father of the gods, father of time. This term is used to describe the long-term course of severe mental illness.

chronically mentally ill—Refers to persons with long-lasting mental illness who may suffer repeated relapses. Recently, the term *chronic,* which carries a negative connotation, has been replaced by *severe and persistent.*

clubhouse—A model of psychiatric rehabilitation day programming also known as the

Fountain House model. Clubhouses are places to congregate for social support and recreation and to address community living needs and problems. Consumers who go to clubhouses are referred to as *members* and are involved in all aspects of the program's operation.

cognition—Thinking and problem-solving processes, or the study of thinking and problem solving.

cognitive-behavioral therapy—Interventions designed to assist persons to solve problems and think about and deal with symptoms in alternative ways that are less distressing.

community support program—A nationwide demonstration project instituted by the National Institute of Mental Health in the 1970s to encourage effective community support systems (case management).

community support system—A comprehensive community-based, case management system designed to ensure that the most comprehensive supports and services are available to consumers.

congregate care—Any community-based residential environment in which groups of people with psychiatric disabilities live together and receive services.

contemplation stage—At this stage the individual is seriously considering making a change.

continuity of care—The provision of services, both according to need and over time.

cortex—The outside or "bark" of the brain, divided into two halves (hemispheres), each of which has four lobes: frontal, temporal, parietal, and occipital.

course—The natural history or sequence of events throughout the length of an illness. For persons experiencing severe and persistent mental illness the course can be lifelong marked by a risk of recurrence of severe symptoms.

crisis residences—Community-based alternatives to psychiatric hospitals, usually small homes designed to provide acute care in a safe, low-stimulation environment.

decompensation—Failure to maintain a stable, relatively symptom-free status.

deinstitutionalization—The movement away from treating and housing people with mental illness in large mental hospitals, accomplished by discharging individuals to live in the community.

delusions—False beliefs that an individual maintains despite an absence of supporting evidence or despite evidence to the contrary.

depressive episode—Episode characterized by feelings of extreme sadness or emptiness lasting most of the day, every day, for a period of 2 or more weeks.

diathesis-stress model—An etiological theory, which proposes that stress can trigger symptoms in individuals with a biological predisposition to severe mental illness.

disability—A functional loss due to the symptoms of mental illness.

dual diagnosis—The simultaneous presence of two distinct psychiatric conditions within one individual; that is, two DSM-IV diagnoses.

dual recovery groups—Groups that offer a 12-step program to people who have both a mental illness and a substance abuse disorder; also known as "Double Trouble" groups.

early intervention team—A multidisciplinary team that provides treatment and sometimes rehabilitative services at the early signs of an acute phase or early in the course of a mental illness; team that visits persons and provides care at the first sign of their illness.

earned income exclusion—Earnings that are excluded from the Social Security Administration's calculation of countable earned income.

emotion—Feelings or the state of reaction to events; how someone feels.

empowerment—A term frequently used in conjunction with the psychiatric rehabilitation value of self-determination. It is often addressed in psychiatric rehabilitation programs via involvement strategies such as sharing knowledge, power, and economic resources with consumers, and it has been recently defined in the literature as being composed of three elements: self-esteem and self-efficacy combined with optimism and a sense of control over the future; possession of actual power; and righteous anger and community activism.

etiology—The cause or origin of a disorder.

evidence-based practice (EBP)—A practice that is well defined with specific interventions that have been tested through rigorous research design, preferably randomized controlled trial experiments. Findings need to be replicated or repeated by more than one independent research group.

exacerbate—To aggravate or worsen.

ex-patient/consumer/survivor movement— Organized efforts by persons with a history of psychiatric illness to advocate for civil rights and humane treatment approaches. The movement has also provided access to a variety of self-help and alternative treatment opportunities.

expressed emotion—Familial psychosocial factors, such as an environment high in criticism, hostility, and levels of emotional over-involvement that may contribute to relapse in some cases.

extended period of eligibility—A period of time following a trial work period during which the worker's eligibility for SSDI cash benefit depends on their earned income. As of 2006, the EPE lasted for 36 consecutive months.

extrapyramidal—A class of motor (movement) side effects cause by antipsychotic medication.

Fairweather Lodge—A residential service model developed by George Fairweather and characterized by groups of people with psychiatric disabilities living and working together on a long-term basis.

family foster care—A situation in which one or more consumers reside with, and are supported by, a family that is not their own.

fidelity scale—An instrument designed to assess a particular service's level of agree-

ment with an ideal service model, typically an evidence-based practice.

functional assessment—An evaluation of a person's level of ability in specific life areas such as vocational, self-care, or education.

GABA—A neurotransmitter.

general income exclusion—Income that is excluded from Social Security Administration's calculation of countable income.

genetic—Inherited, due to the coding on chromosomes.

gentrification—The buying and renovation of homes in deteriorating urban neighborhoods, which may improve property values, but often displaces lower income individuals.

global assessment—An overall assessment of a consumer that does not address ability to function in specific environments.

goals—Desired states or objectives to strive for and achieve.

hallucinations—Sensory perceptions in the absence of appropriate external stimulation, such as hearing voices.

harm reduction—The idea that the important issue in substance abuse treatment is to reduce the harm caused by the substance abuse rather than to require abstinence.

hippocampus—Literally, "sea horse," a sub-cortical brain structure, shaped somewhat like a sea horse, that is involved in important cognitive functions and working memory.

iatrogenic—Refers to the phenomenon of a treatment or environment having unintended negative effects on the persons. "Institutionalized" behavior such as excessive passivity is an example of an iatrogenic effect of long-term hospitalization.

in vivo—Literally "in life"; as opposed to a clinic or service setting, this is the provision of services to clients in the environments where they live, work, and socialize.

Independent Living Movement—The efforts of people with physical disabilities to advocate for civil rights, develop a shared philosophy, and provide peer support in order to recover and maintain control over their lives.

individual written rehabilitation plan (IWRP)—The plan written by a vocational rehabilitation counselor and consumer that describes the consumer's vocational goal and the services that will be accessed to reach that goal.

institutionalized—The negative behavioral effects of long-term stays in institutions such as state psychiatric hospitals, typically manifested by extreme dependency.

integrated services—Services that address dual disorders simultaneously and are provided by staff who are knowledgeable about both disorders affecting the client.

intermediate care—In the context of psychiatric care, a period of several weeks to several months for the management of extended acute episodes and residual phases of the illness.

job development—The tasks involved in job acquisition. These may include generally developing relationships with the business community, investigating the hiring needs of a specific employer, communicating the program's available services to all customers, or more specifically assisting the consumer with job applications, résumé writing, interview skills, and employer contacts.

length of stay—The period of time when an individual is attending a program, a service, or treatment; also, the number days in residence at a psychiatric hospital.

linear continuum model—A residential service approach in which consumers move from a relatively restrictive congregate care setting to a series of progressively less restrictive living environments and eventually to independent living.

longitudinal study—A research study that tracks subjects and relevant outcomes for lengthy periods of time (i.e., 10 or more years).

long-term care—In the context of psychiatric hospitals, a period of several months or longer for the long-term treatment and management of psychiatric illnesses.

maintenance stage—At this stage the individual has changed and is actively maintaining the change.

manic episode—Characterized by an elevated mood, in which the person feels excessively "up" or "high," and occasionally excessively irritable, for a period of a week or more.

medical model—An integral element of the medical system or profession; part of medicine.

meta-analysis—A study or review that combines the findings of previous studies, statistically combining the effects of all studies to determine an average effect.

milieu therapy—*Milieu* is a French term that literally means "environment." Milieu therapy is a technique based on the idea that every aspect (i.e., physical, social, and cultural) of a treatment setting or environment can be used to help achieve therapeutic or rehabilitation goals or results.

mixed episode—Meets the criteria for both depressive and manic episodes simultaneously.

motivational interviewing—A nonconfrontational counseling strategy that focuses on the discrepancy between an individual's stated goals and his or her behavior and attempts to ally itself with the individual's wants, needs, and aspirations rather than confronting the individual about negative behaviors.

multidisciplinary—Literally "many disciplines"; any approach that involves individuals from more than one profession or educational background, for example, physicians, nurses, social workers, and rehabilitation staff working together.

natural supports—Supports provided to persons who have a disability by nonprofessionals such as family members, friends. or coworkers.

negative symptoms—Symptoms that reflect a lessening or loss of functioning; essentially abilities or senses that are lost due to a disease (e.g., restricted emotional expression, reduced productivity of thought) (DSM-IV).

neuroanatomy—The structure of the nerves or neurons composing an individual's brain and nervous system.

neurology—The medical specialty dealing with the nervous system.

neurotransmitter(s)—A group of substances produced by the body that function within the central nervous system to facilitate the passing of impulses between nerve cells.

NIMBY—"Not in my backyard"; an acronym describing community opposition to living near a group home or other residential setting in which people with psychiatric disabilities reside.

normalization—The achievement or acquisition of valued social roles for consumers; normalization is a guiding principle of psychiatric rehabilitation.

normalized—A term used to describe an environment (such as a day program) that is consistent with the psychiatric rehabilitation principle of normalization, which is the creation and maintenance of valued social roles for consumers.

objective burden—Specifically identifiable problems associated with a person's mental illness. The objective burdens of families may include financial hardships due to medical bills, the cost of the consumer's economic dependence, disruptions in household functioning, restriction of social activities, and so on.

outcomes—Specific results, the end of a specific course of treatment, or the end result of the course of an entire illness.

parallel services—Services for two or more conditions that are provided at the same time but by different staff members or by different programs, each of which is knowledgeable about only one of the disorders.

partial hospitalization program—Day programs that are essentially based on the medical model; treatment strategies include medication and medication monitoring; group, individual, and milieu therapies; and recreation and socialization. Some partial hospitals also incorporate psychiatric rehabilitation intervention strategies.

participatory action research—Research carried out by professional researchers working together with the subjects of the research. In psychiatric rehabilitation, studies carried out with persons with severe mental illness participating at all levels of the research process.

peer partnership—An initiative in which consumers collaborate with nonconsumer providers to operate a program that emphasizes peer-delivered services.

peer provider—A psychiatric rehabilitation service provider who has a history of severe mental illness; these individuals have also been called *peer counselors, peer advocates, peer specialists, consumer providers, consumer case managers,* and *prosumers.*

peer support—A term commonly used to describe self-help and other peer-delivered service initiatives in which individuals who are diagnosed with a mental illness assist other consumers.

peer-delivered services—Rehabilitation and support services provided by individuals who identify themselves as having a mental illness. These services encompass peer-operated programs, peer partnership programs, and traditional mental health programs that utilize peer employees.

peer-operated services—Programs that are developed, controlled, and operated by individuals who identify themselves as having a diagnosis of a mental illness. Nonconsumers may also be employed to contribute to service delivery and/or the administration of the program, but consumers clearly direct the entire service delivery process.

person-first language—Intentionally putting the person first in statements about the individual, for example, saying "a person with schizophrenia," as opposed to saying "a schizophrenic."

pharmacology—The study of medications or chemical compounds used to treat disease.

physiological—To do with the body; physical.

polysubstance abuser—An individual who is abusing more than one substance, for example, alcohol and marijuana.

positive symptoms—Indicators or signs of illness that are significant because of the presence (positive status) of something normally not present; hallucinations and delusions are examples.

precontemplation stage—At this stage the individual is not considering making a change.

premorbid—The period of time before a psychiatric illness developed.

preparation stage—At this stage the individual is preparing to make a change.

principles—Specific dictums designed to promulgate values and goals by providing guidelines for addressing specific situations or behaviors.

prodromal phase—"Before the full syndrome"; a period before the full onset of the illness that is characterized by deterioration in functioning and increasing positive and negative symptoms.

prognosis—The probable course or outcome of a disorder.

prosumers—A term used to describe identified consumers of mental health services who are also mental health professionals.

psychoanalytic—A therapeutic approach based on psychological theories proposed by Sigmund Freud; psychoanalytic techniques emphasize the exploration of intrapsychic processes and their relationship to past events.

psychodynamic—A theory that psychopathology arises from conflicts within the psyche or mind of the individual. These conflicts may be rooted in past events.

psychodynamic therapy—An insight-oriented approach that focuses on the interpretation of unconscious material and therapeutic transference. In the treatment of serious mental illnesses, this form of psychotherapy has been found to be generally ineffective.

psychoeducation—A psychiatric rehabilitation intervention that involves connecting with family members by focusing on their current concerns; providing basic information regarding schizophrenia or other major mental illnesses; teaching crisis intervention techniques; and providing other resources that aid families in becoming effective partners in the treatment and rehabilitation process.

psychopharmacology—The study of medication or chemical compounds to the relief of psychiatric symptoms.

psychosis—Incorrect evaluation of reality.

psychosocial treatment—Any approach that attempts to effect change through the manipulation of social or psychological factors.

quality of life—A person's subjective evaluation of the aspects of his or her life that he or she deems important.

reasonable accommodations—Modifications made to a job or work setting to enhance the ability of a qualified worker with a disability to perform the job. The American with Disabilities Act defines *reasonable* as an accommodation that is not excessively expensive compared to the resources of the business and does not fundamentally change the nature of the work being performed.

recidivism—Returning to the psychiatric hospital after discharge (i.e., relapse).

recovery—For a lifelong mental illness, recovery refers to a reformulation of one's self-image and an eventual adaptation to the disease; recovery is one of the goals of psychiatric rehabilitation.

rehabilitation—Any action intended to reduce the negative effects of the disease on the person's everyday life.

relapse—The recurrence of acute phases of an illness, after periods of remission or lack of symptoms.

remission—Time period when an individual with an illness is essentially symptom free.

residential treatment facility—Congregate care settings, such as group homes, that are operated by mental health professionals.

residual phase—The period after the acute phase of an illness when symptoms become milder.

restraint—Prevention of free movement of the individual through physically binding the individual's body, particularly the limbs; can also be achieved through use of medication through sedation (as opposed to symptom relief).

schizoaffective disorder—A psychiatric disorder characterized by both symptoms of schizophrenia and symptoms of affective disorders.

seclusion—Removal of an individual from all social contact to a separate room.

self-advocacy—An individual's efforts to defend his or her own personal or civil rights, including the right to receive quality treatment and rehabilitation services. This term also refers to efforts by an organized group of consumers to rally support for a common cause.

self-contained classroom—A model of supported education in which a group of students, all of whom have a psychiatric disability, take a prescribed curriculum designed to help them achieve postsecondary educational goals.

self-determination—A psychiatric rehabilitation value that is based on the belief that consumers have the right to participate in all decisions that affect their lives; closely related to the concept of empowerment.

self-help—Involvement in nonprofessional activities that provide support and information for oneself and others who share a similar illness or problem.

self-help centers—Alternative programs that offer a variety of mutual support and social and advocacy activities. Sometimes called *drop-in centers,* many of these initiatives now have an expanded focus on wellness, recovery, and employment.

self-medicate—Use by an individual of nonprescribed substances to deal with the symptoms of his or her psychiatric illness.

sequential services—Services provided by one program to address one disorder, followed by services provided by another program to address another disorder.

side effects—Unintended, undesired, or harmful effects of a treatment, usually medication; this is in contrast to therapeutic side effects.

situational assessment—An evaluation of the presence or absence of the skills and resources needed for a consumer to function successfully in the environments (i.e., situations) of their choice; this is in contrast to doing a global assessment, unrelated to specific client goals.

somatic—"Of the body"; biologically based.

staff burnout—A general loss of motivation, meaning, and/or interest in one's job, which may present itself as frustration or hopelessness.

subjective burden—The psychological distress, borne by family members, that is engendered by the severe mental illness of a relative.

substantial gainful activity (SGA)—An amount of earnings designated by the Social Security Administration as an indication of a worker's ability to be self-supporting. As of 2006, this amount was $500 per month.

super-sensitivity hypotheses—Hypothesis that persons with severe mental illness are more sensitive to substances and therefore at greater risk of becoming substance abusers.

supported approaches—Also known as *community-integrated services,* these are psychiatric rehabilitation models that share a common philosophy and strongly emphasize normalization and full inclusion in the community. Collectively, supported employment, supported housing, and supported education have been referred to as *supported approaches.*

supported education (SEd)—Services and supports that are aimed at helping persons diagnosed with severe mental illnesses achieve their postsecondary educational goals.

supported employment (SE)—An individualized approach to assist a consumer to achieve integrated employment. SE emphasizes training and support provided in settings of choice rather than demonstration of skills prior to access to vocational services. Supported employment services provide support to the individual in selecting, obtaining, and maintaining employment. SE is one of the evidence-based practices.

supported housing—Integrated, community-based housing opportunities for people with psychiatric disabilities that emphasize consumer choice and provision of flexible and ongoing supports.

symptoms—Signs or indicators of an illness or disorder.

tardive dyskinesia—Involuntary movements of the mouth and other parts of the body as a consequence of the use of traditional antipsychotics; caused by changes to neurons involving dopamine.

teams—The group of professionals and other staff working together to serve the same consumer.

titrate—To adjust to the right dosage or amount; usually refers to medication, but can be used for any treatment.

transinstitutionalization—Moving from a psychiatric institution to another congregate care setting that allows for minimal involvement in normalized community activities.

transition services—Supports and services provided to teenagers who are diagnosed with a disability. They include assistance with the move from high school to a postsecondary education or training setting and should continue until the age of 21.

transitional employment (TE)—A program of time-limited jobs in regular work settings for real pay. Agency staff acquire the job from an employer and subsequently provide training and support to consumers in that job. Consumers in TE jobs earn the going rate of pay from the employer and remain in the job for a specified period of time. The job will then be filled by another consumer.

treatment—Any action designed to cure a disease or reduce its symptoms; treatment for serious mental illnesses can be broken into two broad categories, biological (somatic) and psychosocial.

trial work period—Nine nonconsecutive months in which an SSDI recipient can earn income while maintaining his or her cash benefit, thus allowing the individual to try working with limited risk.

12-step model—The 12 steps of Alcoholics Anonymous that an alcoholic must complete to remain in recovery.

values—Deeply held beliefs that may inform specific behaviors, attitudes, and ideas.

warm lines—Peer support or assistance offered via the telephone.

Wellness and Recovery Action Plan (WRAP)—A self-help strategy that utilizes a structured tool to help individuals learn to cope with their illnesses and lead healthy, satisfying lives.

word salad—A fairly rare symptom of severe psychosis, in which language has become so impaired, the person attempts to express himself or herself in what sounds like a jumble or mixture of words, rather than coherent sentences.

Index

12-step model, 222, 224, 230, 233, 236, 239, 430

A

Alcoholics Anonymous, 222, 229, 233, 338, 345
Americans with Disabilities Act, 12, 17, 142, 156, 254, 270, 279, 282, 361, 362
American Psychiatric Association, 9, 15, 25, 34, 64, 73, 327
anosognosia, 39–40, 72, 209
Assertive Community Treatment (ACT), 195, 200–201, 215
 criminal justice system, 213–214
 critical ingredients of, 211
 early intervention strategy, 212–213
 fidelity to, 207
 outcomes of, 211–212
 research on, 211–212
 Training in Community Living, 204–206
antipsychotic medication, 79–85, 99–100
 atypicals, 80–81, 83–85
 second generation, 80–81
 side effects, 82–83

B

Bazelon Center for Mental Health Law, 306
Boston University Center for Psychiatric Rehabilitation, 16, 21, 24, 111, 140, 141, 149, 150, 250, 259, 264, 267, 280, 281

C

Carl Perkins Education Act, 282
case management, 196–198
 models of, 199–201
 research on, 203
case manager, 198–199
CAT Scan, 51, 53
Center for Psychiatric Rehabilitation, 16, 21, 24, 111, 140, 141, 149, 150, 250, 259, 264, 267, 280, 281
Certified Psychiatric Rehabilitation Provider (CPRP), 26, 127, 362

choose-get-keep, 259, 264 266, 286
clubhouse model, 168–173
 history of, 166, 168
 research on, 183
 standards, 170–171
 of supported education, 280, 283, 284–285
 transitional employment, 256
community integration, 114–115, 166, 186, 244, 298, 318, 329, 379, 406, 417
community mental health center, 16, 18, 25, 118, 166, 168, 174, 283, 308, 365
continuity of care, 193–195, 197, 412
 also see PsyR principle of *ongoing, accessible, coordinated services,* 123–124, 419–420
course of mental illness, 70, 72–79, 86–87, 93, 95, 97–99, 390, 393
criminal justice, 213–214, 250

D

Depression and Bipolar Support Alliance, 341, 346
developmental disability, 47–49, 99–101, 329, 376, 415
disability (psychiatric), 10–13, 110
Diagnostic and Statistical Manual 3rd Edition (DSM III), 15, 75
Diagnostic and Statistical Manual 4th Edition (DSM IV), 9, 12, 34, 41, 64
Double Trouble groups, 239, 345
drop-in center, 155, 214, 326, 339, 341, 350, 356
dual diagnosis, 9–10, 47–50, 99–101, 220–238
 mental illness/developmental disability, 47–49, 99–101, 329, 376, 415
 mental illness/substance abuse, 49–50, 220–238, 326–327, 376
dual recovery groups, 229–230, 345–346

E

early intervention, 212–213, 296–297, 423–424
empowerment, 115–117, 126, 185, 291, 340, 356, 365
 familial empowerment, 394

environment of choice, 142, 146, 149
environmental assessment, 127, 142
    also see *situational assessment*
environmental modifications, 155–156
etiology, 8, 50–62
    obsolete theories, 62–64
    physiological evidence, 50–52, 54, 62
evidence-based practice, 22–24, 140, 156, 184, 186,
        227, 258, 426
    assertive community treatment, 199, 208,
        210–213
    family psychoeducation, 388, 392–394
    illness management and recovery, 90–93
    integrated dual diagnosis treatment, 224,
        230–233
    medication management (MedMap), 84
    supported education, 294
    supported employment, 231, 268–269
ex-patient movement, 129, 320, 340–342, 343

F
Fair Housing Act, 306
Fairweather Lodge, 309–311, 431
family-to-family, 374, 398
family, 374–401
    as caring agent, 376
    burden, 181, 376, 377, 379, 390, 399
    stigma, 377
    dependence, 377
    dual diagnosis, 377
    dissatisfaction, 379
    levels of involvement, 380
    interventions, 387–394
    psychoeducation, 387–394
    recovery, 395
family foster care, 309, 311
Fountain House, 16, 20, 166, 168, 169, 255, 256,
        270, 280, 338, 430
functional assessment, 145, 146, 159, 160, 200, 431
functional deficits, 101

G
GROW, 338, 353

H
handicap, 110, 111, 117, 283
helper therapy principle, 337
Housing First, 326, 327, 329, 330

I
IAPSRS—see USPRA
Illness Management and Recovery, 24, 90–93, 98

Independent living movement, 323–325, 328, 330,
        343, 431
Individuals with Disabilities Education Act, 282
integrated dual diagnosis services, 186, 224,
        230–233, 292, 432
Individual Placement and Support (IPS), 264–266,
        268, 269, 298

J
job coach, 120, 124, 155, 255, 262–266, 286
job development, 120, 251, 257, 262, 263, 265, 432
John Beard, 168, 169

M
Medicaid, 174, 175, 194, 249, 295, 422
Medicare, 174, 175, 249, 422
MedMap, 84
models of case management, 199, 201, 203
    expanded broker, 199, 200
    rehabilitation, 199, 200, 207
    strengths, 199, 200, 211
    full support, 199–201
    Assertive Community Treatment, 22–24, 73, 93,
        134, 156, 183, 184, 191, 192, 194–196,
        198–200, 204–211, 214, 215
Michigan Supported Education Program, 277, 284,
        286, 291, 296
milieu therapy, 166, 175, 176, 186, 408, 432
modeling, 150, 151, 159, 337, 344 (see role
        modeling)
MRI (Magnetic Resonance Imaging, 10, 14,
        50–52
Myth of Mental Illness, 63

N
NAMI (National Alliance for the Mentally Ill), 141,
        374, 394, 396–398
National Empowerment Center, 341, 343
National Mental Health Consumers Self-Help
        Clearinghouse, 341, 342, 347
natural supports, 76, 265, 283, 287, 318, 321, 375,
        384, 385, 423, 432 399, 431, 433
neurotransmitter, 12, 55, 59, 80, 82, 85, 86, 399,
        431, 433
normalization, 20, 48, 121, 185, 215, 266, 289, 290,
        292, 304, 310, 318, 422, 433

P
Parallel services, 223, 443
Partial hospitalization, 166, 167, 173, 174, 423, 433
Participatory action research, 185, 358, 433
PET Scan, 54

Psychopharmacology, 79–92, 434
  anti depressants, 86–87
  anti psychotics, 79–84, 88–89, 436
  compliance (adherence), 85, 86, 88–90
  mood Stabilizers, 85–86, 88, 429
  side effects, 73, 80–85, 92–93, 101, 247–248, 278, 294, 394
Peer-delivered services, 336, 433
  definition of, 349
  research on, 352–358
Peer employees, 352
Peer-operated services, 349–351
Peer partnerships, 351–352
Peer providers, 207, 321, 353–364, 433
  benefits to service recipients, 353–356
  benefits for, 356–357
  benefits to mental health systems, 357
  challenges of, 358, 361
  professional development of, 362–364
  relationships with non consumer providers, 359–360
  supports for, 362–363
Peer support, 433
  definition of, 337
  history of, 338–342
  studies of, 350
Personal assistance services, 324, 325
Place train approach, 259
President's New Freedom Commission, 365
Psychoeducation
  Family, 388, 391–395
  Evidence-Based Practice, 392–393
  Illness Management, 90–93
Psychosocial Treatments, 93–95

Q
Quality of life, 114, 115

R
Readiness assessment, 143–144
Reasonable accommodations, 142, 254, 434
Recovery concept, 111, 434
Recovery Inc., 338
Rehabilitation readiness, 142–144
Rehabilitation Act, 252–254, 282
Rehabilitation diagnosis, 144–145
Rehabilitation plan, 147
Residential treatment, 434
  history of, 307–309
  facilities, 311–312
  stigma and, 312–313
  linear continuum approach to, 313–318

Resilience
  child, 384
  family, 399
Resource assessment, 145–147
Resource development, 155, 286
Restraints, 416
Role modeling, 112, 159, 281

S
Schizophrenia
  Course, Outcomes, 70–76, 78, 102, 112
  Diagnosed as having, 148
  Differences from Mood Disorders, 45, 77
  Etiology, 50–52, 62
  Phases of, 40
  Symptoms of, 33–39
Schizophrenics Anonymous, 338
seclusion, 128, 129, 342, 416
"Shame of the States", 409
Self-advocacy, 291, 339–341
  definition, 339
  history of, 339–342
self determination, 89, 100, 114–116, 126, 131, 289–290, 310, 321, 324, 395, 418
self-help
  definition of, 336
  history of, 328
  centers, 339, 348, 350, 351
  research on, 353
sequential services, 222
situational assessment, 114, 122, 145, 419
skill development, 154, 200, 256, 264, 292, 318, 357, 376, 384, 421
skill generalization, 153
skill maintenance, 153, 154
skills training, 92, 118, 149, 188, 251, 350, 420
social comparison theory, 337
social learning theory, 112, 151, 154, 188, 337, 420
Social Security (United States), 13, 155, 248–250, 308, 410
Social support, 76, 92, 99, 167–168, 175, 183, 337, 383, 384, 392
social support theory, 337
stages of change, 207, 225–227, 231, 233
stages of treatment, 225, 229
State Hospitals, 406–425
  19th Century Roots, 407
  Length of Stay, 412
  Population, 412
  PSR Models within, 420, 422
  Goals within, 417
Staff Competencies, 26, 92

Stress, 59–60
Stress/Vulnerability/Coping/Competence Model, 61
Symptoms, 33, 45
    Delusions, 34
    Negative, 34
    Persistence, 33, 40, 41
    Positive, 34
    Thought Disorder, 37
super sensitivity hypothesis, 221
supported education
    definition of, 283
    dissemination of, 295
    future directions in, 295, 298
    history of, 280, 282
    models of, 283, 286, 351
    research on, 291, 293–294
supported housing
    at Collaborative Support Programs of NJ, 292
    Principles of, 318–319
    Outcomes of, 322–323
    Implementation of, 319–322
strengths focus, 114, 121–122, 419
strengths model, 199–200

T
Thresholds, 12, 21, 168, 210, 213, 280, 283
transitional employment, 171, 173, 178, 256, 260, 270
Treatment of Psychiatric Disorders, 79–95, 99
    Alternative, 95
    Bipolar (manic depression), 85–86, 95
    Developmental Disorders, 99
    Major Depression, 86–87, 95
    Schizophrenia, 79–84
    Substance Abuse, 99

U
USPRA (United States Psychiatric Rehabilitation Association), formerly IAPSRS, 25–27, 125–127, 130–132, 134, 183–184

W
warm lines, 346
Wellness and Recovery Action Plan (WRAP), 133, 338, 346–347